BASIC IMMUNOLOGY

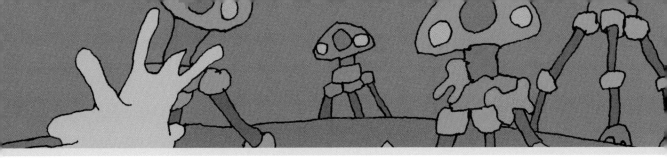

BASIC IMMUNOLOGY

Functions and Disorders of the Immune System

FIFTH EDITION

Abul K. Abbas, MBBS
Distinguished Professor in Pathology
Chair, Department of Pathology
University of California San Francisco
San Francisco, California

Andrew H. Lichtman, MD, PhD
Professor of Pathology
Harvard Medical School
Brigham and Women's Hospital
Boston, Massachusetts

Shiv Pillai, MBBS, PhD
Professor of Medicine and Health Sciences and Technology
Harvard Medical School
Ragon Institute of Massachusetts General Hospital, MIT and Harvard
Boston, Massachusetts

Illustrations by David L. Baker, MA
Alexandra Baker, MS, CMI
DNA Illustrations, Inc.

ELSEVIER

ELSEVIER

3251 Riverport Lane
St. Louis, Missouri 63043

BASIC IMMUNOLOGY: FUNCTIONS AND DISORDERS OF   ISBN: 978-0-323-39082-8
THE IMMUNE SYSTEM, Fifth Edition

Notices

Knowledge and best practice in this field are constantly changing. As new research and experience broaden our understanding, changes in research methods, professional practices, or medical treatment may become necessary.

Practitioners and researchers must always rely on their own experience and knowledge in evaluating and using any information, methods, compounds, or experiments described herein. In using such information or methods they should be mindful of their own safety and the safety of others, including parties for whom they have a professional responsibility.

With respect to any drug or pharmaceutical products identified, readers are advised to check the most current information provided (i) on procedures featured or (ii) by the manufacturer of each product to be administered, to verify the recommended dose or formula, the method and duration of administration, and contraindications. It is the responsibility of practitioners, relying on their own experience and knowledge of their patients, to make diagnoses, to determine dosages and the best treatment for each individual patient, and to take all appropriate safety precautions.

To the fullest extent of the law, neither the Publisher nor the authors, contributors, or editors assume any liability for any injury and/or damage to persons or property as a matter of products liability, negligence or otherwise, or from any use or operation of any methods, products, instructions, or ideas contained in the material herein.

Library of Congress Cataloging-in-Publication Data
Abbas, Abul K., author.
  Basic immunology : functions and disorders of the immune system / Abul K. Abbas, Andrew H. Lichtman, Shiv Pillai ; Illustrations by David L. Baker, Alexandra Baker. -- Fifth edition.
     p. ; cm.
  Includes bibliographical references and index.
  ISBN 978-0-323-39082-8
  I. Lichtman, Andrew H., author. II. Pillai, Shiv, author. III. Title.
  [DNLM: 1. Immunity. 2. Hypersensitivity. 3. Immune System--physiology. 4. Immunologic Deficiency Syndromes. QW 504]
  QR181
  616.07'9--dc23
                                                                    2015029015

Executive Content Strategist: James Merritt
Director, Content Development: Rebecca Gruliow
Publishing Services Manager: Catherine Jackson
Senior Project Manager: Clay S. Broeker
Design Direction: Brian Salisbury

Printed in Canada

Last digit is the print number: 9 8 7 6 5 4 3 2 1

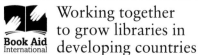

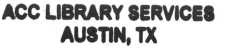

To our students

The fifth edition of *Basic Immunology* has been revised to include recent important advances in our understanding of the immune system and to organize and present information in order to maximize its usefulness to students and teachers. The previous editions have been enthusiastically received by students in the many courses that we and our colleagues teach, and we have not wavered from the guiding principles on which the book has been based through all the past editions. Our experience as immunology teachers and course directors has helped us to judge the amount of detailed information that can be usefully included in introductory medical school and undergraduate courses and the value of presenting the principles of immunology in a succinct and clear manner. We believe a concise and modern consideration of immunology is now a realistic goal, largely because immunology has matured as a discipline and has now reached the stage when the essential components of the immune system and how they interact in immune responses are understood quite well. As a result, we can now teach our students, with reasonable confidence, how the immune system works. In addition, we are better able to relate experimental results, using simple models, to the more complex but physiologically relevant issue of host defense against infectious pathogens. There has also been exciting progress in applying basic principles to understanding and treating human diseases.

This book has been written to address the perceived needs of both medical school and undergraduate curricula and to take advantage of the new understanding of immunology. We have tried to achieve several goals. First, we have presented the most important principles governing the function of the immune system by synthesizing key concepts from the vast amount of experimental data that emerge in the field of immunology. The choice of what is most important is based largely on what is most clearly established by scientific investigation and what has the most relevance to human health and disease. We also have realized that in any concise discussion of complex phenomena it is inevitable that exceptions and caveats cannot be discussed in any detail. Second, we have focused on immune responses against infectious microbes, and most of our discussions of the immune system are in this context. Third, we have made liberal use of illustrations to highlight important principles, but we have reduced factual details that may be found in more comprehensive textbooks. Fourth, we have also discussed immunologic diseases from the perspective of principles, emphasizing their relation to normal immune responses and avoiding details of clinical syndromes and treatments. We have included selected clinical cases in an appendix to illustrate how the principles of immunology may be applied to common human diseases. Finally, in order to make each chapter readable on its own, we have repeated key ideas in different places in the book. We feel such repetition will help students to grasp the most important concepts.

We hope that students will find this new edition of *Basic Immunology* clear, cogent, manageable, and enjoyable to read. We hope the book will convey our sense of wonder about the immune system and excitement about how the field has evolved and how it continues to grow in relevance to human health and disease. Finally, although we were spurred to tackle this project because of our associations with medical school courses, we hope the book will be valued by students of allied health and biology as well. We will have succeeded if the book can answer many of the questions these students have about the immune system and, at the same time, encourage them to delve even more deeply into immunology.

Several individuals played key roles in the writing of this book. Our new editor, James Merritt, has been an enthusiastic source of encouragement and advice. Our talented illustrators, David and Alexandra Baker of DNA Illustrations, have revamped all of the artwork for this new edition and have transformed our ideas into pictures that are informative and aesthetically pleasing. Clay Broeker has moved the book through the production process in an efficient and professional manner. Our development editor, Rebecca Gruliow, has kept the project organized and on track despite pressures of time and logistics. To all of them we owe our many thanks. Finally, we owe an enormous debt of gratitude to our families, whose support and encouragement have been unwavering.

Abul K. Abbas
Andrew H. Lichtman
Shiv Pillai

CONTENTS

BASIC IMMUNOLOGY

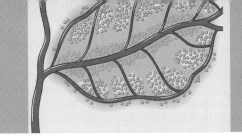

CHAPTER 1

Introduction to the Immune System

Nomenclature, General Properties, and Components

Immunity is defined as resistance to disease, specifically infectious disease. The collection of cells, tissues, and molecules that mediate resistance to infections is called the **immune system,** and the coordinated reaction of these cells and molecules to infectious microbes comprises an **immune response. Immunology** is the study of the immune system, including its responses to microbial pathogens and damaged tissues and its role in disease.

The most important physiologic function of the immune system is to prevent or eradicate infections (Fig. 1-1), and this is the principal context in which immune responses are discussed throughout this book. The importance of the immune system for health is dramatically illustrated by the frequent observation that individuals with defective immune responses are susceptible to serious, often life-threatening infections. Conversely, stimulating immune responses against microbes through vaccination is the most effective method for protecting individuals against infections; this approach has led to the worldwide eradication of smallpox, the only disease that has been eliminated from civilization by human intervention (Fig. 1-2). Unfortunately, interruptions of vaccination programs in developing countries and in regions of social conflict have led to local reemergence of some infectious diseases, such as polio, that have been largely eliminated from other parts of the world. The appearance of acquired immunodeficiency syndrome (AIDS) in the 1980s tragically emphasized the importance of the immune system for defending individuals against infection. The immune system does more than provide

Role of the immune system	Implications
Defense against infections	Deficient immunity results in increased susceptibility to infections; exemplified by AIDS
	Vaccination boosts immune defenses and protects against infections
Defense against tumors	Potential for immunotherapy of cancer
The immune system can injure cells and induce pathologic inflammation	Immune responses are the cause of allergic, autoimmune, and other inflammatory diseases
The immune system recognizes and responds to tissue grafts and newly introduced proteins	Immune responses are barriers to transplantation and gene therapy

FIGURE 1-1 Importance of the immune system in health and disease. This table summarizes some of the physiologic functions of the immune system and its role in disease. *AIDS,* Acquired immunodeficiency syndrome.

protection against infections (see Fig. 1-1). It prevents the growth of some tumors, and some cancers can be treated by stimulating immune responses against tumor cells. Immune responses also participate in the clearance of dead cells and in initiating tissue repair.

In contrast to these beneficial roles, abnormal immune responses cause many inflammatory diseases with serious morbidity and mortality. The immune response is the major barrier to the success of organ transplantation, which is often used to treat organ failure. The products of immune cells can also be of great practical use. For example, antibodies, which are proteins made by certain cells of the immune system, are used in clinical laboratory testing and in research as highly specific reagents for detecting a wide variety of molecules in the circulation and in cells and tissues. Antibodies designed to block or eliminate potentially harmful molecules and cells are used widely for the treatment of immunologic diseases, cancers, and other types of disorders. For all these reasons, the field of immunology has captured

the attention of clinicians, scientists, and the lay public.

This chapter introduces the nomenclature of immunology, important general properties of all immune responses, and the cells and tissues that are the principal components of the immune system. In particular, the following questions are addressed:

- What types of immune responses protect individuals from infections?
- What are the important characteristics of immunity, and what mechanisms are responsible for these characteristics?
- How are the cells and tissues of the immune system organized to find and respond to microbes in ways that lead to their elimination?

We conclude the chapter with a brief overview of immune responses against microbes. The basic principles introduced here set the stage for more detailed discussions of immune responses in later chapters. A glossary of the important terms used in this book is provided in Appendix I.

Disease	Maximum number of cases (year)	Number of cases in 2014	Percent change
Diphtheria	206,939 (1921)	0	−100
Measles	894,134 (1941)	669	−99.93
Mumps	152,209 (1968)	737	−99.51
Pertussis	265,269 (1934)	10,631	−95.99
Polio (paralytic)	21,269 (1952)	0	−100
Rubella	57,686 (1969)	2	−99.99
Tetanus	1560 (1923)	8	−99.48
Hemophilus influenza type B	~20,000 (1984)	34	−99.83
Hepatitis B	26,611 (1985)	1,098	−95.87

FIGURE 1-2 Effectiveness of vaccination for some common infectious diseases. The striking decrease in the incidence of selected infectious diseases in the United States for which effective vaccines have been developed. (Modified from Orenstein WA, Hinman AR, Bart KJ, Hadler SC: Immunization. In Mandell GL, Bennett JE, Dolin R, editors: *Principles and practices of infectious diseases*, 4th edition, New York, 1995, Churchill Livingstone; and *MMWR* 64, No. 20, 2015.)

INNATE AND ADAPTIVE IMMUNITY

Host defenses are grouped under innate immunity, which provides immediate protection against microbial invasion, and adaptive immunity, which develops more slowly and provides more specialized defense against infections (Fig. 1-3). Innate immunity, also called natural immunity or native immunity, is always present in healthy individuals (hence the term *innate*), prepared to block the entry of microbes and to rapidly eliminate microbes that do succeed in entering host tissues. Adaptive immunity, also called specific immunity or acquired immunity, requires expansion and differentiation of lymphocytes in response to microbes before it can provide effective defense; that is, it adapts to the presence of microbial invaders. Innate immunity is phylogenetically older, and the more specialized and powerful adaptive immune response evolved later.

In innate immunity, the first line of defense is provided by epithelial barriers of the skin and mucosal tissues and by cells and natural antibiotics present in epithelia, all of which function to block the entry of microbes. If microbes do breach epithelia and enter the tissues or circulation, they are attacked by phagocytes, specialized lymphocytes called innate lymphoid cells, which include natural killer cells, and several plasma proteins, including the proteins of the complement system. All these mechanisms of innate immunity specifically recognize and react against microbes. In addition to providing early defense against infections, innate immune responses enhance adaptive immune responses against the infectious agents. The components and mechanisms of innate immunity are discussed in detail in Chapter 2.

The adaptive immune system consists of lymphocytes and their products, such as antibodies. Adaptive immune responses are especially important for defense against

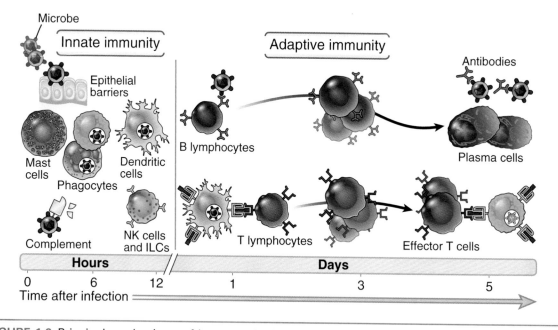

FIGURE 1-3 Principal mechanisms of innate and adaptive immunity. The mechanisms of innate immunity provide the initial defense against infections. Some mechanisms (e.g., epithelial barriers) prevent infections, and other mechanisms (e.g., phagocytes, natural killer [NK] cells and other innate lymphoid cells [ILCs], the complement system) eliminate microbes. Adaptive immune responses develop later and are mediated by lymphocytes and their products. Antibodies block infections and eliminate microbes, and T lymphocytes eradicate intracellular microbes. The kinetics of the innate and adaptive immune responses are approximations and may vary in different infections.

infectious microbes that are pathogenic for humans (i.e., capable of causing disease) and may have evolved to resist innate immunity. Whereas the mechanisms of innate immunity recognize structures shared by classes of microbes, the cells of adaptive immunity (lymphocytes) express receptors that specifically recognize a much wider variety of molecules produced by microbes as well as noninfectious substances. Any substance that is specifically recognized by lymphocytes or antibodies is called an **antigen.** Adaptive immune responses often use the cells and molecules of the innate immune system to eliminate microbes, and adaptive immunity functions to greatly enhance these antimicrobial mechanisms of innate immunity. For example, antibodies (a component of adaptive immunity) bind to microbes, and these coated microbes avidly bind to and activate phagocytes (a component of innate immunity), which ingest and destroy the microbes. Examples of the cooperation between

innate and adaptive immunity are discussed in later chapters.

By convention, the terms *immune response* and *immune system* generally refer to adaptive immunity, and that is the focus of most of this chapter.

TYPES OF ADAPTIVE IMMUNITY

The two types of adaptive immunity, called humoral immunity and cell-mediated immunity, are mediated by different cells and molecules and provide defense against extracellular microbes and intracellular microbes, respectively (Fig. 1-4).

- **Humoral immunity** is mediated by proteins called **antibodies,** which are produced by cells called **B lymphocytes.** Secreted antibodies enter the circulation and mucosal fluids, and they neutralize and eliminate microbes and microbial toxins that are present outside host cells, in the blood, extracellular fluid derived

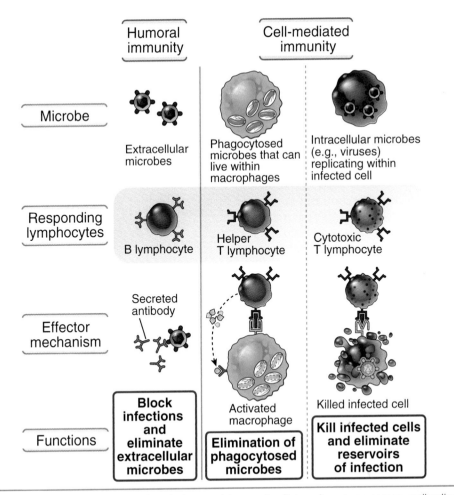

FIGURE 1-4 **Types of adaptive immunity.** In humoral immunity, B lymphocytes secrete antibodies that eliminate extracellular microbes. In cell-mediated immunity, different types of T lymphocytes recruit and activate phagocytes to destroy ingested microbes and kill infected cells.

from plasma, and in the lumens of mucosal organs such as the gastrointestinal and respiratory tracts. One of the most important functions of antibodies is to stop microbes that are present at mucosal surfaces and in the blood from gaining access to and colonizing host cells and connective tissues. In this way, antibodies prevent infections from ever being established. Antibodies cannot gain access to microbes that live and divide inside infected cells.

- Defense against such intracellular microbes is called **cell-mediated immunity** because it is mediated by cells, which are called **T lymphocytes**. Some T lymphocytes activate phagocytes to destroy microbes that have been ingested by the phagocytes into intracellular vesicles. Other T lymphocytes kill any type of host cells that are harboring infectious microbes in the cytoplasm. In both cases, the T cells recognize microbial antigens that are displayed on host cell surfaces, which indicates there is a microbe inside the cell.

The specificities of B and T lymphocytes differ in important respects. Most T cells recognize only protein antigens, whereas B cells and antibodies are able to recognize many different types of molecules, including proteins, carbohydrates, nucleic acids, and lipids. These and other differences are discussed in more detail later.

Immunity may be induced in an individual by infection or vaccination (active immunity) or conferred on an individual by transfer of antibodies or lymphocytes from an actively immunized individual (passive immunity).

- In **active immunity,** an individual exposed to the antigens of a microbe mounts an active response to eradicate the infection and develops resistance to later infection by that microbe. Such an individual is said to be immune to that microbe, in contrast with a naive individual, not previously exposed to that microbe's antigens.
- In **passive immunity,** a naive individual receives antibodies or cells (e.g., lymphocytes, feasible only in animal experiments) from another individual already immune to an infection. The recipient acquires the ability to combat the infection for as long as the transferred antibodies or cells last. Passive immunity is therefore useful for rapidly conferring immunity even before the individual is able to mount an active response, but it does not induce long-lived resistance to the infection. The only physiologic example of passive immunity is seen in newborns, whose immune systems are not mature enough to respond to many pathogens but who are protected against infections by acquiring antibodies from their mothers through the placenta and breast milk. Clinically, passive immunity is limited to treatment of some immunodeficiency diseases with antibodies pooled from multiple donors, and for emergency treatment of some viral infections and snakebites using serum from immunized donors.

PROPERTIES OF ADAPTIVE IMMUNE RESPONSES

Several properties of adaptive immune responses are crucial for the effectiveness of these responses in combating infections (Fig. 1-5).

Specificity and Diversity

The adaptive immune system is capable of distinguishing among millions of different

Feature	Functional significance
Specificity	Ensures that distinct antigens elicit specific responses
Diversity	Enables immune system to respond to a large variety of antigens
Memory	Leads to enhanced responses to repeated exposures to the same antigens
Clonal expansion	Increases number of antigen-specific lymphocytes from a small number of naive lymphocytes
Specialization	Generates responses that are optimal for defense against different types of microbes
Contraction and homeostasis	Allows immune system to respond to newly encountered antigens
Nonreactivity to self	Prevents injury to the host during responses to foreign antigens

FIGURE 1-5 Properties of adaptive immune responses. This table summarizes the important properties of adaptive immune responses and how each feature contributes to host defense against microbes.

antigens or portions of antigens. Specificity is the ability to distinguish between many different antigens. It implies that the total collection of lymphocyte specificities, sometimes called the **lymphocyte repertoire,** is extremely **diverse.** The basis for this remarkable specificity and diversity is that lymphocytes express clonally distributed receptors for antigens, meaning that the total population of lymphocytes consists of many different clones (each made up of one cell and its progeny), and each clone expresses an antigen receptor that is different from the receptors of all other clones. The **clonal selection hypothesis,** formulated in the 1950s, correctly predicted that clones of lymphocytes specific for different antigens develop before an encounter with these antigens, and each antigen elicits an immune response by selecting and activating the lymphocytes of a specific clone (Fig. 1-6). We now

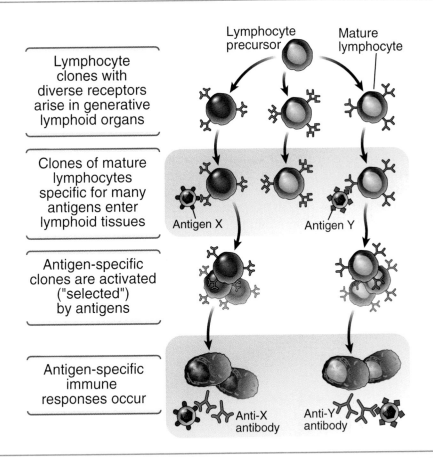

FIGURE 1-6 Clonal selection. Mature lymphocytes with receptors for many antigens develop before encountering these antigens. A clone refers to a population of lymphocytes with identical antigen receptors and therefore specificities; all of these cells are presumably derived from one precursor cell. Each antigen (e.g., X and Y) selects a preexisting clone of specific lymphocytes and stimulates the proliferation and differentiation of that clone. The diagram shows only B lymphocytes giving rise to antibody-secreting cells, but the same principle applies to T lymphocytes. The antigens shown are surface molecules of microbes, but clonal selection also is true for extracellular soluble and intracellular antigens.

know the molecular basis for how the specificity and diversity of lymphocytes are generated (see Chapter 4).

The diversity of the lymphocyte repertoire, which enables the immune system to respond to a vast number and variety of antigens, also means that very few cells, perhaps as few as 1 in 100,000 or 1 in 1,000,000 lymphocytes, are specific for any one antigen. Thus, the total number of naive (unactivated) lymphocytes that can recognize and react against any one antigen ranges from about 1000 to 10,000 cells.

To mount an effective defense against microbes, these few cells have to give rise to a large number of lymphocytes capable of destroying the microbes. The remarkable effectiveness of immune responses is attributable to several features of adaptive immunity, including the marked expansion of the pool of lymphocytes specific for any antigen upon exposure to that antigen, and selection mechanisms that preserve the most useful lymphocytes. These characteristics of the adaptive immune system are described in later chapters.

Memory

The adaptive immune system mounts larger and more effective responses to repeated exposures to the same antigen. This feature of adaptive immune responses implies that the immune system remembers exposure to antigen, and this property of adaptive immunity is therefore called **immunologic memory**. The response to the first exposure to antigen, called the **primary immune response,** is initiated by lymphocytes called naive lymphocytes that are seeing antigen for the first time (Fig. 1-7). The term *naive* refers to these cells being immunologically inexperienced, not having previously responded to antigens. Subsequent encounters with the same antigen lead to responses called **secondary immune responses** that

usually are more rapid, larger, and better able to eliminate the antigen than primary responses. Secondary responses are the result of the activation of memory lymphocytes, which are long-lived cells that were induced during the primary immune response. The term *memory* arose because of the realization that these cells must remember previous encounter with antigen since they respond better upon subsequent encounters. Immunologic memory optimizes the ability of the immune system to combat persistent and recurrent infections, because each exposure to a microbe generates more memory cells and activates previously generated memory cells. Memory also is one of the reasons why vaccines confer long-lasting protection against infections.

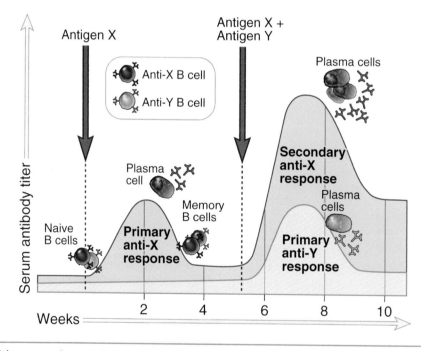

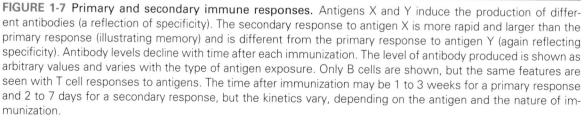

FIGURE 1-7 Primary and secondary immune responses. Antigens X and Y induce the production of different antibodies (a reflection of specificity). The secondary response to antigen X is more rapid and larger than the primary response (illustrating memory) and is different from the primary response to antigen Y (again reflecting specificity). Antibody levels decline with time after each immunization. The level of antibody produced is shown as arbitrary values and varies with the type of antigen exposure. Only B cells are shown, but the same features are seen with T cell responses to antigens. The time after immunization may be 1 to 3 weeks for a primary response and 2 to 7 days for a secondary response, but the kinetics vary, depending on the antigen and the nature of immunization.

Other Features of Adaptive Immunity

Adaptive immune responses have other characteristics that are important for their functions (see Fig. 1-5).

- When lymphocytes are activated by antigens, they undergo proliferation, generating many thousands of clonal progeny cells, all with the same antigen specificity. This process, called **clonal expansion,** rapidly increases the number of cells specific for the antigen encountered and ensures that adaptive immunity keeps pace with rapidly proliferating microbes.
- Immune responses are specialized, and different responses are designed to defend best against different classes of microbes.
- All immune responses are self-limited and decline as the infection is eliminated, allowing the system to return to a resting state, prepared to respond to another infection.
- The immune system is able to react against an enormous number and variety of microbes and other foreign antigens, but it normally does not react against the host's own potentially antigenic substances—so-called self antigens. This unresponsiveness to self is called **immunological tolerance**, referring to the ability of the immune system to coexist with (tolerate) potentially antigenic self molecules, cells, and tissues.

CELLS OF THE IMMUNE SYSTEM

The cells of the immune system are located in different tissues and serve different roles in host defense (Fig. 1-8).

Cell type	Principal function(s)
Lymphocytes: B lymphocytes; T lymphocytes 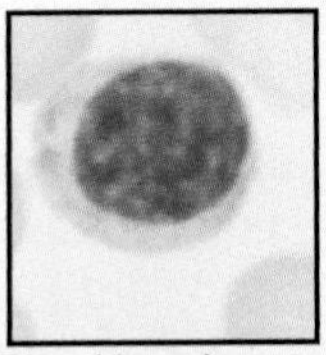 *Blood lymphocyte*	Specific recognition of antigens • B lymphocytes: mediators of humoral immunity • T lymphocytes: mediators of cell-mediated immunity
Antigen-presenting cells: dendritic cells; macrophages; B cells; follicular dendritic cells 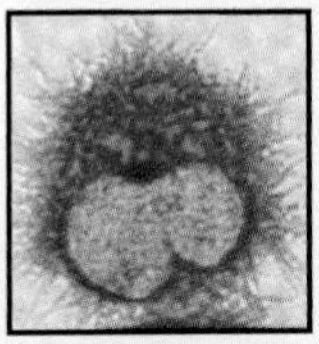 *Dendritic cell*	Capture of antigens for display to lymphocytes: • Dendritic cells: initiation of T cell responses • Macrophages: effector phase of cell-mediated immunity • Follicular dendritic cells: display of antigens to B lymphocytes in humoral immune responses
Effector cells: T lymphocytes; macrophages; granulocytes 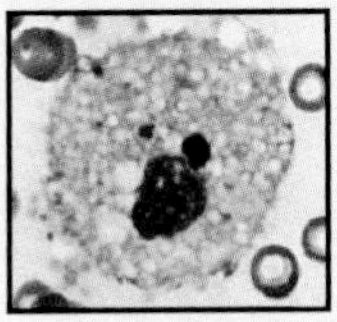 *Macrophage*	Elimination of antigens: • T lymphocytes: activation of phagocytes, killing infected cells • Macrophages: phagocytosis and killing of microbes • Granulocytes: killing microbes

FIGURE 1-8 Principal cells of the immune system. The major cell types involved in immune responses and the key functions of these cells. Micrographs illustrate the morphology of some cells of each type.

- Lymphocytes circulate through lymphoid organs and nonlymphoid tissues. They recognize foreign antigens and initiate adaptive immune responses.
- Cells resident in tissues detect the presence of microbes and react against them. These cells include macrophages, whose function is to ingest and destroy foreign substances; dendritic cells, which capture microbes and display them to lymphocytes to initiate immune responses, and are therefore called **antigen-presenting cells**; and mast cells, which help to recruit other leukocytes to destroy microbes.
- Phagocytes that normally circulate in the blood, including neutrophils and monocytes, are rapidly recruited to sites of infection in the process called inflammation. These leukocytes (white blood cells) ingest and destroy microbes and then start the process of repairing damaged tissues. Because these phagocytes, as well as some T lymphocytes, are responsible for the effect of the immune response, which is to destroy microbes, they are sometimes called **effector cells.**

This section describes the important properties of the major cell populations of adaptive immunity—namely, lymphocytes and antigen-presenting cells. The cells of innate immunity are described in Chapter 2.

Lymphocytes

Lymphocytes are the only cells that produce clonally distributed receptors specific for diverse antigens and are the key mediators of adaptive immunity. A healthy adult contains $0.5-1\times10^{12}$ lymphocytes. Although all lymphocytes are morphologically similar and rather unremarkable in appearance, they are heterogeneous in lineage, function, and phenotype and are capable of complex biologic responses and activities (Fig. 1-9). These cells often are distinguishable by surface proteins that may be identified using panels of monoclonal antibodies. The standard nomenclature for these proteins is the CD (cluster of differentiation) numerical designation, which is used to delineate surface proteins that define a particular cell type or stage of cell differentiation

and that are recognized by a cluster or group of antibodies. (A list of CD molecules mentioned in the book is provided in Appendix II.)

As alluded to earlier, B lymphocytes are the only cells capable of producing antibodies; therefore, they are the cells that mediate humoral immunity. B cells express membrane forms of antibodies that serve as the receptors that recognize antigens and initiate the process of activation of the cells. Soluble antigens and antigens on the surface of microbes and other cells may bind to these B lymphocyte antigen receptors, initiating the process of B cell activation. This leads to the secretion of soluble forms of antibodies with the same antigen specificity as the membrane receptors.

T lymphocytes are responsible for cell-mediated immunity. The antigen receptors of most T lymphocytes recognize only peptide fragments of protein antigens that are bound to specialized peptide display molecules, called major histocompatibility complex (MHC) molecules, on the surface of specialized cells, called antigen-presenting cells (see Chapter 3). Among T lymphocytes, CD4+ T cells are called **helper T cells** because they help B lymphocytes to produce antibodies and help phagocytes to destroy ingested microbes. CD8+ T lymphocytes are called **cytotoxic T lymphocytes** (CTLs) because they kill cells harboring intracellular microbes. Some CD4+ T cells belong to a special subset that functions to prevent or limit immune responses; these are called **regulatory T lymphocytes.**

All lymphocytes arise from stem cells in the bone marrow (Fig. 1-10). **B lymphocytes mature in the bone marrow, and T lymphocytes mature in an organ called the thymus.** These sites in which mature lymphocytes are produced (generated) are called the **generative lymphoid organs.** Mature lymphocytes leave the generative lymphoid organs and enter the circulation and the **peripheral lymphoid organs,** where they may encounter antigen for which they express specific receptors.

When naive lymphocytes recognize microbial antigens and also receive additional signals induced by microbes, the antigen-specific lymphocytes proliferate

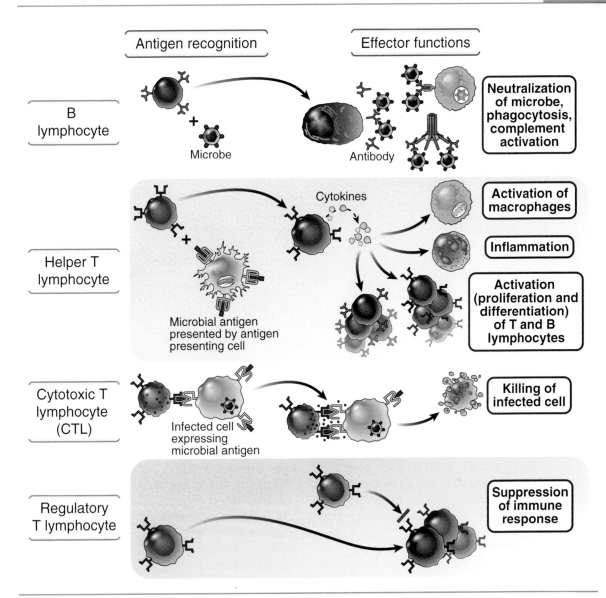

FIGURE 1-9 Classes of lymphocytes. Different classes of lymphocytes in the adaptive immune system recognize distinct types of antigens and differentiate into effector cells whose function is to eliminate the antigens. B lymphocytes recognize soluble or cell surface antigens and differentiate into antibody-secreting cells. Helper T lymphocytes recognize antigens on the surfaces of antigen-presenting cells and secrete cytokines, which stimulate different mechanisms of immunity and inflammation. Cytotoxic T lymphocytes recognize antigens in infected cells and kill these cells. (Note that T lymphocytes recognize peptides that are displayed by MHC molecules, discussed in Chapter 3.) Regulatory T cells limit the activation of other lymphocytes, especially of T cells, and prevent autoimmunity.

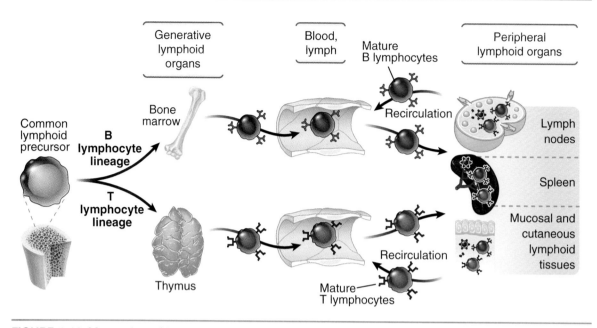

FIGURE 1-10 Maturation of lymphocytes. Lymphocytes develop from precursors in the generative lymphoid organs (bone marrow and thymus). Mature lymphocytes enter the peripheral lymphoid organs, where they respond to foreign antigens and recirculate in the blood and lymph. Some immature B cells leave the bone marrow and complete their maturation in the spleen (not shown).

and differentiate into effector cells and memory cells (Fig. 1-11).

- **Naive lymphocytes** express receptors for antigens but do not perform the functions that are required to eliminate antigens. These cells reside in and circulate between peripheral lymphoid organs and survive for several weeks or months, waiting to find and respond to antigen. If they are not activated by antigen, naive lymphocytes die by the process of apoptosis and are replaced by new cells that have arisen in the generative lymphoid organs. The differentiation of naive lymphocytes into effector cells and memory cells is initiated by antigen recognition, thus ensuring that the immune response that develops is specific for the antigen.
- **Effector lymphocytes** are the differentiated progeny of naive cells that have the ability to produce molecules that function to eliminate antigens. The effector cells in the B lymphocyte lineage are antibody-secreting cells, called **plasma cells.** Plasma cells develop in response to antigenic stimulation in

the peripheral lymphoid organs, where they may stay and produce antibodies. Small numbers of antibody-secreting cells are also found in the blood; these are called plasmablasts. Some of these migrate to the bone marrow, where they mature into long-lived plasma cells and continue to produce small amounts of antibody long after the infection is eradicated, providing immediate protection in case the infection recurs.

Effector CD4+ T cells (helper T cells) produce proteins called **cytokines** that activate B cells, macrophages, and other cell types, thereby mediating the helper function of this lineage. Effector CD8+ T cells (CTLs) have the machinery to kill infected host cells. The development and functions of these effector cells are discussed in later chapters. Effector T lymphocytes are short-lived and die as the antigen is eliminated.
- **Memory cells,** also generated from the progeny of antigen-stimulated lymphocytes, do survive for long periods in the absence of antigen. Therefore, the frequency of memory cells

A

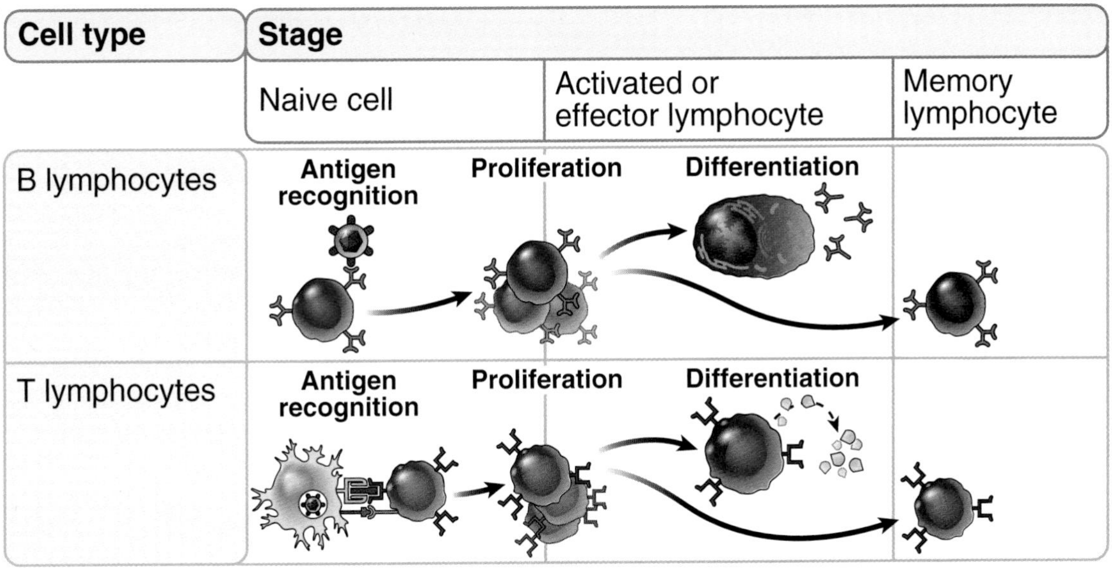

Cell type	Stage		
	Naive cell	Activated or effector lymphocyte	Memory lymphocyte
B lymphocytes	Antigen recognition	Proliferation	Differentiation
T lymphocytes	Antigen recognition	Proliferation	Differentiation

B

	Naive cell	Activated or effector lymphocyte	Memory lymphocyte
T lymphocytes			
Migration	Preferentially to peripheral lymph nodes	Preferentially to inflamed tissues	Heterogenous: one subset to lymph nodes, one subset to mucosa and inflamed tissues
Frequency of cells responsive to particular antigen	Very low	High	Low
Effector functions	None	Cytokine secretion; cytotoxic activity	None
B lymphocytes			
Membrane immunoglobulin (Ig) isotype	IgM and IgD	Frequently IgG, IgA, and IgE	Frequently IgG, IgA, and IgE
Affinity of Ig produced	Relatively low	Increases during immune response	Relatively high
Effector functions	None	Antibody secretion	None

FIGURE 1-11 Stages in the life history of lymphocytes. A, Naive lymphocytes recognize foreign antigens to initiate adaptive immune responses. Naive lymphocytes need signals in addition to antigens to proliferate and differentiate into effector cells; these additional signals are not shown. Effector cells, which develop from naive cells, function to eliminate antigens. The effector cells of the B lymphocyte lineage are antibody-secreting plasma cells (some of which are long-lived). The effector cells of the CD4 T lymphocyte lineage produce cytokines. (The effector cells of the CD8 lineage are CTLs; these are not shown.) Other progeny of the antigen-stimulated lymphocytes differentiate into long-lived memory cells. B, The important characteristics of naive, effector, and memory cells in the B and T lymphocyte lineages are summarized. The generation and functions of effector cells, including changes in migration patterns and types of immunoglobulin produced, are described in later chapters.

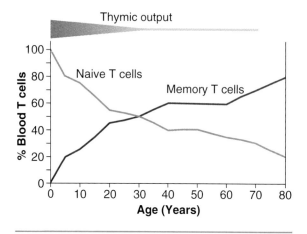

FIGURE 1-12 Change in proportions of naive and memory T cells with age. The proportions of naive and memory T cells are based on data from multiple healthy individuals. The estimate of thymic output is an approximation. (Courtesy of Dr. Donna L. Farber, Columbia University College of Physicians and Surgeons, New York.)

increases with age, presumably because of exposure to environmental microbes. In fact, memory cells make up less than 5% of peripheral blood T cells in a newborn, but 50% or more in an adult (Fig. 1-12). As individuals age, the gradual accumulation of memory cells compensates for the reduced output of new, naive T cells from the thymus, which involutes after puberty (see Chapter 4). Memory cells are functionally inactive; they do not perform effector functions unless stimulated by antigen. When memory cells encounter the same antigen that induced their development, the cells rapidly respond to initiate secondary immune responses. The signals that generate and maintain memory cells are not well understood but include cytokines.

Antigen-Presenting Cells

The common portals of entry for microbes—the skin, gastrointestinal tract, and respiratory tract—contain specialized antigen-presenting cells (APCs) located in the epithelium that capture antigens, transport them to peripheral lymphoid tissues, and display (present) them to lymphocytes.

This function of antigen capture and presentation is best understood for a cell type that is called **dendritic cells** because of their long surface membrane processes. Dendritic cells capture protein antigens of microbes entering through the epithelia and transport the antigens to regional lymph nodes, where the antigen-bearing dendritic cells display portions of the antigens for recognition by T lymphocytes. If a microbe has invaded through the epithelium, it may be phagocytosed and presented by tissue macrophages. Microbes or their antigens that enter lymphoid organs may be captured by dendritic cells or macrophages that reside in these organs and presented to lymphocytes. Dendritic cells are the most effective APCs for initiating T cell responses. The process of antigen presentation to T cells is described in Chapter 3.

Cells that are specialized to display antigens to T lymphocytes have another important feature that gives them the ability to stimulate T cell responses. These specialized cells respond to microbes by producing surface and secreted proteins that are required, together with antigen, to activate naive T lymphocytes to proliferate and differentiate into effector cells. Specialized cells that display antigens to T cells and provide additional activating signals sometimes are called professional APCs. The prototypic professional APCs are dendritic cells, but macrophages, B cells, and a few other cell types may serve the same function in various immune responses.

Less is known about cells that may capture antigens for display to B lymphocytes. B lymphocytes may directly recognize the antigens of microbes (either released or on the surface of the microbes), or macrophages lining lymphatic channels may capture antigens and display them to B cells. A type of cell called the **follicular dendritic cell** (FDC) resides in the germinal centers of lymphoid follicles in the peripheral lymphoid organs and displays antigens that stimulate the differentiation of B cells in the follicles (see Chapter 7). FDCs do not present antigens to T cells and differ from the dendritic cells described earlier that function as APCs for T lymphocytes.

TISSUES OF THE IMMUNE SYSTEM

The tissues of the immune system consist of the generative lymphoid organs, in which T and B lymphocytes mature and become competent to respond to antigens, and the peripheral lymphoid organs, in which adaptive immune responses to microbes are initiated (see Fig. 1-10). Most of the lymphocytes in a healthy human are found in lymphoid organs and other tissues (Fig. 1-13). However, as we discuss later, lymphocytes are unique among the cells of the body because of their ability to circulate among tissues. The generative (also called primary or central) lymphoid organs are described in Chapter 4, when we discuss the process of lymphocyte maturation. The following section highlights some of the features of peripheral (or secondary) lymphoid organs that are important for the development of adaptive immunity.

Peripheral Lymphoid Organs

The peripheral lymphoid organs, which consist of the lymph nodes, the spleen, and the mucosal and cutaneous immune systems, are organized in a way that promotes the development of adaptive immune responses. T and B lymphocytes must locate microbes that enter at any site in the body, then respond to these microbes and eliminate them. In addition, as previously discussed, in the normal immune system, very few of these lymphocytes are specific for any one antigen. It is not possible for the few lymphocytes specific for any antigen to patrol all possible sites of antigen entry. The anatomic organization of peripheral lymphoid organs enables APCs to concentrate antigens in these organs and lymphocytes to locate and respond to the antigens. This organization is complemented by a remarkable ability of lymphocytes to circulate throughout the body in such a way that naive lymphocytes preferentially go to the specialized organs in which antigen is concentrated, and effector cells go to sites of infection where microbes must be eliminated. Furthermore, different types of lymphocytes often need to communicate to generate effective immune responses. For example, helper T cells specific for an antigen interact with and

Tissue	Number of lymphocytes
Spleen	70×10^9
Lymph nodes	190×10^9
Bone marrow	50×10^9
Blood	10×10^9
Skin	20×10^9
Intestines	50×10^9
Liver	10×10^9
Lungs	30×10^9

FIGURE 1-13 Distribution of lymphocytes in lymphoid organs and other tissues. Approximate numbers of lymphocytes in different organs of healthy adults are shown.

help B lymphocytes specific for the same antigen, resulting in antibody production. An important function of lymphoid organs is to bring these rare cells together after stimulation by antigen so they interact.

The major peripheral lymphoid organs share many characteristics but also have some unique features.

- **Lymph nodes** are encapsulated nodular aggregates of lymphoid tissues located along lymphatic channels throughout the body (Fig. 1-14). Fluid constantly leaks out of blood vessels in all epithelia and connective tissues and most parenchymal organs. This fluid, called **lymph,** is drained by lymphatic vessels from the tissues to the lymph nodes and eventually back into the blood circulation. Therefore, the lymph contains a mixture of substances absorbed from epithelia and tissues. As the lymph passes through lymph nodes, APCs in the nodes are able to sample the antigens of microbes that may enter through epithelia into tissues. In addition, dendritic cells pick up antigens of microbes from epithelia and other tissues and transport these antigens to the lymph nodes. The net result of

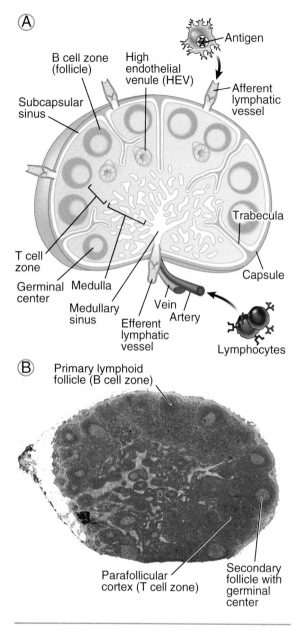

FIGURE 1-14 Morphology of lymph nodes. A, Schematic diagram shows the structural organization of a lymph node. **B,** Light micrograph shows a cross section of a lymph node with numerous follicles in the cortex, some of which contain lightly stained central areas (germinal centers).

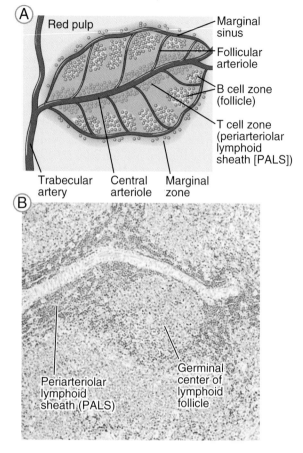

FIGURE 1-15 Morphology of the spleen. A, Schematic diagram shows a splenic arteriole surrounded by the periarteriolar lymphoid sheath (PALS) and attached follicle containing a prominent germinal center. The PALS and lymphoid follicles together constitute the white pulp. **B,** Light micrograph of a section of spleen shows an arteriole with the PALS and a follicle with a germinal center. These are surrounded by the red pulp, which is rich in vascular sinusoids.

these processes of antigen capture and transport is that the antigens of microbes entering through epithelia or colonizing tissues become concentrated in draining lymph nodes.

- The **spleen** is a highly vascularized abdominal organ that serves the same role in immune responses to blood-borne antigens as that of lymph nodes in responses to lymph-borne antigens (Fig. 1-15). Blood entering the spleen flows through a network of channels (sinusoids).

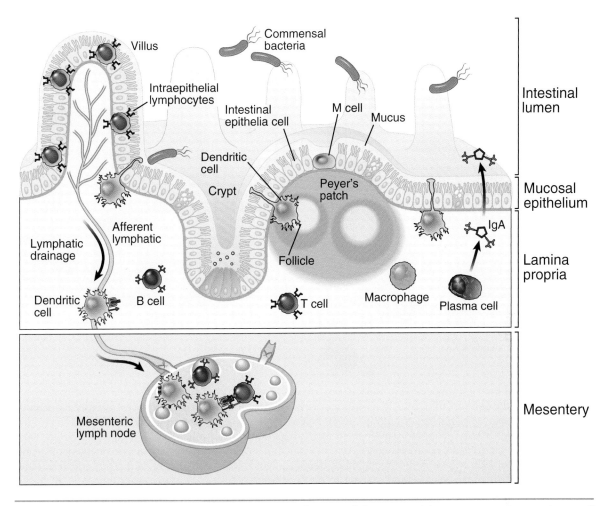

FIGURE 1-16 Mucosal immune system. Schematic diagram of the mucosal immune system uses the small bowel as an example. Many commensal bacteria are present in the lumen. The mucus-secreting epithelium provides an innate barrier to microbial invasion (discussed in Chapter 2). Specialized epithelial cells, such as M cells, promote the transport of antigens from the lumen into underlying tissues. Cells in the lamina propria, including dendritic cells, T lymphocytes, and macrophages, provide innate and adaptive immune defense against invading microbes; some of these cells are organized into specialized structures, such as Peyer's patches in the small intestine. Immunoglobulin A (IgA) is a type of antibody abundantly produced in mucosal tissues that is transported into the lumen, where it binds and neutralizes microbes (see Chapter 8).

Blood-borne antigens are captured and concentrated by dendritic cells and macrophages in the spleen. The spleen contains abundant phagocytes, which ingest and destroy microbes in the blood.

- The **cutaneous immune system** and **mucosal immune system** are specialized collections of lymphoid tissues and APCs located in and under the epithelia of the skin and the gastrointestinal and respiratory tracts, respectively. Although most of the immune cells in these tissues are diffusely scattered beneath the epithelial barriers, there are discrete collections of lymphocytes and APCs organized in a similar way as in lymph nodes. For example, tonsils in the pharynx and Peyer's patches in the intestine are two anatomically defined mucosal lymphoid tissues (Fig. 1-16).

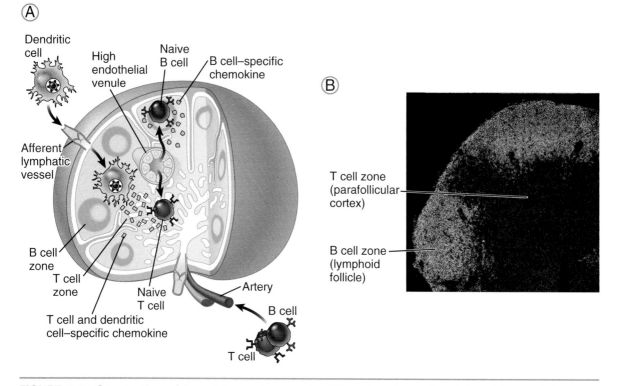

FIGURE 1-17 Segregation of T and B lymphocytes in different regions of peripheral lymphoid organs. A, Schematic diagram illustrates the path by which naive T and B lymphocytes migrate to different areas of a lymph node. Naive B and T lymphocytes enter through a high endothelial venule (HEV), shown in cross section, and are drawn to different areas of the node by chemokines that are produced in these areas and bind selectively to either cell type. Also shown is the migration of dendritic cells, which pick up antigens from epithelia, enter through afferent lymphatic vessels, and migrate to the T cell–rich areas of the node (see Chapter 3). **B,** In this histologic section of a lymph node, the B lymphocytes, located in the follicles, are stained green, and the T cells, in the parafollicular cortex, are stained red using immunofluorescence. In this technique, a section of the tissue is stained with antibodies specific for T or B cells coupled to fluorochromes that emit different colors when excited at the appropriate wavelengths. The anatomic segregation of T and B cells also occurs in the spleen (not shown). (Courtesy Drs. Kathryn Pape and Jennifer Walter, University of Minnesota Medical School, Minneapolis.)

At any time, at least a quarter of the body's lymphocytes are in the mucosal tissues and skin (reflecting the large size of these tissues) (see Fig. 1-13), and many of these are memory cells. Cutaneous and mucosal lymphoid tissues are sites of immune responses to antigens that breach epithelia. A remarkable property of the cutaneous and mucosal immune systems is that they are able to respond to pathogens but do not react to the enormous numbers of usually harmless commensal microbes present at the epithelial barriers. This is accomplished by several mechanisms, including the action of regulatory T cells and other cells that suppress rather than activate T lymphocytes.

Within the peripheral lymphoid organs, T lymphocytes and B lymphocytes are segregated into different anatomic compartments (Fig. 1-17). In lymph nodes, the B cells are concentrated in discrete structures, called **follicles**, located around the periphery, or cortex, of each node. If the B cells in a follicle have recently responded to an antigen, this follicle may contain a central lightly staining region called a **germinal center**. The role of germinal centers in the production of antibodies is described in Chapter 7. The T lymphocytes are concentrated outside but adjacent to the follicles, in the paracortex. The follicles contain the FDCs described earlier that are involved in the activation of B cells, and the paracortex contains the dendritic cells that present antigens to T lymphocytes. In the spleen, T lymphocytes are concentrated in periarteriolar lymphoid sheaths surrounding small arterioles, and B cells reside in the follicles.

The anatomic organization of peripheral lymphoid organs is tightly regulated to allow immune responses to develop after stimulation by antigens. B lymphocytes are attracted to and retained in the follicles because of the action of a class of cytokines called **chemokines** (chemoattractant cytokines; chemokines and other cytokines are discussed in more detail in later chapters). FDCs in the follicles secrete a particular chemokine for which naive B cells express a receptor, called CXCR5. The chemokine that binds to CXCR5 attracts B cells from the blood into the follicles of lymphoid organs. Similarly, T cells are segregated in the paracortex of lymph nodes and the periarteriolar lymphoid sheaths of the spleen, because naive T lymphocytes express a receptor, called CCR7, that recognizes chemokines that are produced in these regions of the lymph nodes and spleen. As a result, T lymphocytes are recruited from the blood into the paracortical region of the lymph node and the periarteriolar lymphoid sheaths of the spleen. When the lymphocytes are activated by antigens, they alter their expression of chemokine receptors. The B cells and T cells then migrate toward each other and meet at the edge of follicles, where helper T cells interact with and help B cells to differentiate into antibody-producing cells (see Chapter 7). Thus, these lymphocyte populations are kept apart from each other until it is useful for them to interact, after exposure to an antigen. This is an excellent example of how the structure of lymphoid organs ensures that the cells that have recognized and responded to an antigen interact and communicate with one another only when necessary.

Many of the activated lymphocytes, especially the effector and memory T cells, ultimately exit the node through efferent lymphatic vessels and leave the spleen through veins. These activated lymphocytes end up in the circulation and can go to distant sites of infection. Some activated T cells remain in the lymphoid organ where they were generated and migrate into lymphoid follicles, where they help B cells to make high-affinity antibodies.

Lymphocyte Recirculation and Migration into Tissues

Naive lymphocytes constantly recirculate between the blood and peripheral lymphoid organs, where they may be activated by antigens to become effector cells, and the effector lymphocytes migrate from lymphoid tissues to sites of infection, where microbes are eliminated (Fig. 1-18). Thus, lymphocytes at distinct stages of their lives migrate to the different sites where they are needed for their functions. Migration of effector lymphocytes to sites of infection is most relevant for T cells, because effector T cells have to locate and eliminate microbes at these sites. By contrast, plasma cells do not need to migrate to sites of infection; instead, they secrete antibodies, and the antibodies enter the blood, where they may bind blood-borne pathogens or toxins. Plasma cells in mucosal organs secrete antibodies that enter the lumens of these organs, where they bind to and combat ingested and inhaled microbes.

• Naive T lymphocytes that have matured in the thymus and entered the circulation migrate to lymph nodes, where they can find antigens that are brought to the lymph nodes through lymphatic vessels that drain epithelia and parenchymal organs. These naive T cells enter lymph nodes through specialized postcapillary venules, called **high endothelial venules** (HEVs). The adhesion molecules used by the T cells to bind to the endothelium are described in Chapter 6. Chemokines produced in the T cell zones of the lymph nodes and displayed on HEV surfaces bind to the chemokine receptor CCR7 expressed on naive T cells, which causes the T cells to bind tightly to HEVs. The naive T cells then migrate into the T cell zone, where antigens are displayed by dendritic cells.

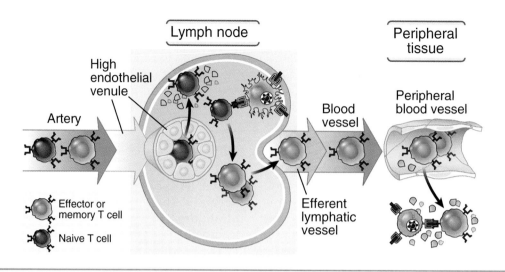

FIGURE 1-18 Migration of T lymphocytes. Naive T lymphocytes migrate from the blood through high endothelial venules into the T cell zones of lymph nodes, where the cells are activated by antigens. Activated T cells exit the nodes, enter the bloodstream, and migrate preferentially to peripheral tissues at sites of infection and inflammation. The adhesion molecules involved in the attachment of T cells to endothelial cells are described in Chapters 5 and 6.

Naive B cells also enter lymphoid tissues but then migrate to follicles in response to chemokines that bind CXCR5, the chemokine receptor expressed on these B cells.

- In the lymph node, if a T cell specifically recognizes an antigen on a dendritic cell, that T cell forms stable conjugates with the dendritic cell and is activated. Such an encounter between an antigen and a specific lymphocyte is likely to be a random event, but most T cells in the body circulate through some lymph nodes at least once a day. As mentioned earlier and described further in Chapter 3, the likelihood of the correct T cell finding its antigen is increased in peripheral lymphoid organs, particularly lymph nodes, because microbial antigens are concentrated in the same regions of these organs through which naive T cells circulate. Thus, T cells find the antigen they can recognize, and these T cells are activated to proliferate and differentiate. Naive cells that have not encountered specific antigens leave the lymph nodes and reenter the circulation.

- The effector cells that are generated upon T cell activation preferentially migrate into the tissues infected by microbes, where the T lymphocytes perform their function of eradicating the infection. Specific signals control these precise patterns of migration of naive and activated T cells (see Chapter 6).
- B lymphocytes that recognize and respond to antigen in lymph node follicles differentiate into antibody-secreting cells, which either remain in the lymph nodes or migrate to the bone marrow (see Chapter 7).
- Memory T cells consist of different populations; some cells recirculate through lymph nodes, where they can mount secondary responses to captured antigens, and other cells migrate to sites of infection, where they can respond rapidly to eliminate the infection.

We know less about lymphocyte circulation through the spleen or other lymphoid tissues. The spleen does not contain HEVs, but the general pattern of naive lymphocyte migration through this organ probably is similar to migration through lymph nodes.

OVERVIEW OF IMMUNE RESPONSES TO MICROBES

Now that we have described the major components of the immune system, it is useful to summarize the key features of immune responses to microbes. The focus here is on the physiologic function of the immune system—defense against infections. In subsequent chapters, each of these features is discussed in more detail.

Early Innate Immune Response to Microbes

In healthy uninfected individuals, the innate immune system is constantly defending against infection by microbial organisms in our environment and against commensal organisms that live on our epithelial barriers, including skin and mucosal barriers (lung, gastrointestinal tract, urogenital tract). In large part, the innate immune system prevents these organisms from getting across the barriers. If microbes do transgress the barriers, the innate immune system is always ready, rapidly responds, and attempts to eliminate the invaders.

The two principal ways the innate immune system deals with microbes is by inducing **inflammation** and by **antiviral mechanisms**. Inflammation, which is triggered by all classes of microbes, is the recruitment of circulating blood leukocytes (e.g., phagocytes and lymphocytes) and various plasma proteins (e.g., complement, antibodies, fibrinogen) to sites of infection, where they function to destroy the microbes and repair damaged tissue. Several different cytokines are involved in the inflammatory response. The antiviral mechanisms render host cells inhospitable for viral infection and reproduction. These innate responses are often sufficient to prevent infection within tissues or the blood.

In order to maintain this state of readiness, the innate immune system populates all tissues with sentinel cells, including macrophages, dendritic cells and mast cells, which express many different cell surface and intracellular molecules that recognize thousands of common features of different classes of microbes, such as bacteria cell walls, or viral nucleic acids. Some of these receptors are also present on epithelial barrier cells. The recognition of microbial products by these cells induces biochemical changes inside the cell that elicit the inflammatory and antiviral responses.

In addition to tissue-resident cells and cells recruited from the circulation, soluble molecules are also present in blood and tissue fluids that can recognize microbes and respond. For example, soluble complement proteins modify the surface of the microbes so the microbes are more readily taken up by phagocytes.

In addition to recognizing microbial structures, the innate immune system also recognizes and responds to dead or injured cells, which may be because of microbial infection or, in the case of sterile injury, may be a site where microbes can readily enter and grow. The innate immune response also initiates the process of tissue repair that is critical for healing damaged tissues and restoring structure and function.

Even though the innate immune system is essential for survival and often sufficient for microbial defense, it may be inadequate to eliminate or control pathogenic microbes that have evolved to evade the innate responses. Innate immunity may also be incapable of defending against organisms if they are introduced in great numbers through damaged barriers, such as in trauma or burns. It is in these situations that the adaptive immune system plays a critical role.

Adaptive Immune Response

The adaptive immune system uses the following strategies to combat the majority of microbes:

- Secreted antibodies bind to extracellular microbes, block their ability to infect host cells, and promote their ingestion and subsequent destruction by phagocytes.
- Phagocytes ingest microbes and kill them, and helper T cells enhance the microbicidal abilities of the phagocytes.
- Helper T cells recruit leukocytes to destroy microbes and enhance epithelial barrier function to prevent the entry of microbes.
- Cytotoxic T lymphocytes kill cells infected by microbes.

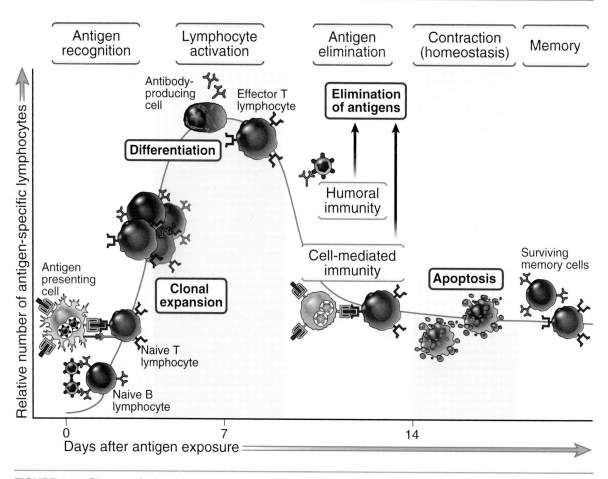

FIGURE 1-19 Phases of adaptive immune response. An adaptive immune response consists of distinct phases; the first three are recognition of antigen, activation of lymphocytes, and elimination of antigen (effector phase). The response declines as antigen-stimulated lymphocytes die by apoptosis, restoring the baseline steady state called homeostasis, and the antigen-specific cells that survive are responsible for memory. The duration of each phase may vary in different immune responses. These principles apply to both humoral immunity (mediated by B lymphocytes) and cell-mediated immunity (mediated by T lymphocytes).

Adaptive immune responses develop in steps, each of which corresponds to particular reactions of lymphocytes (Fig. 1-19).

Initiation of Adaptive Immune Response

If a microbe does get through the initial defenses of the innate immune system, the adaptive immune system is alerted and responds. The adaptive immune system generates and maintains a diverse repertoire of clones of naive B and T lymphocytes, with millions of different specificities for microbial antigens, and all of

these different clones develop prior to exposure to the antigens. These lymphocytes circulate throughout the body, visiting secondary lymphoid organs (lymph nodes, spleen. mucosal lymphoid tissues). Given their diversity, there is a high likelihood that at any time, there will be a small number of naive lymphocyte that can recognize some molecules made by most microbes. In order for the adaptive immune response to be initiated, an antigen made by the microbe selects a naive lymphocyte specific for the antigen (clonal selection), and the lymphocyte responds by proliferating to produce tens of thousands of effector lymphocytes with the identical specificity that are capable of eliminating the microbial infection.

Capture and Display of Microbial Antigens

In order for naive lymphocyte activation by antigen to occur efficiently, the immune system collects antigens from tissue sites of infection or blood and delivers them to the secondary lymphoid organs though which the naive lymphocytes circulate. Microbes that enter through epithelia, as well as their protein antigens, are captured by dendritic cells residing in these epithelia, and the cell-bound antigens are transported to draining lymph nodes. Microbial protein antigens are processed in the dendritic cells to generate peptides that are displayed on the cell surface bound to MHC molecules. Naive T cells recognize these peptide-MHC complexes, and this is the first step in the initiation of T cell responses. Protein antigens also are recognized by B lymphocytes in the lymphoid follicles of the peripheral lymphoid organs. Polysaccharides and other nonprotein antigens are captured in the lymphoid organs and are recognized by B lymphocytes but not by T cells.

As part of the innate immune response, the dendritic cells that present the antigen to naive T cells are activated to express molecules called costimulators and to secrete cytokines, both of which are needed, in addition to the antigen, to stimulate the proliferation and differentiation of T lymphocytes. The innate immune response to some microbes also generates peptide fragments of complement proteins that enhance the response of naive B lymphocytes to antigen. Thus, antigen (often referred to as signal 1) and molecules produced during innate immune responses (signal 2) function cooperatively to activate antigen-specific lymphocytes. The requirement for microbe-triggered signal 2 ensures that the adaptive immune response is induced by microbes and not by harmless substances. Signals generated in lymphocytes by the engagement of antigen receptors and receptors for costimulators lead to the transcription of various genes, which encode cytokines, cytokine receptors, effector molecules, and proteins that control cell survival and cycling. All of these molecules are involved in the responses of the lymphocytes.

Cell-Mediated Immunity: Activation of T Lymphocytes and Elimination of Cell-Associated Microbes

When activated by antigen and costimulators in lymphoid organs, naive T cells secrete cytokines that function as growth factors and respond to other cytokines secreted by dendritic cells. The combination of signals (antigen, costimulation, and cytokines) stimulates the proliferation of the T cells and their differentiation into effector T cells. Some of the effector T cells generated in the lymphoid organ may migrate back into the blood and then into any site where the antigen (or microbe) is present. These effector cells are reactivated by antigen at sites of infection and perform the functions responsible for elimination of the microbes. Helper T cells secrete cytokines and express surface molecules that mediate their functions. Helper T cells differentiate into different subsets of effector cells with distinct functions. Some of these helper cells recruit neutrophils and other leukocytes to sites of infection; other helper cells activate macrophages to kill ingested microbes; and still others stay in the lymphoid organs and help B lymphocytes to produce antibodies. CTLs directly kill cells harboring microbes in the cytoplasm. By destroying the infected cells, CTLs eliminate the reservoirs of infection.

Humoral Immunity: Activation of B Lymphocytes and Elimination of Extracellular Microbes

On activation, B lymphocytes proliferate and then differentiate into plasma cells that secrete different classes of antibodies with distinct functions. Many nonprotein antigens, such as polysaccharides and lipids, have multiple identical antigenic determinants (epitopes) that are able to engage many antigen receptor molecules on each B cell and initiate the process of B cell activation. Protein antigens are typically folded and do not contain multiple identical epitopes, so they are not able to simultaneously bind to many antigen receptors, and the full response of B cells to protein antigens requires help from CD4+ T cells. B cells ingest protein antigens, degrade them, and display peptides bound to MHC molecules for recognition by and activation of helper T cells. The helper T cells then express cytokines and cell surface proteins, which work together to activate the B cells.

Some of the progeny of the expanded B cell clones differentiate into antibody-secreting plasma cells. Each B cell secretes antibodies that have the same antigen-binding site as the cell surface antibodies (B cell antigen receptors) that first recognized the antigen. Nonprotein antigens stimulate secretion of antibodies with a limited range of functions and low affinity for the antigen. Protein antigens, by engaging the help of T cells, stimulate the production of several different kinds of antibodies with different functions and high affinity for antigen. In addition, protein antigens induce very long-lived antibody secreting cells and memory B cells.

The humoral immune response defends against microbes in many ways. Antibodies bind to microbes and prevent them from infecting cells, thereby neutralizing the microbes. Antibodies coat (opsonize) microbes and target them for phagocytosis, because phagocytes (neutrophils and macrophages) express receptors for the antibodies. Additionally, antibodies activate the complement system, generating protein fragments that promote phagocytosis and destruction of microbes. Specialized types of antibodies and specialized transport mechanisms for antibodies serve distinct roles at particular anatomic sites, including the lumens of the respiratory and gastrointestinal tracts and the placenta and fetus.

Decline of Immune Responses and Immunologic Memory

The majority of effector lymphocytes induced by an infectious pathogen die by apoptosis after the microbe is eliminated, thus returning the immune system to its basal resting state, called **homeostasis.** This occurs because microbes provide essential stimuli for lymphocyte survival and activation, and effector cells are short-lived. Therefore, as the stimuli are eliminated, the activated lymphocytes are no longer kept alive.

The initial activation of lymphocytes generates long-lived memory cells, which may survive for years after the infection and mount rapid and robust responses to a repeat encounter with the antigen.

▮ SUMMARY

- ▪ The physiologic function of the immune system is to protect individuals against infections.
- ▪ Innate immunity is the early line of defense, mediated by cells and molecules that are always present and ready to eliminate infectious microbes.
- ▪ Adaptive immunity is mediated by lymphocytes stimulated by microbial antigens, requires clonal expansion and differentiation of the lymphocytes before it is effective, and responds more effectively against each successive exposure to a microbe.
- ▪ Lymphocytes are the cells of adaptive immunity and are the only cells with clonally distributed receptors with fine specificities for different antigens.
- ▪ Adaptive immunity consists of humoral immunity, in which antibodies neutralize and eradicate extracellular microbes and toxins, and cell-mediated immunity, in which T lymphocytes eradicate intracellular microbes.
- ▪ Adaptive immune responses consist of sequential phases: antigen recognition by lymphocytes, activation of the lymphocytes to proliferate and to differentiate into effector and memory cells, elimination of the microbes, decline of the immune response, and long-lived memory.
- ▪ Different populations of lymphocytes serve distinct functions and may be distinguished by the surface expression of particular membrane molecules.
- ▪ B lymphocytes are the only cells that produce antibodies. B lymphocytes express membrane antibodies that recognize antigens, and the progeny of activated B cells, called plasma cells, secrete the antibodies that neutralize and eliminate the antigen.
- ▪ T lymphocytes recognize peptide fragments of protein antigens displayed on other cells.

Helper T lymphocytes produce cytokines that activate phagocytes to destroy ingested microbes, recruit leukocytes, and activate B lymphocytes to produce antibodies. Cytotoxic T lymphocytes (CTLs) kill infected cells harboring microbes in the cytoplasm.

- Antigen-presenting cells (APCs) capture antigens of microbes that enter through epithelia, concentrate these antigens in lymphoid organs, and display the antigens for recognition by T cells.
- Lymphocytes and APCs are organized in peripheral lymphoid organs, where immune responses are initiated and develop.
- Naive lymphocytes circulate through peripheral lymphoid organs, searching for foreign antigens. Effector T lymphocytes migrate to peripheral sites of infection, where they function to eliminate infectious microbes. Plasma cells remain in lymphoid organs and the bone marrow, where they secrete antibodies that enter the circulation and find and eliminate microbes.

REVIEW QUESTIONS

1. What are the two types of adaptive immunity, and what types of microbes do these adaptive immune responses combat?
2. What are the principal classes of lymphocytes, and how do they differ in function?
3. What are the important differences among naive, effector, and memory T and B lymphocytes?
4. Where are T and B lymphocytes located in lymph nodes, and how is their anatomic separation maintained?
5. How do naive and effector T lymphocytes differ in their patterns of migration?

Answers to and discussion of the Review Questions are available at https://studentconsult.inkling.com.

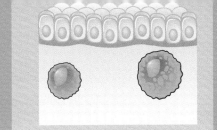

CHAPTER 2

Innate Immunity

The Early Defense Against Infections

As multicellular organisms such as plants, invertebrates, and vertebrates arose during evolution, they had to develop mechanisms for defending themselves against microbial infections and for eliminating damaged and necrotic cells. The defense mechanisms that evolved first are always present in the organism, ready to recognize and eliminate microbes and dead cells; therefore, this type of host defense is known as **innate immunity,** also called natural immunity or native immunity. The cells and molecules that are responsible for innate immunity make up the innate immune system.

Innate immunity is the critical first step in host defense against infections. It blocks microbial invasion through epithelial barriers, destroys many microbes that do enter the body, and is capable of controlling and even eradicating infections. The innate immune response is able to combat microbes immediately upon infection; in contrast, the adaptive immune response needs to be induced by antigen and therefore is delayed. The innate immune response also instructs the adaptive immune system to respond to different microbes in ways that are effective for combating these microbes. In addition, innate immunity is a key participant in the clearance of dead tissues and the initiation of repair after tissue damage.

Before we consider adaptive immunity, the main topic of this book, we discuss the early defense reactions of innate immunity in this chapter. The discussion focuses on the following three questions:

1. How does the innate immune system recognize microbes and damaged cells?

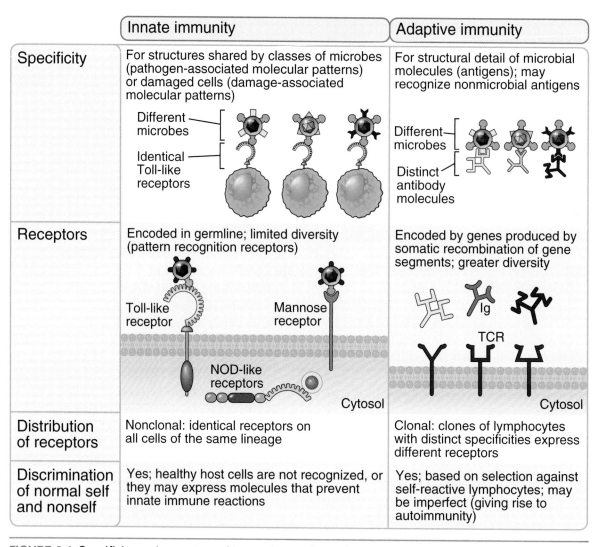

	Innate immunity	Adaptive immunity
Specificity	For structures shared by classes of microbes (pathogen-associated molecular patterns) or damaged cells (damage-associated molecular patterns) Different microbes Identical Toll-like receptors	For structural detail of microbial molecules (antigens); may recognize nonmicrobial antigens Different microbes Distinct antibody molecules
Receptors	Encoded in germline; limited diversity (pattern recognition receptors) Toll-like receptor Mannose receptor NOD-like receptors Cytosol	Encoded by genes produced by somatic recombination of gene segments; greater diversity Ig TCR Cytosol
Distribution of receptors	Nonclonal: identical receptors on all cells of the same lineage	Clonal: clones of lymphocytes with distinct specificities express different receptors
Discrimination of normal self and nonself	Yes; healthy host cells are not recognized, or they may express molecules that prevent innate immune reactions	Yes; based on selection against self-reactive lymphocytes; may be imperfect (giving rise to autoimmunity)

FIGURE 2-1 Specificity and receptors of innate immunity and adaptive immunity. This figure summarizes the important features of the specificity and receptors of innate and adaptive immunity, with select examples illustrated. *Ig*, Immunoglobulin (antibody); *TCR*, T cell receptor.

2. How do the different components of innate immunity function to combat different types of microbes?

3. How do innate immune reactions stimulate adaptive immune responses?

GENERAL FEATURES AND SPECIFICITY OF INNATE IMMUNE RESPONSES

The innate immune system performs its defensive functions with a restricted set of reactions, which are more limited than the more varied and specialized responses of adaptive immunity. The specificity of innate immunity is also different in several respects from the specificity of lymphocytes, the antigen-recognizing cells of adaptive immunity (Fig. 2-1).

The two principal types of reactions of the innate immune system are inflammation and antiviral defense. Inflammation consists of the accumulation and activation of leukocytes and plasma proteins at sites of infection or tissue injury. These cells and proteins act together to kill mainly extracellular microbes and to eliminate damaged tissues. Innate immune defense against intracellular viruses is mediated by natural killer (NK) cells, which kill virus-infected cells, and by cytokines called type I interferons, which block viral replication within host cells.

The innate immune system responds in essentially the same way to repeat encounters with a microbe, whereas the adaptive immune system mounts stronger and more effective responses to each successive encounter with a microbe. In other words, the innate immune system does not remember prior encounters with microbes and resets to baseline after each such encounter, whereas memory is a cardinal feature of the adaptive immune response. There is emerging evidence that some cells of innate immunity (such as macrophages and natural killer cells) are altered by encounters with microbes such that they respond better upon repeat encounters. But it is not clear if this process results in improved protection against recurrent infections or is specific for different microbes.

The innate immune system recognizes structures that are shared by various classes of microbes and are not present on normal host cells. The mechanisms of innate immunity recognize and respond to a limited number of microbial molecules, much less than the almost unlimited number of microbial and nonmicrobial antigens that are recognized by the adaptive immune system. Each component of innate immunity may recognize many bacteria, viruses, or fungi. For example, phagocytes express receptors for bacterial endotoxin, also called lipopolysaccharide (LPS), and other receptors for peptidoglycans, each of which is present in the cell walls of many bacterial species but is not produced by mammalian cells. Other receptors of phagocytes recognize terminal mannose residues, which are typical of bacterial but not mammalian glycoproteins. Mammalian cells recognize and respond to double-stranded ribonucleic acid (dsRNA), which is found in many viruses but not in mammalian cells, and to unmethylated CG-rich (CpG) oligonucleotides, which are common in microbial DNA but are not abundant in mammalian DNA. The microbial molecules that stimulate innate immunity are often called **pathogen-associated molecular patterns** (PAMPs) to indicate that they are present in infectious agents (pathogens) and shared by microbes of the same type (i.e., they are molecular patterns). The receptors of innate immunity that recognize these shared structures are called **pattern recognition receptors**.

The components of innate immunity have evolved to recognize structures of microbes that are often essential for the survival and infectivity of these microbes. This characteristic of innate immunity makes it a highly effective defense mechanism because a microbe cannot evade innate immunity simply by mutating or not expressing the targets of innate immune recognition. Microbes that do not express functional forms of these structures lose their ability to infect and colonize the host. In contrast, microbes frequently evade adaptive immunity by mutating the antigens that are recognized by lymphocytes, because these antigens are usually not required for the life of the microbes.

The innate immune system also recognizes molecules that are released from damaged or necrotic host cells. Such molecules are called **damage-associated molecular patterns (DAMPs)**. The subsequent responses to DAMPs serve to eliminate the damaged cells and to initiate the process of tissue repair. Thus, innate responses occur even following sterile injury, such as infarction, the death of tissue due to loss of its blood supply.

The receptors of the innate immune system are encoded by inherited genes that are identical in all cells. The pattern recognition receptors of the innate immune system are nonclonally distributed; that is, identical receptors are expressed on all the cells of a particular type, such as macrophages. Therefore, many cells of innate immunity may recognize and respond to the same microbe. This is in contrast to the antigen receptors of the adaptive immune system, which are encoded by genes formed by somatic rearrangement of gene segments during lymphocyte development, resulting in unique receptors in each clone of B and T lymphocytes. It is estimated that there are about 100 types of innate immune receptors that are capable of recognizing about 1000 PAMPs and DAMPs. In striking contrast, there are only two kinds of specific receptors in the adaptive immune system (immunoglobulin [Ig] and T cell receptors [TCRs]), but because of their diversity they are able to recognize millions of different antigens.

The innate immune system does not react against the normal host. Several features of the innate immune system account for its inability to react against an individual's own, or self, cells and molecules. First, the receptors of innate immunity have evolved to be specific for microbial structures (and products of damaged cells) but not for substances in healthy cells. Second, some pattern recognition receptors can recognize substances such as nucleic acids that are present in normal cells, but these receptors are located in cellular compartments (such as endosomes; see below) from where components of healthy cells are excluded. Third, normal mammalian cells express regulatory molecules that prevent innate immune reactions. The adaptive immune system also discriminates between self and nonself; in the adaptive immune system, lymphocytes capable of recognizing self antigens are produced, but they die or are inactivated on encounter with self antigens.

The innate immune response can be considered as a series of reactions that provide defense at the following stages of microbial infections:

- At the portals of entry for microbes: Most microbial infections are acquired through the epithelia of the skin and gastrointestinal and respiratory systems. The earliest defense mechanisms active at these sites are epithelia, providing physical barriers and antimicrobial molecules and lymphoid cells.
- In the tissues: Microbes that breach epithelia, as well as dead cells in tissues, are detected by resident macrophages, dendritic cells, and mast cells. Some of these cells react by secreting cytokines, which initiate the process of inflammation, and phagocytes residing in the tissues or recruited from the blood destroy the microbes and eliminate the damaged cells.
- In the blood: Plasma proteins, including proteins of the complement system, react against microbes and promote their destruction.
- Viruses elicit special reactions, including the production of interferons from infected cells that inhibit infection of other cells and the killing of infected cells by NK cells.

We will return to a more detailed discussion of these components of innate immunity and their reactions later in the chapter. We start with a consideration of how microbes, damaged cells, and other foreign substances are detected, and how innate immune responses are triggered.

CELLULAR RECEPTORS FOR MICROBES AND DAMAGED CELLS

The receptors used by the innate immune system to react against microbes and damaged cells are expressed on phagocytes, dendritic cells, and many other cell types, and are expressed in different cellular compartments where microbes may be located. These receptors are present on the cell surface, where they detect extracellular microbes; in vesicles (endosomes) into which microbial products are ingested; and in the cytosol, where they function as sensors of cytoplasmic microbes (Fig. 2-2). These receptors for PAMPs and DAMPs belong to several protein families.

Toll-Like Receptors

Toll-like receptors (TLRs) are homologous to a *Drosophila* protein called *Toll*, which was discovered for its role in the development of the fly and later shown to be essential for protecting flies against infections. Different TLRs are specific for different components of microbes (Fig. 2-3). TLR-2 recognizes several bacterial and parasitic glycolipids and peptidoglycans; TLR-3, -7, and -8 are specific for viral single-stranded and double-stranded RNAs; TLR-4 is specific for bacterial LPS (endotoxin); TLR-5 is specific for a bacterial flagellar protein called flagellin; and TLR-9 recognizes unmethylated CpG DNA, which is more abundant in microbial genomes than in mammalian DNA. TLRs specific for microbial proteins, lipids, and polysaccharides (many of which are present in bacterial cell walls) are located on cell surfaces, where they recognize these products of extracellular microbes. TLRs that recognize nucleic acids are in endosomes, into which microbes are ingested and where the microbes are digested and their nucleic acids are released.

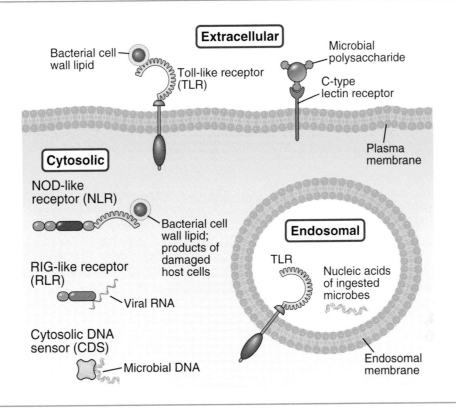

FIGURE 2-2 Cellular locations of receptors of the innate immune system. Some receptors, such as certain Toll-like receptors (TLRs) and lectins, are located on cell surfaces; other TLRs are in endosomes. Some receptors for viral nucleic acids, bacterial peptides, and products of damaged cells are in the cytoplasm. NOD and RIG refer to the founding members of families of structurally homologous cytosolic receptors for bacterial and viral products, respectively. (Their full names are complex and do not reflect their functions.) There are five major families of cellular receptors in innate immunity: TLRs, CLRs (C-type lectin receptors), NLRs (NOD-like receptors), RLRs (RIG-like receptors), and CDSs (cytosolic DNA sensors). Formylpeptide receptors (not shown) are involved in migration of leukocytes in response to bacteria.

Signals generated by engagement of TLRs activate transcription factors that stimulate expression of genes encoding cytokines, enzymes, and other proteins involved in the antimicrobial functions of activated phagocytes and other cells (Fig. 2-4). Among the most important transcription factors activated by TLR signals are members of the nuclear factor κB (NF-κB) family, which promote expression of various cytokines and endothelial adhesion molecules, and interferon regulatory factors (IRFs), which stimulate production of the antiviral cytokines, type I interferons.

Rare inherited mutations of signaling molecules downstream of TLRs are associated with recurrent and severe infections, highlighting the importance of these pathways in host defense against microbes.

NOD-Like Receptors and the Inflammasome

The NOD-like receptors (NLRs) are a large family of cytosolic receptors that sense DAMPs and PAMPs in the cytoplasm. All NLRs contain a central NOD (nucleotide oligomerization domain) but have different N-terminal domains. Three important NLRs are NOD-1, NOD-2, and NLRP-3.

- NOD-1 and NOD-2 are cytosolic proteins containing N-terminal CARD (caspase related) domains. They are specific for bacterial

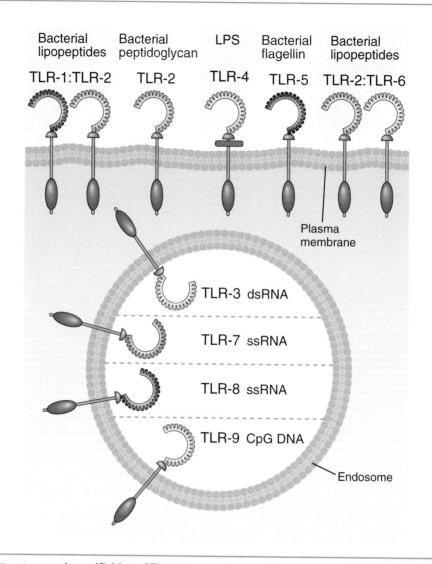

FIGURE 2-3 Structure and specificities of Toll-like receptors. Different TLRs respond to many different, structurally diverse products of microbes. Endosomal TLRs respond only to nucleic acids. All TLRs contain a ligand-binding domain composed of leucine-rich motifs and a cytoplasmic signaling, Toll-like interleukin-1 (IL-1) receptor (TIR) domain. *ds*, Double-stranded; *LPS*, lipopolysaccharide; *ss*, single-stranded.

peptidoglycans, which are common components of bacterial cell walls. They both activate the NF-κB transcription factor. Some polymorphisms of the *NOD2* gene are associated with inflammatory bowel disease; the underlying mechanisms remain poorly understood.

• NLRP-3 (NOD-like receptor family, pyrin domain containing 3) is a cytosolic NLR that responds to many unrelated microbial structures or pathologic changes in the cytosol and reacts by enhancing production mainly of the inflammatory cytokine IL-1β. It contains an N-terminal pyrin domain (so named because it is present in receptors that induce the production of fever-causing cytokines; Greek, *pyro* meaning burn). NLRP-3 recognizes microbial products; substances that indicate cell damage and death, including released adenosine

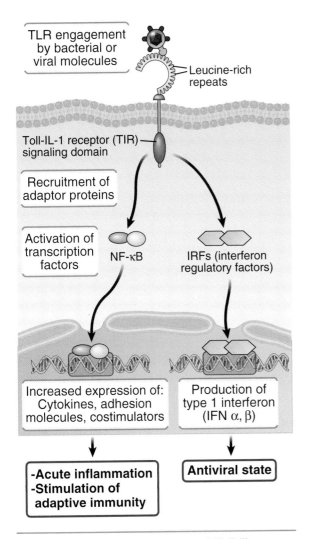

FIGURE 2-4 Signaling functions of Toll-like receptors. TLRs activate similar signaling mechanisms, which involve adaptor proteins and lead to the activation of transcription factors. These transcription factors stimulate the production of proteins that mediate inflammation and antiviral defense. *NF-κB*, Nuclear factor κB.

triphosphate (ATP), uric acid crystals derived from nucleic acids, and changes in intracellular potassium ion (K+) concentration; and endogenous substances that are deposited in cells and tissues in excessive amounts (e.g., cholesterol crystals and free fatty acids). After recognition of these varied substances, NLRP-3 oligomerizes with an adaptor

protein and an inactive (pro) form of the enzyme caspase-1, resulting in generation of the active form of the enzyme (Fig. 2-5). Active caspase-1 cleaves a precursor form of the cytokine interleukin-1β (IL-1β) to generate biologically active IL-1β. As discussed later, IL-1 induces acute inflammation and causes fever. This cytosolic complex of NLRP-3 (the sensor), an adaptor protein, and caspase-1 is known as the **inflammasome.** There are also other caspase-1 activating inflammasomes that contain different sensor proteins besides NLRP3.

The inflammasome is important not only for host defense but also because of its role in several diseases. Gain-of-function mutations in NLRP-3 are the cause of rare **autoinflammatory syndromes,** characterized by uncontrolled and spontaneous inflammation. IL-1 antagonists are effective treatments for these diseases. The common joint disease **gout** is caused by deposition of urate crystals, and subsequent inflammation mediated by inflammasome recognition of the crystals and IL-1β production. The inflammasome may also contribute to atherosclerosis, in which inflammation caused by cholesterol crystals may play a role, and obesity-associated type 2 diabetes, in which IL-1 produced on recognition of lipids may contribute to insulin resistance of tissues.

Other Cellular Receptors of Innate Immunity

Many other receptor types are involved in innate immune responses to microbes (see Fig. 2-2):
- The RIG-like receptor (RLR) family recognizes RNA produced by viruses in the cytosol and activates signaling pathways that lead to the production of type I interferon (IFN).
- Cytosolic DNA sensors (CDSs) include several structurally related proteins that recognize cytosolic viral DNA and also induce type I IFN production.
- Lectin (carbohydrate-recognizing) receptors in the plasma membrane are specific for fungal glycans (these receptors are called dectins) and for terminal mannose residues (called mannose receptors); they are involved in the

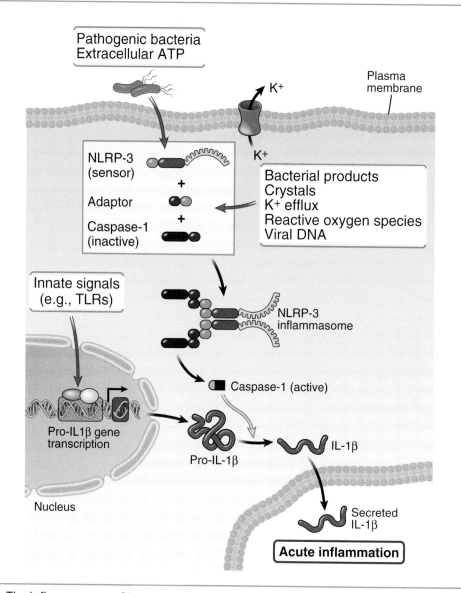

FIGURE 2-5 The inflammasome. Shown is the activation of the NLRP-3 inflammasome, which processes pro–interleukin-1β (pro–IL-1β) to active IL-1. The synthesis of pro–IL-1β is induced by various PAMPs or DAMPs through pattern recognition receptor signaling. Subsequent production of biologically active IL-1β is mediated by the inflammasome. Note that the inflammasome consists of several molecules of NLRP-3, an adaptor protein, and caspase-1 Other forms of the inflammasome exist which contain sensors other than NLRP-3, including NLRP1, NLRC4, or AIM2. *ATP,* Adenosine triphosphate; *NLRP-3,* NOD-like receptor family, pyrin domain containing 3; *TLRs,* Toll-like receptors.

phagocytosis of fungi and bacteria and in inflammatory responses to these pathogens.

- A cell surface receptor expressed mainly on phagocytes recognizes peptides that begin with *N*-formylmethionine, which is specific

to bacterial proteins, and promotes the migration as well as the antimicrobial activities of the phagocytes.

Although our emphasis thus far has been on cellular receptors, the innate immune system also contains several circulating molecules that recognize and provide defense against microbes, as discussed later.

COMPONENTS OF INNATE IMMUNITY

The components of the innate immune system include epithelial cells; sentinel cells in tissues (macrophages, dendritic cells, mast cells, and others); innate lymphoid cells, including NK cells; and a number of plasma proteins. We next discuss the properties of these cells and soluble proteins and their roles in innate immune responses.

Epithelial Barriers

The major interfaces between the body and the external environment—the skin, gastrointestinal tract, respiratory tract, and genitourinary tract—are protected by continuous epithelia that provide physical and chemical barriers against infection (Fig. 2-6). Microbes may enter hosts through these interfaces by physical contact, ingestion, and inhalation. All these portals of entry are lined by continuous epithelia consisting of tightly adherent cells that form a mechanical barrier against microbes. Keratin on the surface of the skin and mucus secreted by mucosal epithelial cells prevent microbes from coming in contact with and infecting the epithelia. Epithelial cells also produce peptide antibiotics, called defensins and cathelicidins, which kill bacteria and thus provide a chemical barrier against infection. In addition, epithelia contain lymphocytes called intraepithelial T lymphocytes that belong to the T cell lineage but express antigen receptors of limited diversity. Some of these T cells express receptors composed of two chains, γ and δ, that are similar but not identical to the $\alpha\beta$ T cell receptors expressed on the majority of T lymphocytes (see Chapters 4 and 5). Intraepithelial lymphocytes often recognize microbial lipids and other structures that are shared by microbes of the same type. Intraepithelial T lymphocytes presumably react against infectious agents that attempt to breach the epithelia, but the specificity and functions of these cells are poorly understood.

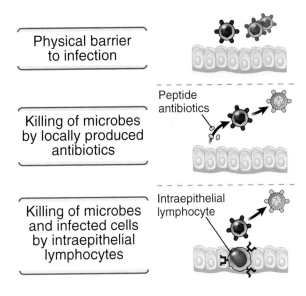

FIGURE 2-6 Functions of epithelia in innate immunity. Epithelia present at the portals of entry of microbes provide physical barriers formed by keratin (in the skin) or secreted mucus (in the gastrointestinal, bronchopulmonary and genitourinary systems) and by tight junctions between epithelial cells. Epithelia also produce antimicrobial substances (e.g., defensins) and harbor lymphocytes that kill microbes and infected cells.

Phagocytes: Neutrophils and Monocytes/Macrophages

The two types of circulating phagocytes, neutrophils and monocytes, are blood cells that are recruited to sites of infection, where they recognize and ingest microbes for intracellular killing.

- **Neutrophils,** also called polymorphonuclear leukocytes (PMNs), are the most abundant leukocytes in the blood, numbering 4000 to 10,000 per µL (Fig. 2-7, *A*). In response to infections, the production of neutrophils from the bone marrow increases rapidly, and their number may rise to as high as 20,000 per µL of blood. The production of neutrophils is stimulated by cytokines, known as colony-stimulating factors (CSFs), which are secreted by many cell types in response to infections and act on hematopoietic stem cells to stimulate proliferation and maturation of neutrophil precursors.

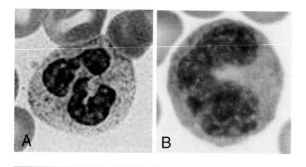

FIGURE 2-7 Morphology of neutrophils and monocytes. **A,** Light micrograph of blood neutrophil shows the multilobed nucleus, which is why these cells are also called polymorphonuclear leukocytes, and the faint cytoplasmic granules, most of which are lysosomes. **B,** Light micrograph of blood monocyte shows the typical horseshoe-shaped nucleus.

Neutrophils are the first cell type to respond to most infections, particularly bacterial and fungal infections, and thus are the dominant cells of acute inflammation, as discussed later. Neutrophils ingest microbes in the circulation, and they rapidly enter extravascular tissues at sites of infection, where they also phagocytose (ingest) and destroy microbes. Neutrophils express receptors for products of complement activation and for antibodies that coat microbes. These receptors enhance phagocytosis, and also transduce activating signals that enhance the ability of the neutrophils to kill ingested microbes. The process of phagocytosis and intracellular destruction of microbes is described later. These cells are also recruited to sites of tissue damage in the absence of infection, where they initiate the clearance of cell debris. Neutrophils live for only a few hours in tissues, so they are the early responders, but they do not provide prolonged defense.

- **Monocytes** are less abundant in the blood than neutrophils, numbering 500 to 1000 per μL (Fig. 2-7, *B*). They also ingest microbes in the blood and in tissues. During inflammatory reactions, monocytes enter extravascular tissues and differentiate into cells called **macrophages**, which, unlike neutrophils, survive in these sites for long periods. Thus, blood monocytes and tissue macrophages are two stages of the same cell lineage, which often is called the mononuclear

phagocyte system (Fig. 2-8). (This has been called the reticuloendothelial system, for historical reasons, but this name is a misnomer and should be avoided.) Some macrophages that are resident in different tissues, such as the brain, liver, and lungs, are derived not from circulating monocytes but from progenitors in the yolk sac or fetal liver early during the development of the organism. Macrophages are also found in all connective tissues and organs of the body.

Macrophages serve several important roles in host defense: they produce cytokines that induce and regulate inflammation, they ingest and destroy microbes, and they clear dead tissues and initiate the process of tissue repair (Fig. 2-9). A number of receptor families are expressed in macrophages and involved in the activation and functions of these cells. Pattern recognition receptors discussed earlier, including TLRs and NLRs, recognize products of microbes and damaged cells and activate the macrophages. Phagocytosis is mediated by cell surface receptors, such as mannose receptors and scavenger receptors, which directly bind microbes (and other particles), and receptors for products of complement activation and antibodies that are also expressed by neutrophils. Some of these phagocytic receptors activate the microbial killing functions of macrophages, as well. In addition, macrophages respond to various cytokines.

Macrophages may be activated by two different pathways that serve distinct functions (see Fig. 6-9, Chapter 6). These pathways of activation have been called classical and alternative. **Classical macrophage activation** is induced by innate immune signals, such as from TLRs, and by the cytokine IFN-γ, which may be produced in both innate and adaptive immune responses. Classically activated macrophages, also called M1, are involved in destroying microbes and in triggering inflammation. **Alternative macrophage activation** occurs in the absence of strong TLR signals and is induced by the cytokines IL-4 and IL-13; these macrophages, called M2, appear to be more important for tissue repair and to terminate inflammation. The relative abundance of these two forms of activated macrophages may influence the outcome of host reactions and contribute

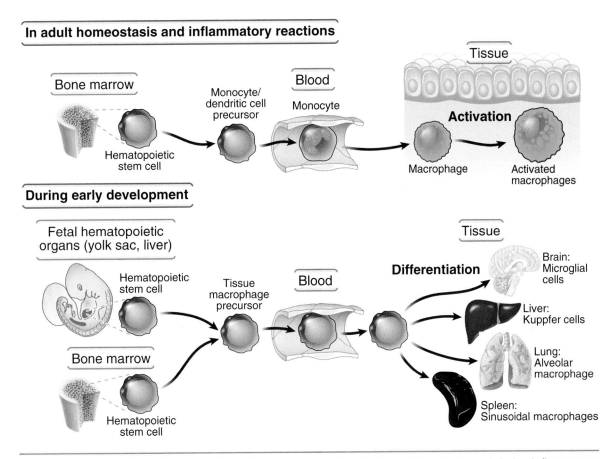

FIGURE 2-8 Maturation of mononuclear phagocytes. In the steady state in adults, and during inflammatory reactions, precursors in the bone marrow give rise to circulating monocytes, which enter peripheral tissues, mature to form macrophages, and are activated locally. In early development, as in fetal life, precursors in the yolk sac and fetal liver give rise to cells that seed tissues to generate specialized tissue-resident macrophages.

to various disorders. We will return to the functions of these macrophage populations in Chapter 6, when we discuss cell-mediated immunity.

Although our discussion has been limited to the role of phagocytes in innate immunity, macrophages are also important effector cells in both the cell-mediated arm and the humoral arm of adaptive immunity, as discussed in Chapters 6 and 8, respectively.

Dendritic Cells

Dendritic cells respond to microbes by producing numerous cytokines that serve two main functions: they initiate inflammation and they stimulate adaptive immune responses. By sensing microbes and interacting with lymphocytes, especially T cells, dendritic cells constitute an important bridge between innate and adaptive immunity. We discuss the properties and functions of dendritic cells further in Chapter 3, in the context of antigen display, which is a major function of dendritic cells.

Mast Cells

Mast cells are bone marrow–derived cells with abundant cytoplasmic granules that are present in the skin and mucosal epithelium. Mast cells can be activated by microbial products binding to TLRs, as part of innate immunity, or by a special antibody-dependent mechanism. Mast cell granules contain vasoactive amines such as histamine that cause vasodilation and

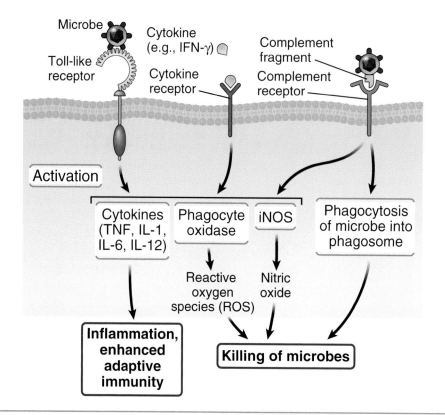

FIGURE 2-9 **Activation and functions of macrophages.** In innate immune responses, macrophages are activated by microbial products binding to TLRs and by cytokines, such as NK cell–derived interferon-γ (IFN-γ), which lead to the production of proteins that mediate inflammatory and microbicidal functions of these cells. Cell surface complement receptors promote the phagocytosis of complement-coated microbes as well as activation of the macrophages. (Macrophage Fc receptors for IgG [not shown] bind antibody-coated microbes and perform similar functions as the complement receptors.) *IL*, Interleukin; *iNOS*, inducible nitric oxide synthase; *TNF*, tumor necrosis factor.

increased capillary permeability, as well as proteolytic enzymes that can kill bacteria or inactivate microbial toxins. Mast cells also synthesize and secrete lipid mediators (e.g., prostaglandins) and cytokines (e.g., tumor necrosis factor [TNF]), which stimulate inflammation. Mast cell products provide defense against helminths and other pathogens and are responsible for symptoms of allergic diseases (see Chapter 11).

Innate Lymphoid Cells

Innate lymphoid cells (ILCs) are lymphocyte-like cells that produce cytokines and **perform functions similar to those of T lymphocytes but do not express T cell antigen receptors (TCRs).** ILCs have been divided into three major groups based on their secreted cytokines; these groups correspond to the Th1, Th2, and Th17 subsets of CD4+ T cells that we describe in Chapter 6. How ILCs recognize microbes and damaged cells is not defined. The responses of ILCs are often stimulated by cytokines produced by epithelial and other cells at sites of infection. ILCs provide early defense against infections and also guide the subsequent T cell response. NK cells, described next, are related to group 1 ILCs.

Natural Killer Cells

Natural killer (NK) cells recognize infected and stressed cells and respond by killing these cells and by secreting the macrophage-activating cytokine IFN-γ (Fig. 2-10). NK cells make up approximately 10% of the lymphocytes in the blood and peripheral lymphoid organs. NK cells contain abundant cytoplasmic granules and express some unique surface proteins but do not express immunoglobulins or T cell receptors, the antigen receptors of B and T lymphocytes, respectively.

On activation by infected cells, NK cells empty the contents of their cytoplasmic granules into the extracellular space at the point of contact with the infected cell. The granule proteins then enter infected cells and activate enzymes that induce apoptosis. The cytotoxic mechanisms of NK cells, which are the same as the mechanisms used by cytotoxic T lymphocytes (CTLs; see Chapter 6), result in the death of infected cells. Thus, as with CTLs, NK cells function to eliminate cellular reservoirs of infection and eradicate infections by obligate intracellular microbes, such as viruses.

Activated NK cells also synthesize and secrete the cytokine interferon-γ. IFN-γ activates macrophages to become more effective at killing phagocytosed microbes. Cytokines secreted by macrophages and dendritic cells that have encountered microbes enhance the ability of NK cells to protect against infections. Three of these NK cell–activating cytokines are interleukin-15 (IL-15), type I interferons (type I IFNs), and interleukin-12 (IL-12). IL-15 is important for the development and maturation of NK cells, and type I IFNs and IL-12 enhance the killing functions of NK cells. Thus, NK cells and macrophages are examples of two cell types that function cooperatively to eliminate intracellular microbes: Macrophages ingest microbes and produce IL-12, IL-12 activates NK cells to secrete IFN-γ, and IFN-γ in turn activates the macrophages to kill the ingested microbes. As discussed in Chapter 6, essentially the same sequence of reactions involving macrophages and T lymphocytes is central to the cell-mediated arm of adaptive immunity.

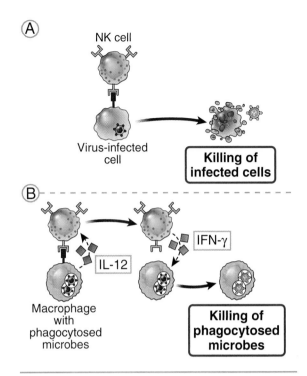

FIGURE 2-10 Functions of natural killer (NK) cells. **A,** NK cells kill host cells infected by intracellular microbes, thus eliminating reservoirs of infection. **B,** NK cells respond to interleukin-12 (IL-12) produced by macrophages and secrete interferon-γ (IFN-γ), which activates the macrophages to kill phagocytosed microbes.

The activation of NK cells is determined by a balance between engagement of activating and inhibitory receptors (Fig. 2-11). The activating receptors recognize cell surface molecules typically expressed on cells infected with viruses and intracellular bacteria, as well as cells stressed by DNA damage and malignant transformation. These receptors enable NK cells to eliminate cells infected with intracellular microbes, as well as irreparably injured cells and tumor cells. One of the well-defined activating receptors of NK cells is called NKG2D; it recognizes molecules that resemble class I major histocompatibility complex (MHC) proteins and are expressed in response to many types of cellular stress. Another activating receptor, called CD16, is specific for immunoglobulin G (IgG) antibodies

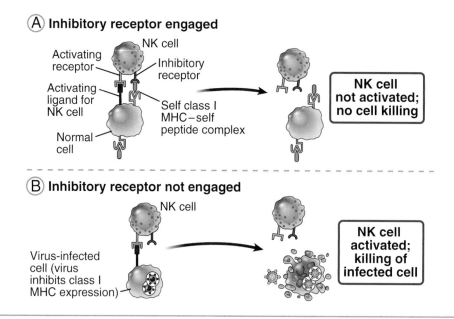

FIGURE 2-11 Activating and inhibitory receptors of natural killer (NK) cells. **A,** Healthy host cells express self class I major histocompatibility complex (MHC) molecules, which are recognized by inhibitory receptors, thus ensuring that NK cells do not attack normal host cells. Note that healthy cells may express ligands for activating receptors (as shown) or may not express such ligands, but they are not attacked by NK cells because they engage the inhibitory receptors. **B,** NK cells are activated by infected cells in which ligands for activating receptors are expressed (often at high levels) and class I MHC expression is reduced so that the inhibitory receptors are not engaged. The result is that the infected cells are killed.

bound to cells. The recognition of antibody-coated cells results in killing of these cells, a phenomenon called **antibody-dependent cellular cytotoxicity** (ADCC). NK cells are the principal mediators of ADCC. The role of this reaction in antibody-mediated immunity is described in Chapter 8. Activating receptors on NK cells have signaling subunits that contain immunoreceptor tyrosine-based activation motifs (ITAMs) in their cytoplasmic tails. ITAMs, which also are present in subunits of lymphocyte antigen receptor–associated signaling molecules, become phosphorylated on tyrosine residues when the receptors recognize their activating ligands. The phosphorylated ITAMs bind and promote the activation of cytosolic protein tyrosine kinases, and these enzymes phosphorylate, and thereby activate, other substrates in several different downstream signal transduction pathways, eventually leading to cytotoxic granule exocytosis and production of IFN-γ.

The inhibitory receptors of NK cells, which block signaling by activating receptors, are specific for self class I MHC molecules, which are expressed on all healthy nucleated cells. Therefore, class I MHC expression protects healthy cells from destruction by NK cells. (In Chapter 3 we describe the important function of MHC molecules in displaying peptide antigens to T lymphocytes.) Two major families of NK cell inhibitory receptors in humans are the killer cell immunoglobulin-like receptors (KIRs), so called because they share structural homology with Ig molecules (see Chapter 4), and receptors consisting of a protein called CD94 and a lectin subunit called NKG2. Both families of inhibitory receptors contain in their cytoplasmic domains structural motifs called immunoreceptor tyrosine-based inhibitory motifs (ITIMs), which become phosphorylated on tyrosine residues when the receptors bind class I MHC molecules. The phosphorylated ITIMs bind and promote activation of cytosolic protein tyrosine phosphatases. These enzymes remove phosphate groups from the tyrosine residues of various signaling molecules, thereby counteracting the function of the ITAMs and blocking the activation of NK cells through activating receptors. Therefore, when the inhibitory receptors of NK cells encounter self MHC molecules on normal host cells, the NK cells are shut off (see Fig. 2-11). Many viruses have developed mechanisms to block expression of class I molecules in infected cells, which allows them to evade killing by virus-specific CD8+ CTLs. When this happens, the NK cell inhibitory receptors are not engaged, and if the virus induces expression of activating ligands at the same time, the NK cells become activated and eliminate the virus-infected cells.

The role of NK cells and CTLs in defense illustrates how hosts and microbes are engaged in a constant struggle for survival. The host uses CTLs to recognize MHC-displayed viral antigens, viruses inhibit MHC expression to evade killing of the infected cells by CTLs, and NK cells can compensate for the defective CTL response because the NK cells are more effective in the absence of MHC molecules. The winner of this struggle, the host or the microbe, determines the outcome of the infection. The same principles may apply to the functions of NK cells in eradication of tumors, many of which also attempt to escape from CTL-mediated killing by reducing expression of class I MHC molecules.

Lymphocytes with Limited Diversity

Several types of lymphocytes that have some features of T and B lymphocytes also function in the early defense against microbes and may be considered part of the innate immune system. A unifying characteristic of these lymphocytes is that they express somatically rearranged antigen receptors (as do classical T and B cells), but the receptors have limited diversity.

- As mentioned earlier, γδ T cells are present in epithelia.
- NK-T cells express TCRs with limited diversity and surface molecules typically found on NK cells. They are present in epithelia and lymphoid organs. They recognize microbial lipids bound to a class I MHC–related molecule called CD1.

- B-1 cells are a population of B lymphocytes that are found mostly in the peritoneal cavity and mucosal tissues, where they produce antibodies in response to microbes and microbial toxins that pass through the walls of the intestine. Most of the circulating IgM antibodies found in the blood of normal individuals, called natural antibodies, are the products of B-1 cells, and many of these antibodies are specific for carbohydrates that are present in the cell walls of many bacteria.
- Another type of B lymphocyte, marginal-zone B cells, is present at the edges of lymphoid follicles in the spleen and other organs and also is involved in rapid antibody responses to blood-borne polysaccharide-rich microbes.

NK-T cells, γδ T cells, B-1 cells and marginal-zone B lymphocytes all respond to infections in ways that are characteristic of adaptive immunity (e.g., cytokine secretion or antibody production) but have features of innate immunity (rapid responses, limited diversity of antigen recognition).

Complement System

The complement system is a collection of circulating and membrane-associated proteins that are important in defense against microbes. Many complement proteins are proteolytic enzymes, and complement activation involves the sequential activation of these enzymes. The complement cascade may be activated by any of three pathways (Fig. 2-12):

- The alternative pathway is triggered when some complement proteins are activated on microbial surfaces and cannot be controlled, because complement regulatory proteins are not present on microbes (but are present on host cells). The alternative pathway is a component of innate immunity.
- The classical pathway is most often triggered by antibodies that bind to microbes or other antigens and is thus a component of the humoral arm of adaptive immunity.
- The lectin pathway is activated when a carbohydrate-binding plasma protein, mannose-binding lectin (MBL), binds to terminal mannose residues on the surface glycoproteins

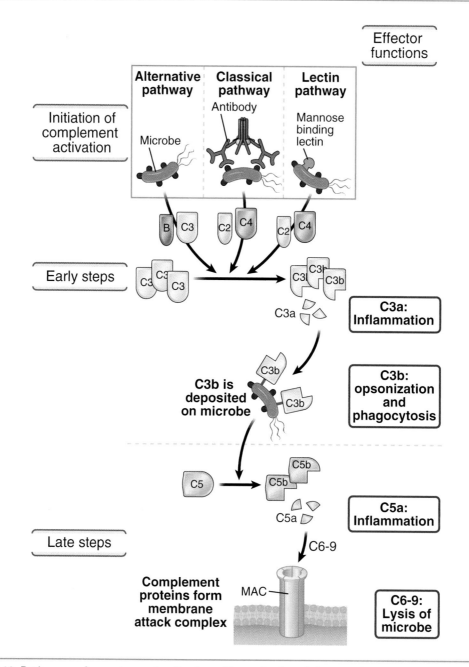

FIGURE 2-12 Pathways of complement activation. The activation of the complement system (the early steps) may be initiated by three distinct pathways, all of which lead to the production of C3b. C3b initiates the late steps of complement activation, culminating in the formation of a multiprotein complex called the membrane attack complex (MAC), which is a transmembrane channel composed of polymerized C9 molecules that causes lysis of thin-walled microbes. Peptide by-products released during complement activation are the inflammation-inducing C3a and C5a. The principal functions of proteins produced at different steps are shown. The activation, functions, and regulation of the complement system are discussed in more detail in Chapter 8.

of microbes. This lectin activates proteins of the classical pathway, but because it is initiated by a microbial product in the absence of antibody, it is a component of innate immunity.

Activated complement proteins function as proteolytic enzymes to cleave other complement proteins. Such an enzymatic cascade can be rapidly amplified because each proteolytic step generates many molecules that are substrates for another enzyme in the cascade. The central component of complement is a plasma protein called C3, which is cleaved by enzymes generated in the early steps. The major proteolytic fragment of C3, called C3b, becomes covalently attached to microbes and is able to recruit and activate downstream complement proteins on the microbial surface. The three pathways of complement activation differ in how they are initiated, but they share the late steps and perform the same effector functions.

The complement system serves three main functions in host defense:

- *Opsonization and phagocytosis.* C3b coats microbes and promotes the binding of these microbes to phagocytes, by virtue of receptors for C3b that are expressed on the phagocytes. Thus, microbes that are coated with complement proteins are rapidly ingested and destroyed by phagocytes. This process of coating a microbe with molecules that are recognized by receptors on phagocytes is called **opsonization.**
- *Inflammation.* Some proteolytic fragments of complement proteins, especially C5a and C3a, are chemoattractants for leukocytes (mainly neutrophils and monocytes), so they promote leukocyte recruitment (inflammation) at the site of complement activation.
- *Cell lysis.* Complement activation culminates in the formation of a polymeric protein complex that inserts into the microbial cell membrane, disturbing the permeability barrier and causing either osmotic lysis or apoptosis of the microbe.

A more detailed discussion of the activation and functions of complement is presented in

Chapter 8, where we consider the effector mechanisms of humoral immunity.

Other Plasma Proteins of Innate Immunity

Several circulating proteins in addition to complement proteins are involved in innate immune defense against infections. Plasma MBL recognizes microbial carbohydrates and can coat microbes for phagocytosis or activate the complement cascade by the lectin pathway, as discussed earlier. MBL belongs to a family of proteins called the collectins, because they are structurally similar to collagen and contain a carbohydrate-binding (lectin) domain. Surfactant proteins in the lung also belong to the collectin family and protect the airways from infection. C-reactive protein (CRP) is a pentraxin (five-headed molecule) that binds to phosphorylcholine on microbes and opsonizes the microbes for phagocytosis by macrophages, which express a receptor for CRP. CRP can also activate proteins of the classical complement pathway.

The circulating levels of many of these plasma proteins increase rapidly after infection. This protective response is called the **acute-phase response** to infection.

Cytokines of Innate Immunity

In response to microbes, dendritic cells, macrophages, mast cells, and other cells secrete cytokines that mediate many of the cellular reactions of innate immunity (Fig. 2-13). As mentioned earlier, cytokines are soluble proteins that mediate immune and inflammatory reactions and are responsible for communications between leukocytes and between leukocytes and other cells. Most of the molecularly defined cytokines are called **interleukins**, by convention, implying that these molecules are produced by leukocytes and act on leukocytes. (In reality, this is too limited a definition, because many cytokines are produced by or act on cells other than leukocytes, and many cytokines that do mediate communications between leukocytes are given other names for historical reasons.) In innate

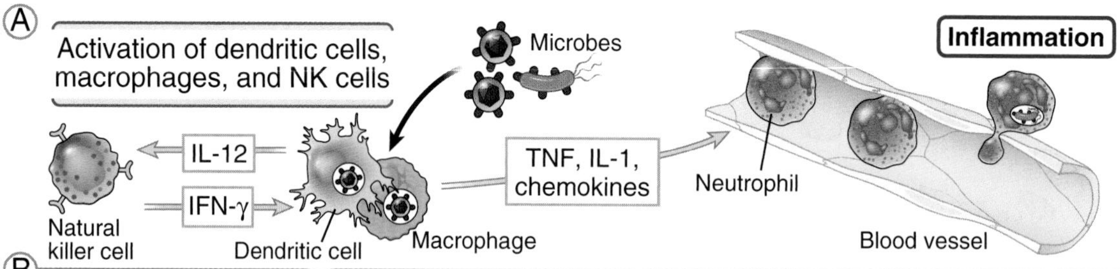

Ⓐ

Activation of dendritic cells, macrophages, and NK cells

Microbes

| Inflammation |

IL-12

IFN-γ

TNF, IL-1, chemokines

Natural killer cell

Dendritic cell   Macrophage

Neutrophil

Blood vessel

Ⓑ

Cytokine	Principal cell source(s)	Principal cellular targets and biologic effects
Tumor necrosis factor (TNF)	Macrophages, T cells, mast cells	Endothelial cells: activation (inflammation, coagulation) Neutrophils: activation Hypothalamus: fever Liver: synthesis of acute-phase proteins Muscle, fat: catabolism (cachexia) Many cell types: apoptosis
Interleukin-1 (IL-1)	Macrophages, dendritic cells, endothelial cells, some epithelial cells, mast cells	Endothelial cells: activation (inflammation, coagulation) Hypothalamus: fever Liver: synthesis of acute-phase proteins T cells: Th17 differentiation
Chemokines	Macrophages, dendritic cells, endothelial cells, T lymphocytes, fibroblasts, platelets	Leukocytes: increased integrin affinity, chemotaxis, activation
Interleukin-12 (IL-12)	Dendritic cells, macrophages,	Natural killer (NK) cells and T cells: IFN-γ production, increased cytotoxic activity T cells: Th1 differentiation
Interferon-γ (IFN-γ)	NK cells, T lymphocytes	Activation of macrophages Stimulation of some antibody responses
Type I IFNs (IFN-α, IFN-β)	IFN-α: Dendritic cells, macrophages IFN-β: Fibroblasts	All cells: antiviral state, increased class I major histocompatibility complex (MHC) expression NK cells: activation
Interleukin-10 (IL-10)	Macrophages, dendritic cells, T cells	Macrophages, dendritic cells: inhibition of cytokine and chemokine production, reduced expression of costimulators and class II MHC molecules
Interleukin-6 (IL-6)	Macrophages, endothelial cells, T cells	Liver: synthesis of acute-phase proteins B cells: proliferation of antibody-producing cells
Interleukin-15 (IL-15)	Macrophages, others	NK cells: proliferation T cells: proliferation
Interleukin-18 (IL-18)	Macrophages	NK cells and T cells: IFN-γ synthesis
TGF-β	Many cell types	Inhibition of inflammation T cells: differentiation of Th17, regulatory T cells

immunity, the principal sources of cytokines are mast cells, dendritic cells, and macrophages activated by recognition of microbes, although epithelial cells and other cell types also secrete cytokines. Recognition of bacterial components such as LPS or of viral molecules such as dsRNA by TLRs and other microbial sensors is a powerful stimulus for cytokine secretion by macrophages and dendritic cells. In adaptive immunity, helper T lymphocytes are a major source of cytokines (see Chapters 5 and 6).

Cytokines are secreted in small amounts in response to an external stimulus and bind to high-affinity receptors on target cells. Most cytokines act on the cells that produce them (autocrine actions) or on adjacent cells (paracrine actions). In innate immune reactions against infections, enough dendritic cells and macrophages may be activated that large amounts of cytokines are produced, and they may be active distant from their site of secretion (endocrine actions).

The cytokines of innate immunity serve various functions in host defense. Tumor necrosis factor (TNF), interleukin-1 (IL-1), and chemokines (chemoattractant cytokines) are the principal cytokines involved in recruiting blood neutrophils and monocytes to sites of infection (described later). TNF and IL-1 also have systemic effects, including inducing fever by acting on the hypothalmus, and these cytokines as well as IL-6 stimulate liver cells to produce various proteins of the acute phase response, such as C-reactive protein, and fibrinogen, which contribute to microbial killing and walling off infectious sites. At high concentrations, TNF promotes thrombus formation on the endothelium and reduces blood pressure by a combination of reduced myocardial contractility and vascular dilation and leakiness. Severe, disseminated bacterial infections sometimes lead to a potentially lethal clinical syndrome called **septic shock,** which is characterized by low blood pressure (the defining feature of shock), disseminated intravascular coagulation, and metabolic disturbances. The early clinical and pathologic manifestations of septic shock may be caused by high levels of TNF, which is produced in response to the bacteria. Dendritic cells and macrophages also produce IL-12 in response to LPS and other microbial molecules. The role of IL-12 in activating NK cells, ultimately leading to macrophage activation, was mentioned previously. NK cells produce IFN-γ, whose function as a macrophage-activating cytokine was also described earlier. Because IFN-γ is produced by T cells as well, it is considered a cytokine of both innate immunity and adaptive immunity. In viral infections, a subset of dendritic cells, and, to a lesser extent, other infected cells, produce type I IFNs, which inhibit viral replication and prevent spread of the infection to uninfected cells.

INNATE IMMUNE REACTIONS

The innate immune system eliminates microbes mainly by inducing the acute inflammatory response and by antiviral defense mechanisms. Different microbes may elicit different types of innate immune reactions, each type being particularly effective in eliminating a particular kind of microbe. The major

---

FIGURE 2-13 Cytokines of innate immunity. **A,** Dendritic cells, macrophages, and other cells (such as mast cells and ILCs, not shown) respond to microbes by producing cytokines that stimulate inflammation (leukocyte recruitment) and activate natural killer (NK) cells to produce the macrophage-activating cytokine interferon-γ (IFN-γ). **B,** Some important characteristics of the major cytokines of innate immunity are listed. Note that IFN-γ and transforming growth factor beta (TGF-β) are cytokines of both innate and adaptive immunity (see Chapters 5 and 6). More information about these cytokines and their receptors is provided in Appendix II. *MHC,* Major histocompatibility complex.

protective innate immune responses to different microbes are the following:

- Extracellular bacteria and fungi are combated mainly by the acute inflammatory response, in which neutrophils and monocytes are recruited to the site of infection, and by the complement system.
- Intracellular bacteria, which can survive inside phagocytes, are eliminated by phagocytes that are activated by Toll-like receptors and other sensors as well as by cytokines.
- Defense against viruses is provided by type I interferons and natural killer cells.

Inflammation

Inflammation is a tissue reaction that delivers mediators of host defense—circulating cells and proteins—to sites of infection and tissue damage (Fig. 2-14). The process of inflammation consists of recruitment of cells and leakage of plasma proteins through blood vessels and activation of these cells and proteins in the extravascular tissues. The initial release of histamine, substance P, and other mediators by mast cells and macrophages causes an increase in local blood flow, exudation of plasma proteins, and triggering of nerve endings. These contribute to redness, warmth, swelling, and pain, which are the characteristic features of inflammation. This is often followed by a local accumulation in the tissue of phagocytes, mainly neutrophils, in response to cytokines, discussed below. Activated phagocytes engulf microbes and dead material and destroy these potentially harmful substances. We next describe the steps in a typical inflammatory reaction.

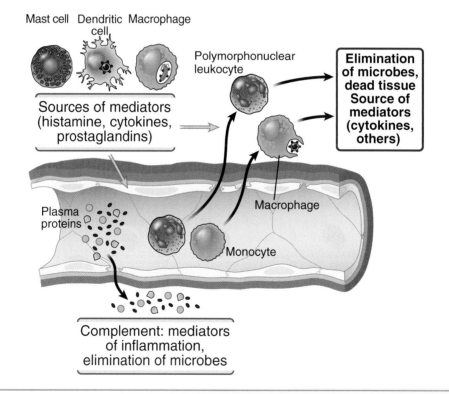

FIGURE 2-14 Acute inflammatory response. Cytokines and other mediators are produced by macrophages, dendritic cells, mast cells, and other cells in tissues in response to microbial products and damaged host cells. These mediators increase the permeability of blood vessels, leading to the entry of plasma proteins (e.g., complement proteins) into the tissues and promote the movement of leukocytes from the blood into the tissues, where the leukocytes destroy microbes, clear damaged cells, and promote more inflammation and repair.

Recruitment of Phagocytes to Sites of Infection and Tissue Damage

Neutrophils and monocytes migrate to extravascular sites of infection or tissue damage by binding to venular endothelial adhesion molecules and in response to chemoattractants produced by tissue cells reacting to infection or injury. Leukocyte migration from the blood into tissues is a multi-step process in which initial weak adhesive interactions of the leukocytes with endothelial cells are followed by firm adhesion and then transmigration through the endothelium (Fig. 2-15).

If an infectious microbe breaches an epithelium and enters the subepithelial tissue, resident dendritic cells, macrophages and other cells recognize the microbe and respond by producing cytokines. Two of these cytokines, TNF and IL-1, act on the endothelium of venules near the site of infection and initiate the sequence of events in leukocyte migration into tissues.

- *Rolling of leukocytes.* In response to TNF and IL-1, endothelial cells express an adhesion molecule of the **selectin** family called E-selectin. Other stimuli, including thrombin, cause rapid translocation of P-selectin to the endothelial surface. (The term selectin refers to the carbohydrate-binding, or lectin, property of these molecules). Circulating neutrophils and monocytes express surface carbohydrates that bind specifically to

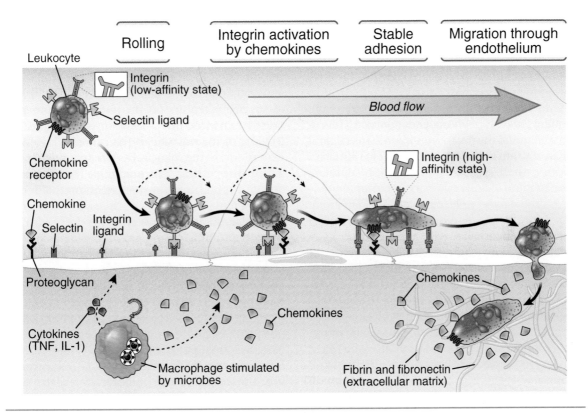

FIGURE 2-15 Sequence of events in migration of blood leukocytes to sites of infection. At sites of infection, macrophages, dendritic cells, and other cells that have encountered microbes produce cytokines such as tumor necrosis factor (TNF) and interleukin-1 (IL-1) that activate the endothelial cells of nearby venules to express selectins and ligands for integrins and to secrete chemokines. Selectins mediate weak tethering and rolling of blood neutrophils on the endothelium, integrins mediate firm adhesion of neutrophils, and chemokines activate the neutrophils and stimulate their migration through the endothelium to the site of infection. Blood monocytes and activated T lymphocytes use the same mechanisms to migrate to sites of infection.

the selectins. The neutrophils become tethered to the endothelium, flowing blood disrupts this binding, the bonds reform downstream, and this repetitive process results in the rolling of the leukocytes along the endothelial surface.

- *Firm adhesion.* Leukocytes express another set of adhesion molecules that are called **integrins** because they integrate extrinsic signals into cytoskeletal alterations. Leukocyte integrins, such as LFA-1 and VLA-4, are present in a low-affinity state on unactivated cells. Within a site of infection, tissue macrophages and endothelial cells produce **chemokines**, which bind to proteoglycans on the luminal surface of endothelial cells and are thus displayed at a high concentration to the leukocytes that are rolling on the endothelium. These chemokines stimulate a rapid increase in the affinity of the leukocyte integrins for their ligands on the endothelium. Concurrently, TNF and IL-1 act on the endothelium to stimulate expression of ligands for integrins, including ICAM-1 and VCAM-1. The firm binding of integrins to their ligands arrests the rolling leukocytes on the endothelium. The cytoskeleton of the leukocytes is reorganized, and the cells spread out on the endothelial surface.
- *Leukocyte migration.* Chemokines also stimulate the motility of leukocytes, as do bacterial products and products of complement activation. As a result, the leukocytes begin to migrate between endothelial cells, through the vessel wall, and along the concentration gradient of these chemoattractants to the site of infection.

The sequence of selectin-mediated rolling, chemokine-dependent integrin-mediated firm adhesion, and chemokine-mediated motility leads to the migration of blood leukocytes to an extravascular site of infection within minutes after the infection. (As discussed in Chapters 5 and 6, the same sequence of events is responsible for the migration of activated T lymphocytes into infected tissues.) Inherited deficiencies in integrins and selectin ligands lead to defective leukocyte recruitment to sites of infection and increased susceptibility to infections. These disorders are called **leukocyte adhesion deficiencies** (LADs).

Microbial products and inflammatory cytokines such as TNF cause capillaries to become leaky, allowing circulating proteins, including complement proteins and antibodies, to exit the blood vessels and enter the tissue site of infection. These proteins work together with phagocytes to destroy the offending agents. In some infections, blood leukocytes other than neutrophils and macrophages, such as eosinophils, may be recruited to sites of infection and provide defense against the pathogens.

Phagocytosis and Destruction of Microbes

Neutrophils and macrophages ingest (phagocytose) microbes and destroy the ingested microbes in intracellular vesicles (Fig. 2-16). **Phagocytosis** is a process of ingestion of particles larger than 0.5 μm in diameter. It begins with membrane receptors binding to the microbe. The principal phagocytic receptors are some pattern recognition receptors, such as mannose receptors and other lectins, and receptors for antibodies and complement. Microbes opsonized with antibodies and complement fragments are able to bind avidly to specific receptors on phagocytes, resulting in greatly enhanced internalization (see Chapter 8). Binding of the microbe to the cell is followed by extension of the phagocyte plasma membrane around the particle. The membrane then closes up and pinches off, and the microbe is internalized in a membrane-bound vesicle, called a phagosome. The phagosomes fuse with lysosomes to form phagolysosomes.

At the same time that the microbe is being bound by the phagocyte's receptors and ingested, the phagocyte receives signals from various receptors that activate several enzymes in the phagolysosomes. One of these enzymes, called phagocyte oxidase, rapidly converts molecular oxygen into superoxide anion and free radicals, a process called the oxidative burst (or respiratory burst). These free radicals are called **reactive oxygen species** (ROS) and are toxic to the ingested microbes. A second enzyme, inducible nitric oxide synthase (iNOS), catalyzes the conversion of arginine to **nitric oxide** (NO), also a microbicidal substance. The third set of enzymes, the lysosomal proteases, break down microbial proteins. All these microbicidal substances are produced mainly within lysosomes and

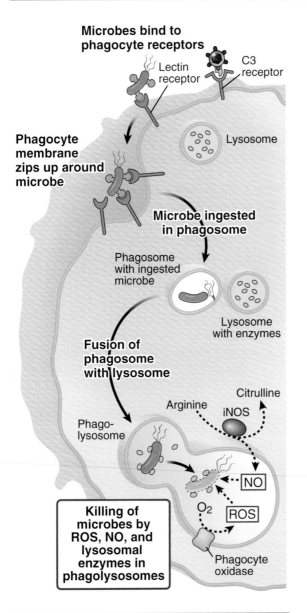

Microbes bind to phagocyte receptors

Lectin receptor

C3 receptor

Lysosome

Phagocyte membrane zips up around microbe

Microbe ingested in phagosome

Phagosome with ingested microbe

Lysosome with enzymes

Fusion of phagosome with lysosome

Citrulline

Arginine   iNOS

Phago-lysosome

NO

O_2 ROS

Phagocyte oxidase

Killing of microbes by ROS, NO, and lysosomal enzymes in phagolysosomes

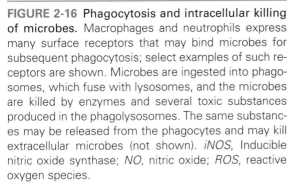

FIGURE 2-16 Phagocytosis and intracellular killing of microbes. Macrophages and neutrophils express many surface receptors that may bind microbes for subsequent phagocytosis; select examples of such receptors are shown. Microbes are ingested into phagosomes, which fuse with lysosomes, and the microbes are killed by enzymes and several toxic substances produced in the phagolysosomes. The same substances may be released from the phagocytes and may kill extracellular microbes (not shown). *iNOS*, Inducible nitric oxide synthase; *NO*, nitric oxide; *ROS*, reactive oxygen species.

phagolysosomes, where they act on the ingested microbes but do not damage the phagocytes.

In addition to intracellular killing, neutrophils use additional mechanisms to destroy microbes. They can release microbicidal granule contents into the extracellular environment. In response to pathogens and inflammatory mediators, neutrophils die, and during this process they extrude their nuclear contents to form networks of chromatin called neutrophil extracellular traps (NETs), which contain antimicrobial substances that are normally sequestered in neutrophil granules. These NETs trap bacteria and fungi and kill the organisms. In some cases, the enzymes and ROS that are liberated into the extracellular space may injure host tissues. This is the reason why inflammation, normally a protective host response to infections, may cause tissue injury as well.

Inherited deficiency of the phagocyte oxidase enzyme is the cause of an immunodeficiency disorder called **chronic granulomatous disease** (CGD). In CGD, phagocytes are unable to eradicate intracellular microbes, and the host tries to contain the infection by calling in more macrophages and lymphocytes, resulting in collections of cells around the microbes called granulomas.

Antiviral Defense

Defense against viruses is a special type of host response that involves interferons, NK cells, and other mechanisms.

Type I interferons inhibit viral replication, and induce an antiviral state, in which cells become resistant to infection. Type I IFNs, which include several forms of IFN-α and one of IFN-β, are secreted by many cell types infected by viruses. A major source of these cytokines is a type of dendritic cell called the plasmacytoid dendritic cell (so named because these cells morphologically resemble plasma cells; see Chapter 3), which secretes type I IFNs when activated by recognition of viral nucleic acids by TLRs and other receptors. When type I IFNs secreted from dendritic cells or other infected cells bind to the IFN receptor on the infected or adjacent uninfected cells, signaling pathways are activated that inhibit viral replication and destroy viral genomes (Fig. 2-17). This action is the basis for

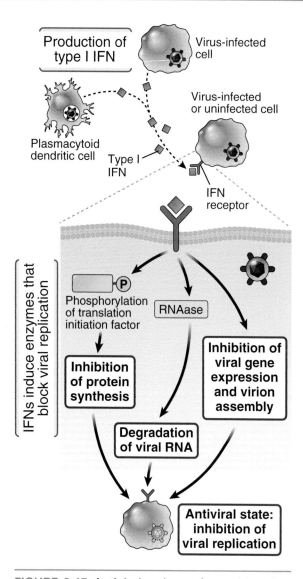

FIGURE 2-17 Antiviral actions of type I interferons. Type I interferons (IFN-α, IFN-β) are produced by plasmacytoid dendritic cells and virus-infected cells in response to intracellular TLR signaling and other sensors of viral nucleic acids. Type I interferons bind to receptors on the infected and uninfected cells and activate signaling pathways that induce expression of enzymes that interfere with viral replication at different steps, including inhibition of viral protein translation, increasing viral RNA degradation, and inhibition of viral gene expression and virion assembly. Type I IFNs also increase the infected cell's susceptibility to CTL-mediated killing (not shown).

the use of IFN-α to treat some forms of chronic viral hepatitis.

Virus-infected cells may be destroyed by NK cells, as described earlier. Type I IFNs enhance the ability of NK cells to kill infected cells. In addition, part of the innate response to viral infections includes increased apoptosis of infected cells, which also helps to eliminate the reservoir of infection.

Regulation of Innate Immune Responses

Innate immune responses are regulated by a variety of mechanisms that are designed to prevent excessive damage to tissues. These regulatory mechanisms include the production of antiinflammatory cytokines by macrophages and dendritic cells, including interleukin-10 (IL-10), which inhibits the microbicidal and pro-inflammatory functions of macrophages (classical pathway of macrophage activation), and IL-1 receptor antagonist, which blocks the actions of IL-1. There are also many feedback mechanisms in which signals that induce proinflammatory cytokine production also induce expression of inhibitors of cytokine signaling. For example, TLR signaling stimulates expression of proteins called suppressors of cytokine signaling (SOCS), which block the responses of cells to various cytokines, including IFNs.

Microbial Evasion of Innate Immunity

Pathogenic microbes have evolved to resist the mechanisms of innate immunity and are thus able to enter and colonize their hosts (Fig. 2-18). Some intracellular bacteria resist destruction inside phagocytes. *Listeria monocytogenes* produces a protein that enables it to escape from phagocytic vesicles and enter the cytoplasm of infected cells, where it is no longer susceptible to ROS or NO (which are produced mainly in phagolysosomes). The cell walls of mycobacteria contain a lipid that inhibits fusion of phagosomes containing ingested bacteria with lysosomes. Other microbes have cell walls that are resistant to the actions of complement proteins. As discussed in Chapters 6 and 8, these mechanisms also enable microbes to resist the effector mechanisms of cell-mediated and humoral immunity, the two arms of adaptive immunity.

Mechanism of immune evasion	Organism (example)	Mechanism
Resistance to phagocytosis	Pneumococci	Capsular polysaccharide inhibits phagocytosis
Resistance to reactive oxygen intermediates in phagocytes	Staphylococci	Production of catalase, which breaks down reactive oxygen intermediates
Resistance to complement activation (alternative pathway)	*Neisseria meningitidis*	Sialic acid expression inhibits C3 and C5 convertases
	Streptococci	M protein blocks C3 binding to organism, and C3b binding to complement receptors
Resistance to antimicrobial peptide antibiotics	*Pseudomonas*	Synthesis of modified LPS that resists action of peptide antibiotics

FIGURE 2-18 **Evasion of innate immunity by microbes.** Selected examples of the mechanisms by which microbes may evade or resist innate immunity. *LPS,* Lipopolysaccharide.

ROLE OF INNATE IMMUNITY IN STIMULATING ADAPTIVE IMMUNE RESPONSES

So far we have focused on how the innate immune system recognizes microbes and combats infections. We mentioned at the beginning of this chapter that, in addition to its roles in host defense, the innate immune response to microbes serves an important warning function by alerting the adaptive immune system that an effective immune response is needed. In this final section, we summarize some of the mechanisms by which innate immune responses stimulate adaptive immune responses.

Innate immune responses generate molecules that provide signals, in addition to antigens, that are required to activate naive T and B lymphocytes. In Chapter 1 we introduced the concept that full activation of antigen-specific lymphocytes requires two signals. Antigen may be referred to as signal 1, and innate immune responses to microbes and to host cells damaged by microbes may provide signal 2 (Fig. 2-19). The stimuli that warn the adaptive immune system that it needs to respond have also been called danger signals. This requirement for microbe-dependent second signals ensures that lymphocytes respond to infectious agents and not to harmless, noninfectious substances. In experimental situations or for vaccination, adaptive immune responses may be induced by antigens without microbes. In all such instances, the antigens need to be administered with substances called adjuvants that elicit the same innate immune reactions as microbes do. In fact, many potent adjuvants are the products of microbes. The nature and mechanisms of action of second signals are described in the discussion of the activation of T and B lymphocytes in Chapters 5 and 7, respectively. Here we describe two illustrative examples of second signals that are generated during innate immune reactions.

Microbes (or IFN-γ produced by NK cells in response to microbes) stimulate dendritic cells and macrophages to produce two types of second signals that can activate T lymphocytes. First, dendritic cells increase their expression of surface molecules called **costimulators,** which bind to receptors on naive T cells and function together with antigen recognition to activate the T cells. Second, the

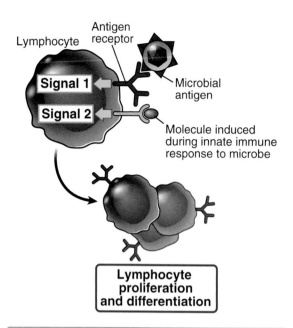

FIGURE 2-19 Two-signal requirement for lymphocyte activation. Antigen recognition by lymphocytes provides signal 1 for activation of the lymphocytes, and substances produced during innate immune responses to microbes (or components of microbes) provide signal 2. In this illustration, the lymphocytes could be T cells or B cells. By convention, the major second signals for T cells are called costimulators because they function together with antigens to stimulate the cells. The nature of second signals for T and B lymphocytes is described further in later chapters.

dendritic cells and macrophages secrete cytokines such as IL-12, IL-1, and IL-6, which stimulate the differentiation of naive T cells into effector cells of cell-mediated adaptive immunity.

Blood-borne microbes activate the complement system by the alternative pathway. One of the proteins produced during complement activation by proteolysis of C3b, called C3d, is covalently attached to the microbe. At the same time that B lymphocytes recognize microbial antigens by their antigen receptors, the B cells recognize the C3d bound to the microbe by a receptor for C3d. The combination of antigen recognition and C3d recognition initiates the process of B cell differentiation into antibody-secreting cells. Thus, a complement product serves as the second signal for humoral immune responses.

These examples illustrate an important feature of second signals: these signals not only stimulate adaptive immunity, but they also guide the nature of the adaptive immune response. Intracellular and phagocytosed microbes need to be eliminated by cell-mediated immunity, the adaptive response mediated by T lymphocytes. Microbes that are encountered and ingested by dendritic cells or macrophages induce the second signals—that is, costimulators and cytokines—that stimulate T cell responses. By contrast, blood-borne microbes need to be combated by antibodies, which are produced by B lymphocytes during humoral immune responses. Blood-borne microbes activate the plasma complement system, which in turn stimulates B cell activation and antibody production. Thus, different types of microbes induce different innate immune responses, which then stimulate the types of adaptive immunity that are best able to combat different infectious pathogens.

SUMMARY

- All multicellular organisms have intrinsic mechanisms of defense against infections, which constitute innate immunity.
- The innate immune system uses germline-encoded receptors to respond to structures that are characteristic of various classes of microbes and also recognizes products of dead cells. Innate immune reactions are not enhanced by repeat exposures to microbes.
- Toll-like receptors (TLRs), expressed on plasma membranes and in endosomes of many cell types, are a major class of innate immune system receptors that recognize different microbial products, including bacterial cell wall constituents and viral nucleic acids. Some receptors of the NLR family recognize microbes, products of damaged cells, and other substances, and these receptors signal through a cytosolic multiprotein complex, the inflammasome, to induce secretion of the proinflammatory cytokine interleukin-1 (IL-1).
- The principal components of innate immunity are epithelia, phagocytes, dendritic cells,

natural killer cells, cytokines, and plasma proteins, including the proteins of the complement system.

- Epithelia provide physical barriers against microbes, produce antibiotics, and contain lymphocytes that may prevent infections.
- The principal phagocytes—neutrophils and monocytes/macrophages—are blood cells that are recruited to sites of infection, where they are activated by engagement of different receptors. Some activated macrophages destroy microbes and dead cells and other macrophages limit inflammation and initiate tissue repair.
- Innate lymphoid cells (ILCs) secrete various cytokines that induce inflammation. Natural killer (NK) cells kill host cells infected by intracellular microbes and produce the cytokine interferon-γ, which activates macrophages to kill phagocytosed microbes.
- The complement system is a family of proteins that are activated on encounter with some microbes (in innate immunity) and by antibodies (in the humoral arm of adaptive immunity). Complement proteins coat (opsonize) microbes for phagocytosis, stimulate inflammation, and lyse microbes.
- Cytokines of innate immunity function to stimulate inflammation (TNF, IL-1, chemokines), activate NK cells (IL-12), activate macrophages (IFN-γ), and prevent viral infections (type I IFNs).
- In inflammation, phagocytes are recruited from the circulation to sites of infection and tissue damage. The cells bind to endothelial adhesion molecules that are induced by the cytokines TNF and IL-1, and migrate in response to soluble chemoattractants, including chemokines, complement fragments, and bacterial peptides. The leukocytes are activated, and they ingest and destroy microbes and damaged cells.
- Antiviral defense is mediated by type I interferons, which inhibit viral replication, and NK cells, which kill infected cells.
- In addition to providing early defense against infections, innate immune responses provide signals that work together with antigens to activate B and T lymphocytes. The requirement for these second signals ensures that adaptive immunity is elicited by microbes (the inducers of innate immune reactions) and not by non-microbial substances.

REVIEW QUESTIONS

1. How does the specificity of innate immunity differ from that of adaptive immunity?
2. What are examples of microbial substances recognized by the innate immune system, and what are the receptors for these substances?
3. What is the inflammasome, and how is it stimulated?
4. What are the mechanisms by which the epithelium of the skin prevents the entry of microbes?
5. How do phagocytes ingest and kill microbes?
6. What is the role of MHC molecules in the recognition of infected cells by NK cells, and what is the physiologic significance of this recognition?
7. What are the roles of the cytokines TNF, IL-12, and type I interferons in defense against infections?
8. How do innate immune responses enhance adaptive immunity?

Answers to and discussion of the Review Questions are available at https://studentconsult.inkling.com.

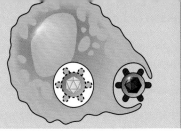

CHAPTER 3

Antigen Capture and Presentation to Lymphocytes

What Lymphocytes See

Adaptive immune responses are initiated by the recognition of antigens by antigen receptors of lymphocytes. B and T lymphocytes differ in the types of antigens they recognize. The antigen receptors of B lymphocytes—namely, membrane-bound antibodies—can recognize a variety of macromolecules (proteins, polysaccharides, lipids, nucleic acids), in soluble form or cell surface–associated form, as well as small chemicals. Therefore, B cell–mediated humoral immune responses may be generated against many types of microbial cell wall and soluble antigens. The antigen receptors of most T lymphocytes, on the other hand, can see only peptide fragments of protein antigens, and only when these peptides are presented by specialized molecules that bind peptides generated inside a host cell and then display them on the cell surface. Therefore, T cell–mediated immune responses may be generated only against protein antigens that are either produced in or taken up by host cells. This chapter focuses on the nature of the antigens that are recognized by lymphocytes. Chapter 4 describes the receptors used by lymphocytes to detect these antigens.

The induction of immune responses by antigens is a highly orchestrated process with a number of remarkable features. The first is that very few naive lymphocytes are specific for any one antigen, as few as 1 in 10^5 or 10^6 circulating lymphocytes, and this small fraction of the body's lymphocytes needs to locate and react rapidly to the antigen, wherever it is introduced. Second, different types of adaptive immune responses are required to defend against different types of microbes. In fact, the immune system has to react in different ways even to the same microbe at different stages of its life. For example, defense against a microbe (e.g., a virus) that has entered the circulation and is free in the blood depends on antibodies that bind the microbe, prevent it from infecting host cells, and help to eliminate it. The production of potent antibodies requires the activation of CD4+ helper T cells. After it has infected host cells, however, the microbe is safe from antibodies, which cannot enter the cells. As a result, activation of CD8+ cytotoxic T lymphocytes (CTLs) may be necessary to kill the infected cells and eliminate the reservoir of infection. Thus, we are faced with two important questions:

- How do the rare lymphocytes specific for any microbial antigen find that microbe, especially considering that microbes may enter anywhere in the body?
- How do different types of immune cells and molecules recognize microbes in different locations, such that helper T cells and antibodies respond to extracellular microbes and CTLs kill infected cells harboring microbes in their cytoplasm?

The answer to both questions is that the immune system has developed a highly specialized system for capturing and displaying antigens to lymphocytes. Research by immunologists, cell biologists, and biochemists has led to a sophisticated understanding of how protein antigens are captured, broken down, and displayed for recognition by T lymphocytes. This is the major topic of discussion in this chapter.

ANTIGENS RECOGNIZED BY T LYMPHOCYTES

The majority of T lymphocytes recognize peptide antigens that are bound to and displayed by major histocompatibility complex (MHC) molecules of antigen-presenting cells. The MHC is a genetic locus whose principal protein products function as the peptide display molecules of the immune system. In every individual, different clones of CD4+ and CD8+ T cells can see peptides only when these peptides are displayed by that individual's MHC molecules.

This property of T cells is called **MHC restriction**. The T cell receptor (TCR) recognizes some amino acid residues of the peptide antigen and simultaneously also recognizes residues of the MHC molecule that is displaying that peptide (Fig. 3-1). The properties of MHC molecules and the significance of MHC restriction are described later in this chapter. How we generate T cells that recognize peptides presented only by self MHC molecules is described in Chapter 4. Also, some small populations of T cells recognize lipid and other nonpeptide antigens either presented by nonpolymorphic class I MHC–like molecules or without a requirement for a specialized antigen display system.

The cells that capture microbial antigens and display them for recognition by T lymphocytes are called **antigen-presenting cells** (APCs). Naive T lymphocytes must see protein antigens presented by dendritic cells to initiate clonal expansion and differentiation of the T cells into effector and memory cells. For this reason, dendritic cells are considered the most efficient and specialized APCs, and are therefore sometimes called professional APCs. Differentiated effector T cells again need to see antigens, which may be

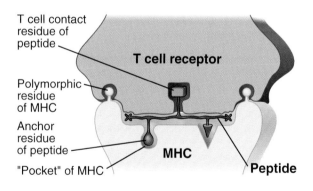

FIGURE 3-1 Model showing how a T cell receptor recognizes a complex of peptide antigen displayed by an MHC molecule. Major histocompatibility complex (MHC) molecules are expressed on antigen-presenting cells and function to display peptides derived from protein antigens. Peptides bind to the MHC molecules by anchor residues, which attach the peptides to pockets in the MHC molecules. The antigen receptor of every T cell recognizes some amino acid residues of the peptide and some (polymorphic) residues of the MHC molecule.

presented by various kinds of APCs besides dendritic cells, to activate the effector functions of the T cells in both humoral and cell-mediated immune responses. We first describe the way in which APCs capture and present antigens to trigger immune responses and then examine the role of MHC molecules in antigen presentation to T cells.

CAPTURE OF PROTEIN ANTIGENS BY ANTIGEN-PRESENTING CELLS

Protein antigens of microbes that enter the body are captured mainly by dendritic cells and concentrated in the peripheral lymphoid organs, where immune responses are initiated (Fig. 3-2). Microbes usually enter the body

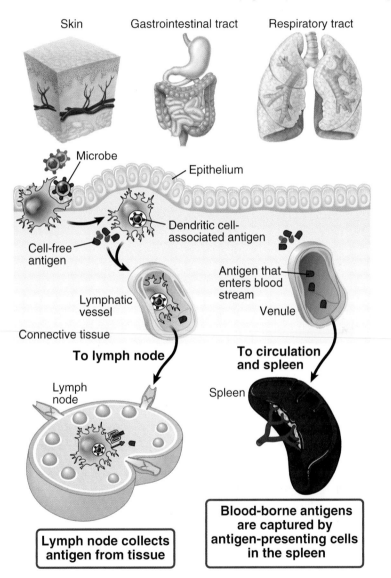

FIGURE 3-2 **Capture and display of microbial antigens.** Microbes enter through an epithelial barrier and are captured by antigen-presenting cells resident in the tissue or microbes enter lymphatic vessels or blood vessels. The microbes and their antigens are transported to peripheral lymphoid organs, the lymph nodes and the spleen, where protein antigens are displayed for recognition by T lymphocytes.

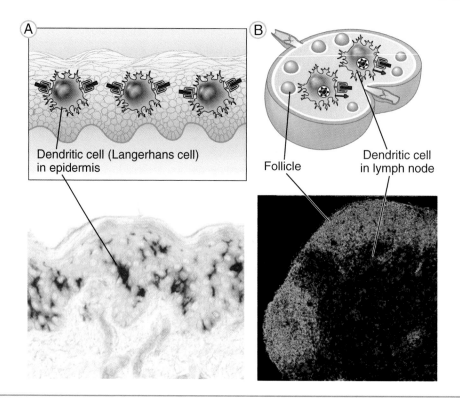

FIGURE 3-3 Dendritic cells. A, Immature dendritic cells reside in tissues including epithelia, such as the skin, and form a network of cells with interdigitating processes, seen as blue cells on the section of skin stained with an antibody that recognizes dendritic cells. **B,** Mature dendritic cells reside in the T cell–rich areas of lymph nodes (and spleen, not shown) and are seen in the section of a lymph node stained with fluorochrome-conjugated antibodies against dendritic cells (red) and B cells in follicles (green). Note that the dendritic cells are in the same regions of the lymph node as T cells (see Fig. 1-15, *B*). (*A,* Micrograph of skin courtesy Dr. Y-J. Liu, MD, Anderson Cancer Center, Houston; *B,* courtesy of Drs. Kathryn Pape and Jennifer Walter, University of Minnesota Medical School, Minneapolis.)

through the skin (by contact), the gastrointestinal tract (by ingestion), and the respiratory tract (by inhalation). Some insect-borne microbes may be injected into the bloodstream as a result of insect bites, and some infections are acquired through the genitourinary tract. Microbial antigens can also be produced in any infected tissue. Because of the vast surface area of the epithelial barriers and the large volume of blood, connective tissues, and internal organs, it would be impossible for lymphocytes of all possible specificities to efficiently patrol all these sites searching for foreign invaders; instead, antigens are taken to the lymphoid organs through which lymphocytes recirculate. This process involves a series of events following the encounter of dendritic cells with microbes—capture of antigens, activation of the dendritic

cells, migration of the antigen-carrying cells to lymph nodes, and display of the antigen to T cells.

All the interfaces between the body and the external environment are lined by continuous epithelia, whose principal function is to provide a barrier to infection. The epithelia and subepithelial tissues contain a network of **dendritic cells;** the same cells are present in the T cell–rich areas of peripheral lymphoid organs and, in smaller numbers, in most other organs (Fig. 3-3). There are two major populations of dendritic cells, called classical and plasmacytoid, which differ in their locations and responses (Fig. 3-4). The majority of dendritic cells in tissues and lymphoid organs belong to the classical subset. In the skin, the epidermal dendritic cells are called Langerhans cells. Plasmacytoid dendritic cells are named because

Feature	Classical dendritic cells	Plasmacytoid dendritic cells
Surface markers	CD11c high CD11b high	CD11c low CD11b negative B220 high
Major location	Tissues	Blood and tissue
Expression of Toll-like receptors	TLRs 4, 5, 8 high	TLRs 7, 9 high
Major cytokines produced	TNF, IL-6, IL-12	Type I interferons
Postulated major functions	Induction of T cell responses against most antigens	Antiviral innate immunity and induction of T cell responses against viruses

FIGURE 3-4 **Populations of dendritic cells.** This figure lists the properties of two major classes of dendritic cell: classical (or conventional) and plasmacytoid. Many subsets of classical dendritic cells have been described (not shown) that may perform specialized functions in different tissues. The surface markers listed in the table are best defined in mice. *IL*, Interleukin; *TLRs*, toll-like receptors; *TNF*, tumor necrosis factor.

of their morphologic resemblance to plasma cells; they are present in the blood and tissues. Plasmacytoid dendritic cells are also the major source of type I interferons in innate immune responses to viral infections (see Chapter 2).

Dendritic cells use various membrane receptors to bind microbes, such as lectin receptors for carbohydrate structures typical of microbial but not mammalian glycoproteins. These microbes or their antigens enter the dendritic cells by phagocytosis or receptor-mediated endocytosis. At the same time that the dendritic cells are capturing antigens, products of the microbes stimulate innate immune reactions by binding to Toll-like receptors (TLRs) and other innate pattern recognition receptors in the dendritic cells, tissue epithelial cells, and resident macrophages (see Chapter 2). This results in production of inflammatory cytokines such as tumor necrosis factor (TNF) and interleukin-1 (IL-1). The combination of TLR signaling and cytokines activates the dendritic cells, resulting in several changes in phenotype, migration, and function.

Upon activation by these signals, classical dendritic cells lose their adhesiveness for epithelia and begin to express the chemokine receptor CCR7, which is specific for chemoattracting cytokines (chemokines) produced by lymphatic endothelium and by stromal cells in the T cell zones of lymph nodes. These chemokines direct the dendritic cells to exit the epithelium and migrate through lymphatic vessels to the lymph nodes draining that epithelium (Fig. 3-5). During the process of migration, the dendritic cells mature from cells designed to capture antigens into APCs capable of stimulating T lymphocytes. This maturation is reflected by increased synthesis and stable expression of MHC molecules, which display antigens to T cells, and of costimulators, which were introduced in Chapter 2, that are required for full T cell responses. Soluble antigens in the lymph are picked up by dendritic cells that reside in the lymph nodes, and blood-borne antigens are handled in essentially the same way by dendritic cells in the spleen.

The net result of this sequence of events is that the protein antigens of microbes that enter the body are transported to and concentrated in the regions of lymph nodes where the antigens are most likely to encounter T lymphocytes.

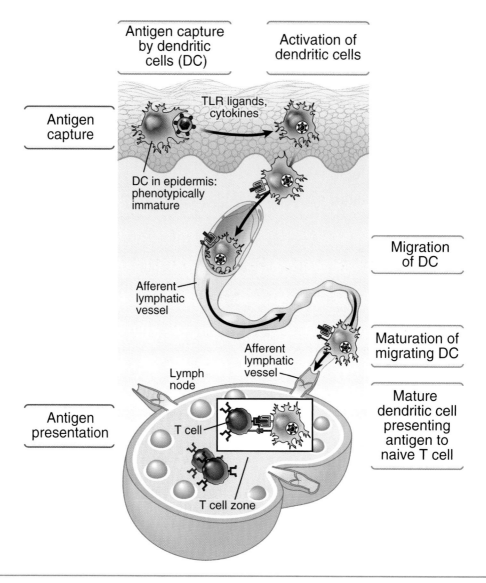

FIGURE 3-5 Capture and presentation of protein antigens by dendritic cells. Immature dendritic cells in the epithelium (skin, as shown here, where the dendritic cells are called Langerhans cells) capture microbial antigens, are activated, and leave the epithelium. The dendritic cells migrate to draining lymph nodes, being attracted there by chemokines produced in the lymphatic vessels and nodes. In response to signals induced by the microbe, such as Toll-like receptor (TLR) signals and cytokines, the dendritic cells mature and acquire the ability to present antigens to naive T lymphocytes in the lymph nodes. Dendritic cells at different stages of their maturation may express different membrane proteins. Immature dendritic cells express surface receptors that capture microbial antigens, whereas mature dendritic cells express high levels of major histocompatibility complex molecules and costimulators, which function to stimulate T cells.

| Cell type | Expression of | | Principal function |
	Class II MHC	Costimulators	
Dendritic cells	Constitutive; increases with maturation; increased by IFN-γ	Constitutive; increases with maturation; increased by TLR ligands, IFN-γ, and T cells (CD40-CD40L interactions)	Antigen presentation to naive T cells in the initiation of T cell responses to protein antigens (priming)
Macrophages	Low or negative; inducible by IFN-γ	Low, inducible by TLR ligands, IFN-γ, and T cells (CD40-CD40L interactions)	Antigen presentation to CD4+ effector T cells in the effector phase of cell-mediated immune responses
B lymphocytes	Constitutive; increased by cytokines (e.g., IL-4)	Induced by T cells (CD40-CD40L interactions), antigen receptor cross-linking	Antigen presentation to CD4+ helper T cells in humoral immune responses (T cell–B cell interactions)

FIGURE 3-6 Major antigen-presenting cells (APCs). The properties of the principal class II major histocompatibility complex (MHC)–expressing APCs, which present antigens to CD4+ helper T cells. Other cell types, such as vascular endothelial cells, also express class II MHC, but their roles in initiating immune responses to microbes are not established. In the thymus, epithelial cells express class II MHC molecules and play a role in the maturation and selection of T cells. All nucleated cells can present class I MHC–associated peptides to CD8+ T cells. *IFN-γ*, Interferon-γ; *IL-4*, interleukin-4; *TLR*, Toll-like receptor.

Recall that naive T lymphocytes continuously recirculate through lymph nodes and also express CCR7, which promotes their entry into the T cell zones of lymph nodes (see Chapter 1). Therefore, dendritic cells bearing captured antigen and naive T cells poised to recognize antigens come together in lymph nodes. This process is remarkably efficient; it is estimated that if a microbial antigen is introduced at any site in the body, a T cell response to the antigen begins in the lymph nodes draining that site within 12 to 18 hours.

Different types of APC serve distinct functions in T cell–dependent immune responses (Fig. 3-6).

- Dendritic cells are the principal inducers of such responses, because these cells are located at sites of microbe entry and are the most potent APCs for activating naive T lymphocytes.
- One important type of APC for effector T cells is the macrophage, which is abundant in all

tissues. In cell-mediated immune reactions, macrophages phagocytose microbes and display the antigens of these microbes to effector T cells, which activate the macrophages to kill the microbes (see Chapter 6).

- B lymphocytes ingest protein antigens and display them to helper T cells within lymphoid tissues; this process is important for the development of humoral immune responses (see Chapter 7).
- As discussed later in this chapter, all nucleated cells can present antigens derived from microbes in the cytoplasm to CD8+ T cells.

Now that we know how protein antigens are captured, transported to, and concentrated in peripheral lymphoid organs, we next ask, how are these antigens displayed to T lymphocytes? To answer this question, we first need to understand what MHC molecules are and how they function in immune responses.

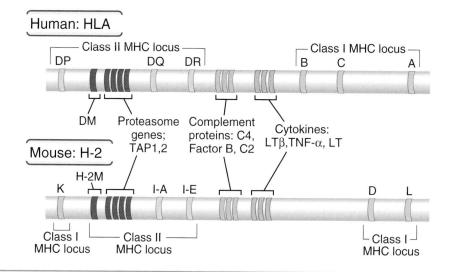

FIGURE 3-7 Genes of the major histocompatibility complex (MHC) locus. Schematic maps show the human MHC, called the human leukocyte antigen (HLA) complex, and the mouse MHC, called the H-2 complex, illustrating the major genes that code for molecules involved in immune responses. Sizes of genes and intervening DNA segments are not drawn to scale. Class II loci are shown as single blocks, but each consists of at least two genes encoding the α and β chains, respectively. The products of some of the genes (DM, proteasome components, TAP) are involved in antigen processing. The MHC locus also contains genes that encode molecules other than peptide display molecules, including some complement proteins and cytokines; this region is sometimes called "class III MHC." In addition, there are multiple class I–like genes and pseudogenes (not shown). *LT,* Lymphotoxin; *TAP,* transporter associated with antigen processing; *TNF,* tumor necrosis factor.

STRUCTURE AND FUNCTION OF MAJOR HISTOCOMPATIBILITY COMPLEX MOLECULES

MHC molecules are membrane proteins on APCs that display peptide antigens for recognition by T lymphocytes. The MHC was discovered as the genetic locus that is the principal determinant of acceptance or rejection of tissue grafts exchanged between individuals (tissue, or *histo*, compatibility). In other words, individuals who are identical at their MHC locus (inbred animals and identical twins) will accept grafts from one another, and individuals who differ at their MHC loci will reject such grafts. Because graft rejection is not a natural biologic phenomenon, MHC genes and the molecules they encode must have evolved to perform other functions. We now know that the physiologic role of MHC molecules is to display peptides derived from microbial protein antigens to antigen-specific T lymphocytes as a first step in protective T cell–mediated immune responses to microbes. This function of MHC molecules is the explanation for the phenomenon of MHC restriction of T cells, as mentioned earlier.

The collection of genes that make up the MHC locus is found in all mammals (Fig. 3-7) and includes genes that encode MHC molecules and other proteins. Human MHC proteins are called **human leukocyte antigens** (HLAs) because they were discovered as antigens of leukocytes that could be identified with specific antibodies. In all mammals, the MHC locus contains two sets of highly polymorphic genes, called the class I and class II MHC genes. (As discussed later, polymorphism refers to the presence of many variants of these genes in the population.) These genes encode the class I and class II MHC molecules that display peptides to T cells. In addition to the polymorphic genes, the MHC locus contains many nonpolymorphic genes, some of which code for proteins involved in antigen presentation.

Structure of MHC Molecules

Class I and class II MHC molecules are membrane proteins that each contains a peptide-binding cleft at the amino-terminal end. Although the two classes of molecules differ in subunit composition, they are very similar in overall structure (Fig. 3-8).

Class I MHC Molecules

Each **class I MHC molecule** consists of an α chain noncovalently associated with a protein called β_2-microglobulin that is encoded by a gene outside the MHC. The α chain consists of three extracellular domains followed by short transmembrane and cytoplasmic domains.

- The amino-terminal α1 and α2 domains of the α chain molecule form a peptide-binding cleft, or groove, that can accommodate peptides typically 8 to 9 amino acids long. The floor of the peptide-binding cleft is the region that binds peptides for display to T lymphocytes, and the walls of the cleft are the regions that make contact with the T cell receptor (which also contacts part of the displayed peptide; see Fig. 3-1). The polymorphic residues of class I molecules—that is, the amino acids that differ among different individuals' MHC molecules—are located in the α1 and α2 domains of the α chain. Some of these polymorphic residues contribute to variations in the floor of the peptide-binding cleft and thus in the ability of different MHC molecules to bind peptides. Other polymorphic residues contribute to variations in the walls of the clefts and thus influence recognition by T cells.
- The α3 domain is invariant and contains a site that binds the CD8 T cell coreceptor but not CD4. As discussed in Chapter 5, T cell activation requires recognition of MHC-associated peptide antigen by the TCR and simultaneous recognition of the MHC molecule by the coreceptor. Therefore, CD8+ T cells can only

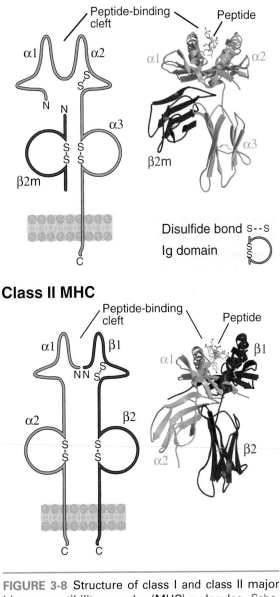

Class I MHC

Class II MHC

FIGURE 3-8 Structure of class I and class II major histocompatibility complex (MHC) molecules. Schematic diagrams (at left) and models of the crystal structures (at right) of class I MHC and class II MHC molecules illustrate the domains of the molecules and the fundamental similarities between them. Both types of MHC molecules contain peptide-binding clefts and invariant portions that bind CD8 (the α3 domain of class I) or CD4 (the β2 domain of class II). *β2m*, β_2-microglobulin; *Ig*, immunoglobulin. (Crystal structures courtesy of Dr. P. Bjorkman, California Institute of Technology, Pasadena.)

respond to peptides displayed by class I MHC molecules, the MHC molecules to which the CD8 coreceptor binds.

Class II MHC Molecules

Each **class II MHC molecule** consists of two transmembrane chains, called α and β. Each chain has two extracellular domains, followed by the transmembrane and cytoplasmic regions.

- The amino-terminal regions of both chains, called the α1 and β1 domains, contain polymorphic residues and form a cleft that is large enough to accommodate peptides of 10 to 30 residues.
- The nonpolymorphic α2 and β2 domains contain the binding site for the CD4 T cell coreceptor. Because CD4 binds to class II MHC molecules but not to class I, CD4+ T cells can only respond to peptides presented by class II MHC molecules.

Properties of MHC Genes and Proteins

Several features of MHC genes and molecules are important for the normal function of these molecules (Fig. 3-9):

- **MHC genes are highly polymorphic,** meaning that many different alleles (variants) are present among the different individuals in the population. The total number of HLA alleles in the population is estimated to be more than 10,000 for class I and over 3000 for class II, with about 3000 for the HLA-B locus alone, making MHC genes the most polymorphic of all genes in mammals. The polymorphism of MHC genes is so great that any two individuals in an outbred population are extremely unlikely to have exactly the same MHC genes and molecules. These different polymorphic variants are inherited and not generated de novo in individuals by somatic gene recombination, as are antigen receptor genes (see Chapter 4). Because the polymorphic residues determine which peptides are presented by which MHC molecules, the existence of multiple alleles ensures that there are always some members of the population who will be able to pres-

ent any particular microbial protein antigen. Therefore, MHC polymorphism ensures that a population will be able to deal with the diversity of microbes and at least some individuals will be able to mount effective immune responses to the peptide antigens of these microbes. Thus, everyone will not succumb to a newly encountered or mutated microbe.

- **MHC genes are codominantly expressed, meaning that the alleles inherited from both parents are expressed equally.** Codominant inheritance maximizes the number of HLA genes, and therefore proteins, present in each individual and thus enables each individual to display a large number of peptides. Because every individual expresses both sets of MHC alleles inherited from each parent, there is a 1 in 4 chance of siblings expressing all the same MHC molecules.
- **Class I molecules are expressed on all nucleated cells, but class II molecules are expressed mainly on dendritic cells, macrophages, and B lymphocytes.** The physiologic significance of this strikingly different expression pattern is described later. Class II molecules also are expressed on thymic epithelial cells and endothelial cells and can be induced on other cell types by the cytokine interferon-γ.

Nomenclature of HLA Genes and Proteins

Three polymorphic class I gene loci, called HLA-A, HLA-B, and HLA-C, exist in humans, and each person inherits one set of these genes from each parent, so any cell can express six different class I molecules. In the class II locus, every individual inherits from each parent two genes encoding the α chain and the β chain of HLA-DP, two encoding DQα and DQβ, one or two for DRβ (HLA-DRB1 and HLA-DRB3, 4 or 5), and one for DRα. The polymorphism resides mainly in the β chains. Because of the extra DRβ genes, because of the production of two isoforms from each DQβ gene, and because some α chains encoded on one chromosome can associate with β chains encoded from the other chromosome, the total number of expressed class II molecules may be considerably more than six.

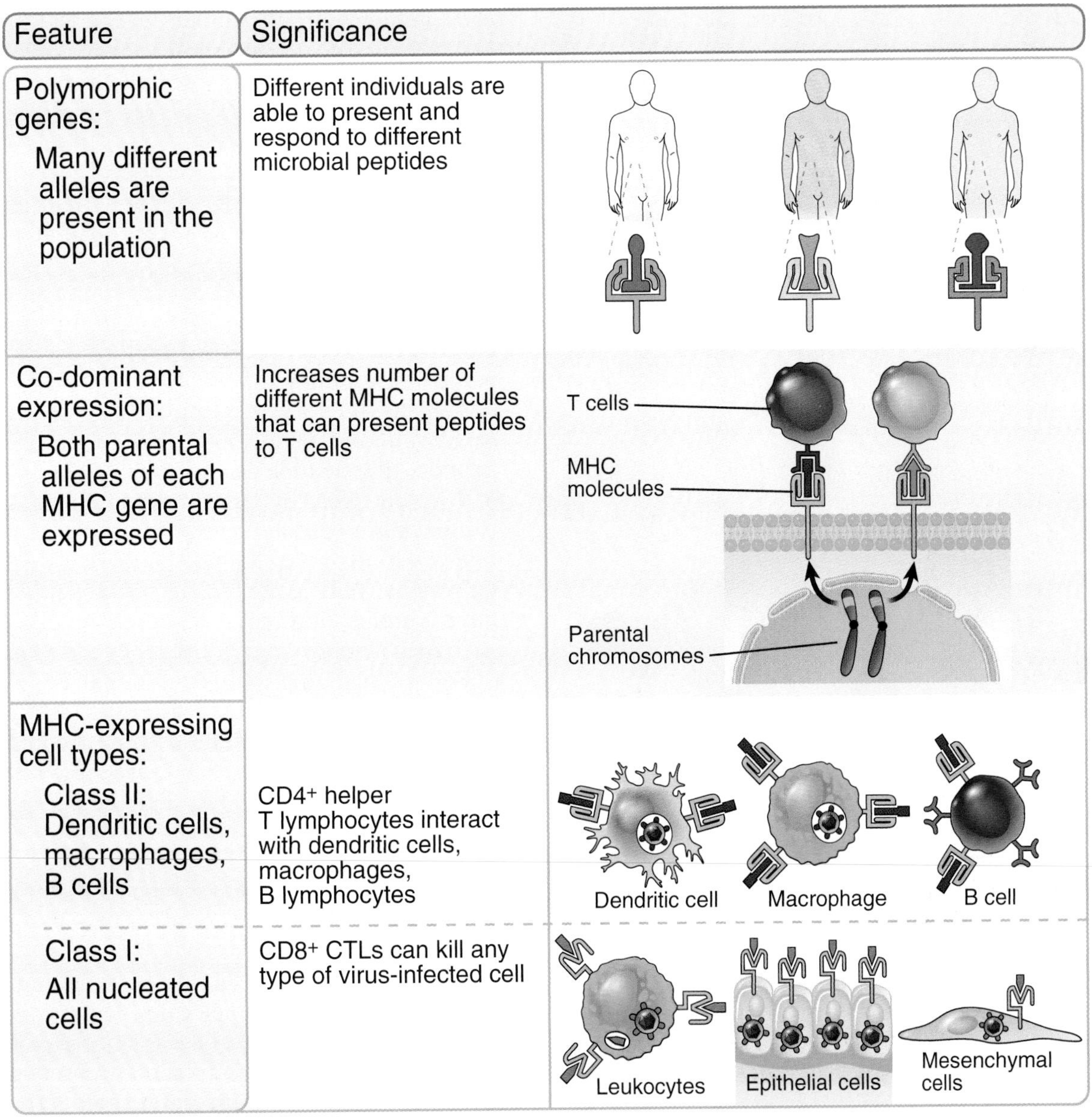
Feature
Significance
Polymorphic genes:
Many different alleles are present in the population
Different individuals are able to present and respond to different microbial peptides
Co-dominant expression:
Both parental alleles of each MHC gene are expressed
Increases number of different MHC molecules that can present peptides to T cells
T cells
MHC molecules
Parental chromosomes
MHC-expressing cell types:
Class II:
Dendritic cells, macrophages, B cells
CD4+ helper T lymphocytes interact with dendritic cells, macrophages, B lymphocytes
Dendritic cell
Macrophage
B cell
Class I:
All nucleated cells
CD8+ CTLs can kill any type of virus-infected cell
Leukocytes
Epithelial cells
Mesenchymal cells

FIGURE 3-9 **Properties of major histocompatibility complex (MHC) molecules and genes.** Some of the important features of MHC molecules and their significance for immune responses. *CTLs*, Cytotoxic T lymphocytes.

The set of MHC alleles present on each chromosome is called an **MHC haplotype.** In humans, each HLA allele is given a numeric designation. For example, an HLA haplotype of an individual could be HLA-A2, B5, DR3, and so on. In the modern terminology, based on molecular typing, individual alleles may be called HLA-A*0201, referring to the 01 subtype of HLA-A2, or HLA-DRB1*0401, referring to the 01 subtype of the DR4B1 gene, and so on.

Peptide Binding to MHC Molecules

The peptide-binding clefts of MHC molecules bind peptides derived from protein

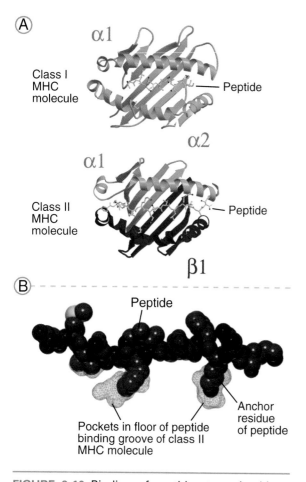

FIGURE 3-10 Binding of peptides to major histocompatibility complex (MHC) molecules. **A,** The top views of the crystal structures of MHC molecules show how peptides (in yellow) lie on the floors of the peptide-binding clefts and are available for recognition by T cells. **B,** The side view of a cutout of a peptide bound to a class II MHC molecule shows how anchor residues of the peptide hold it in the pockets in the cleft of the MHC molecule. (*A,* courtesy of Dr. P. Bjorkman, California Institute of Technology, Pasadena, California; *B,* from Scott CA, Peterson PA, Teyton L, Wilson IA: Crystal structures of two I-Ad-peptide complexes reveal that high affinity can be achieved without large anchor residues. *Immunity* 8: 319–329, 1998. © Cell Press; with permission.)

antigens and display these peptides for recognition by T cells (Fig. 3-10). There are pockets in the floors of the peptide-binding clefts of most MHC molecules. Some of the amino acids in the peptide antigens fit into these MHC

pockets and anchor the peptides in the cleft of the MHC molecule; these amino acids are called anchor residues. Other residues of the bound peptide project upward and are recognized by the antigen receptors of T cells.

Several features of the interaction of peptide antigens with MHC molecules are important for understanding the peptide display function of MHC molecules (Fig. 3-11):

- Each MHC molecule can present only one peptide at a time, because there is only one binding cleft, but each MHC molecule is capable of presenting many different peptides. As long as the pockets of the MHC molecule can accommodate the anchor residues of the peptide, that peptide can be displayed by the MHC molecule. Therefore, only one or two residues in a peptide determine if that peptide will bind in the cleft of a particular MHC molecule. Thus, MHC molecules are said to have a broad specificity for peptide binding; each MHC molecule can bind many peptides of the optimal length range but not all possible peptides. This feature is essential for the antigen display function of MHC molecules, because each individual has only a few different MHC molecules that must be able to present a vast number and variety of protein antigens.
- MHC molecules bind mainly peptides and not other types of antigens. Among various classes of molecules, only peptides have the structural and charge characteristics that permit binding to the clefts of MHC molecules. This is why MHC-restricted CD4+ T cells and CD8+ T cells can recognize and respond mainly to protein antigens, the natural source of peptides. The MHC is also involved in the reactions of T cells to some nonpeptide antigens, such as small molecules and metal ions. The recognition of such antigens is discussed briefly later in the chapter.
- MHC molecules acquire their peptide cargo during their biosynthesis, assembly, and transport inside cells. Therefore, MHC molecules display peptides derived from protein antigens that are inside host cells (produced inside cells or ingested from the

Feature	Significance	
Broad specificity	Many different peptides can bind to the same MHC molecule	
Each MHC molecule displays one peptide at a time	Each T cell responds to a single peptide bound to an MHC molecule	
MHC molecules bind only peptides	MHC-restricted T cells respond mainly to protein antigens	
Peptides are acquired during intracellular assembly	Class I and class II MHC molecules display peptides from different cellular compartments	
Stable surface expression of MHC molecule requires bound peptide	Only peptide-loaded MHC molecules are expressed on the cell surface for recognition by T cells	
Very slow off-rate	MHC molecule displays bound peptide for long enough to be located by T cell	

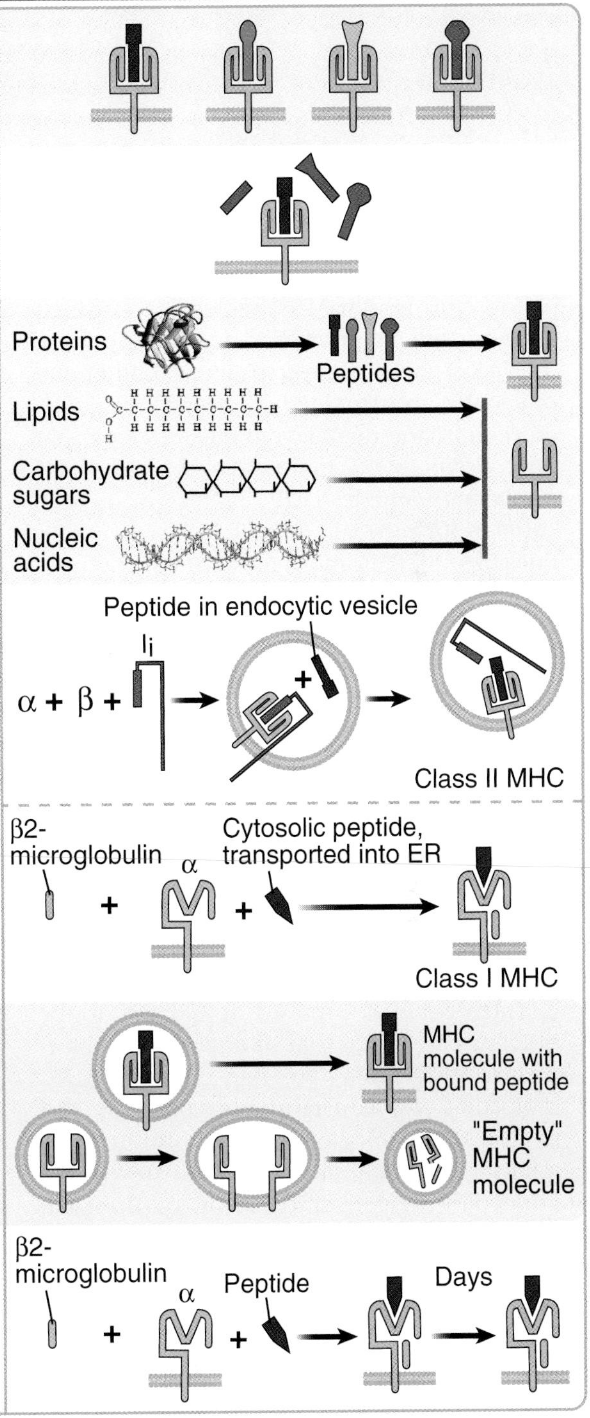

FIGURE 3-11 Features of peptide binding to MHC molecules. Some of the important features of peptide binding to MHC molecules, with their significance for immune responses. *ER*, Endoplasmic reticulum; *I$_i$*, invariant chain.

extracellular environment). This explains why MHC-restricted T cells recognize cell-associated microbes. Class I MHC molecules acquire peptides from cytosolic proteins and class II molecules from proteins that are taken up into intracellular vesicles. The mechanisms and significance of these pathways of peptide-MHC association are discussed later.

- Only peptide-loaded MHC molecules are stably expressed on cell surfaces. The reason for this is that MHC molecules must assemble both their chains and bound peptides to achieve a stable structure, and empty molecules are degraded inside cells. This requirement for peptide binding ensures that only useful MHC molecules—that is, those displaying peptides—are expressed on cell surfaces for recognition by T cells. Once peptides bind to MHC molecules, they stay bound for a long time, up to days for some peptides. The slow off-rate ensures that after an MHC molecule has acquired a peptide, it will display the peptide long enough that a particular T cell that can recognize the peptide will find it and initiate a response.

- In each individual, the MHC molecules can display peptides derived from the individual's own proteins, as well as peptides from foreign (i.e., microbial) proteins. This inability of MHC molecules to discriminate between self antigens and foreign antigens raises two questions. First, at any time, the quantity of self proteins is certain to be much greater than that of any microbial antigens. Why, then, are the available MHC molecules not constantly occupied by self peptides and unable to present foreign antigens? The likely answer is that new MHC molecules are constantly being synthesized, ready to accept peptides, and they are adept at capturing any peptides that are present in cells. Also, a single T cell may need to see a peptide displayed by only as few as 0.1% to 1% of the approximately 10^5 MHC molecules on the surface of an APC, so that even rare MHC molecules displaying a peptide

are enough to initiate an immune response. The second problem is that if MHC molecules are constantly displaying self peptides, why do we not develop immune responses to self antigens, so-called autoimmune responses? The answer is that T cells specific for self antigens are either killed or inactivated (see Chapter 9). Thus, T cells are constantly patrolling the body looking at MHC-associated peptides, and if there is an infection, only those T cells that recognize microbial peptides will respond, while self peptide–specific T cells will either be absent or will have been previously inactivated.

MHC molecules are capable of displaying peptides but not intact microbial protein antigens, which are too large to fit into the MHC cleft. Therefore, mechanisms must exist for converting naturally occurring proteins into peptides able to bind to MHC molecules. This conversion, called **antigen processing,** is described next.

PROCESSING AND PRESENTATION OF PROTEIN ANTIGENS

Extracellular proteins that are internalized by specialized APCs (dendritic cells, macrophages, B cells) are processed in late endosomes and lysosomes and displayed by class II MHC molecules, whereas proteins in the cytosol of any nucleated cell are processed in proteolytic structures called proteasomes and displayed by class I MHC molecules (Fig. 3-12). These two pathways of antigen processing involve different cellular proteins (Fig. 3-13). They are designed to sample all the proteins present in the extracellular and intracellular environments. The segregation of antigen-processing pathways also ensures that different classes of T lymphocytes recognize antigens from different compartments. Next we discuss the mechanisms of antigen processing, beginning with the class II MHC pathway because it was defined first and was the basis for much of our understanding of antigen processing.

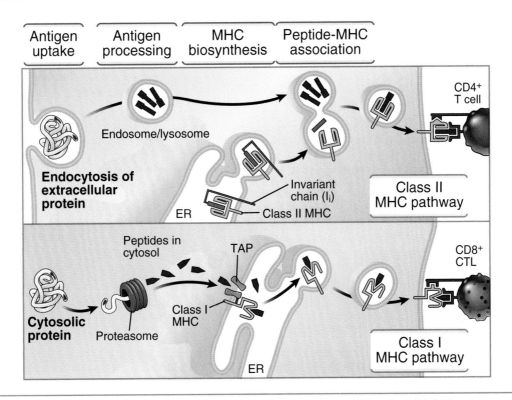

FIGURE 3-12 Pathways of intracellular processing of protein antigens. The class II MHC pathway converts protein antigens that are endocytosed into vesicles of antigen-presenting cells into peptides that bind to class II MHC molecules for recognition by CD4+ T cells. The class I MHC pathway converts proteins in the cytosol into peptides that bind to class I MHC molecules for recognition by CD8+ T cells. *CTL*, Cytotoxic T lymphocyte; *ER*, endoplasmic reticulum; *TAP*, transporter associated with antigen processing.

Processing of Internalized Antigens for Display by Class II MHC Molecules

The main steps in the presentation of peptides by class II MHC molecules include internalization of the antigen, proteolysis in endocytic vesicles, and association of peptides with class II molecules (Fig. 3-14):

- *Internalization and digestion of antigens.* **Antigens destined for the class II MHC pathway are usually internalized from the extracellular environment.** Dendritic cells and macrophages may ingest extracellular microbes or microbial proteins by several mechanisms, including phagocytosis and receptor-mediated endocytosis. Microbes may bind to surface receptors specific for microbial products or to receptors that recognize

antibodies or products of complement activation (opsonins) attached to the microbes. B lymphocytes efficiently internalize proteins that specifically bind to the cells' antigen receptors (see Chapter 7). These APCs may also pinocytose proteins without any specific recognition event. After internalization into APCs by any of these pathways, the microbial proteins enter acidic intracellular vesicles, called endosomes or phagosomes, which may fuse with lysosomes. In these vesicles the proteins are broken down by proteolytic enzymes, generating many peptides of varying lengths and sequences.

- *Binding of peptides to MHC molecules.* **Peptides bind to newly synthesized MHC molecules in specialized vesicles.** Class II

Feature	Class II MHC Pathway	Class I MHC pathway
Composition of stable peptide-MHC complex	Polymorphic α and β chains of MHC, peptide 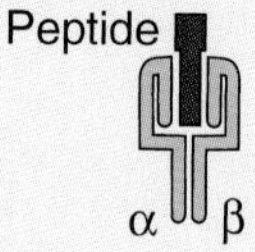	Polymorphic α chain of MHC, β2-microglobulin, peptide 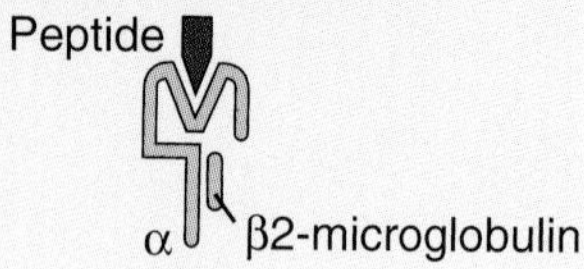
Cells that express that MHC	Dendritic cells, mononuclear phagocytes, B lymphocytes; endothelial cells, thymic epithelium	All nucleated cells
Responsive T cells	CD4+ T cells 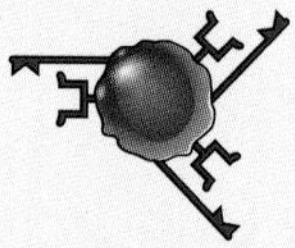	CD8+ T cells 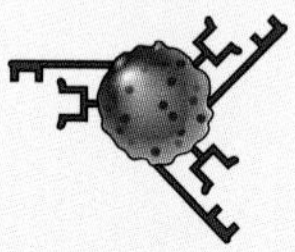
Source of protein antigens	Endosomal/lysosomal proteins (mostly internalized from extracellular environment)	Cytosolic proteins (mostly synthesized in the cell; may enter cytosol from phagosomes)
Enzymes responsible for peptide generation	Endosomal and lysosomal proteases (e.g., cathepsins)	Enzymatic components of cytosolic proteasome
Site of peptide loading of MHC	Late endosomes and lysosomes	Endoplasmic reticulum
Molecules involved in transport of peptides and loading of MHC molecules	Invariant chain, DM	TAP

FIGURE 3-13 **Features of the pathways of antigen processing.** Some of the comparative features of the two major antigen processing pathways. *MHC*, Major histocompatibility complex; *TAP*, transporter associated with antigen processing.

MHC–expressing APCs constantly synthesize these MHC molecules in the endoplasmic reticulum (ER). Each newly synthesized class II molecule carries with it an attached protein called the **invariant chain** (I$_i$), which contains a sequence called the class II invariant chain peptide (CLIP) that binds to the peptide-binding cleft of the class II molecule. Thus, the cleft of the newly synthesized class II molecule is occupied and prevented from accepting peptides in the ER that are destined to bind to class I MHC molecules (see below). This class II molecule with its associated I$_i$ is targeted to the late endosomal/lysosomal vesicles that contain peptides derived from ingested extracellular proteins. In these vesicles, the invariant chain is degraded, leaving only CLIP in the peptide-binding cleft. Late endosomes/lysosomes also contain a class II MHC–like protein called DM, whose function is to exchange CLIP in the class II MHC molecule with other peptides that may be available in this compartment and can bind to the MHC molecule with higher affinity.

• *Transport of peptide-MHC complexes to the cell surface.* **Peptide loading stabilizes class II MHC molecules, which are exported**

Uptake of extracellular proteins into vesicular compartments of APC	Processing of internalized proteins in endosomal/ lysosomal vesicles	Biosynthesis and transport of class II MHC molecules to endosomes	Association of processed peptides with class II MHC molecules in vesicles	Expression of peptide-MHC complexes on cell surface

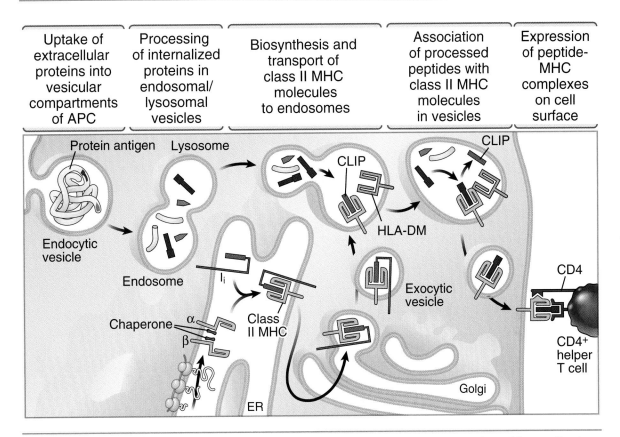

FIGURE 3-14 Class II major histocompatibility complex (MHC) pathway of processing of internalized vesicular antigens. Protein antigens are ingested by antigen-presenting cells (APCs) into vesicles, where they are degraded into peptides. Class II MHC molecules enter the same vesicles, where the class II invariant chain peptide (CLIP) that occupies the cleft of newly synthesized class II molecules is removed. These class II molecules are then able to bind peptides derived from the endocytosed protein. The DM molecule facilitates the removal of CLIP and subsequent binding of the antigenic peptide. The peptide–class II MHC complexes are transported to the cell surface and are recognized by CD4+ T cells. *ER,* Endoplasmic reticulum; *l*$_i$, invariant chain.

to the cell surface. Once the class II MHC molecule binds tightly to one of the peptides generated from the ingested proteins, this peptide-MHC complex becomes stable and is delivered to the cell surface. If the MHC molecule does not find a peptide it can bind, the empty molecule is unstable and is eventually degraded by lysosomal proteases. One protein antigen may give rise to many peptides, only a few of which (perhaps only one or two) can bind to the MHC molecules present in the individual and have the potential to stimulate immune responses in that individual.

Processing of Cytosolic Antigens for Display by Class I MHC Molecules

The main steps in antigen presentation by class I MHC molecules include the tagging of antigens in the cytosol or nucleus, proteolysis by a specialized enzymatic complex and transport into the ER, and binding of peptides to newly synthesized class I molecules (Fig. 3-15):

- *Proteolysis of cytosolic proteins.* **The peptides that bind to class I MHC molecules are derived from cytosolic proteins following digestion by the ubiquitin-proteasome pathway.** Antigenic proteins may be produced

Production of proteins in the cytosol	Proteolytic degradation of proteins	Transport of peptides from cytosol to ER	Assembly of peptide-class I complexes in ER	Surface expression of peptide-class I complexes

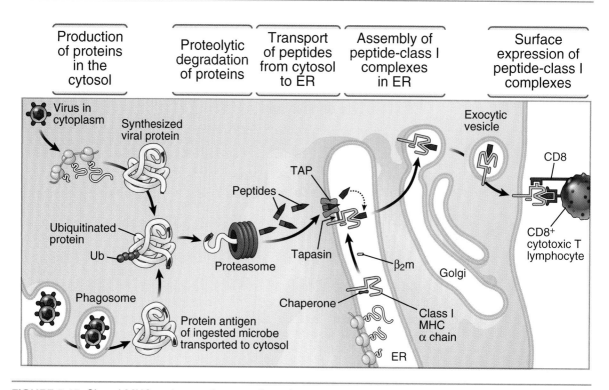

FIGURE 3-15 **Class I MHC pathway of processing of cytosolic antigens.** Proteins enter the cytoplasm of cells either from endogenous synthesis by microbes, such as viruses, that reside in the cytosol (or nucleus, not shown) of infected cells or from microbes that are ingested but whose antigens are transported into the cytosol (the process of cross-presentation, described later). Cytoplasmic proteins are unfolded, ubiquitinated, and degraded in proteasomes. The peptides that are produced are transported by the transporter associated with antigen processing (TAP) into the endoplasmic reticulum (ER), where the peptides may be further trimmed. Newly synthesized class I MHC molecules are initially stabilized by chaperones and attached to TAP by a linker protein called tapasin, so the MHC molecules are strategically located to receive peptides that are transported into the ER by TAP. The peptide–class I MHC complexes are transported to the cell surface and are recognized by CD8+ T cells. $\beta_2 m$, β_2-microglobulin; *Ub*, ubiquitin.

in the cytoplasm from viruses that are living inside infected cells, from some phagocytosed microbes that may leak from or be transported out of phagosomes into the cytosol, and from mutated or altered host genes that encode cytosolic or nuclear proteins, as in tumors. All of these proteins, as well as the cell's own misfolded cytosolic and nuclear proteins, are targeted for destruction by proteolysis by the ubiquitin-proteasome pathway. These proteins are unfolded, covalently tagged with multiple copies of a peptide called ubiquitin, and threaded through a protein complex called the **proteasome** that is composed of stacked rings of proteolytic enzymes. The unfolded proteins are degraded by the proteasomes into peptides. In cells that have been exposed to inflammatory cytokines (as in an infection), the enzymatic composition of the proteasomes changes. As a result, these cells become very efficient at cleaving cytosolic and nuclear proteins into peptides with the size and sequence properties that enable the peptides to bind well to class I MHC molecules.

- *Binding of peptides to class I MHC molecules.* **In order to form peptide-MHC complexes, the peptides must be transported into the endoplasmic reticulum.** The peptides produced by proteasomal digestion are in the cytosol, while the MHC molecules are being synthesized in the ER, and the two need to come together. This transport function is provided by a molecule, called the **transporter associated with antigen processing** (TAP), located in the ER membrane. TAP binds proteasome-generated peptides on the cytosolic side of the ER membrane, then actively pumps them into the interior of the ER. Newly synthesized class I MHC molecules, which do not contain bound peptides, associate with a bridging protein called tapasin that links them to TAP molecules in the ER membrane. Thus, as peptides enter the ER, they can easily be captured by the empty class I molecules. (Recall that in the ER, the class II MHC molecules are not able to bind peptides because of the associated invariant chain.)

- *Transport of peptide-MHC complexes to the cell surface.* If a class I molecule finds a peptide with the right fit, the complex is stabilized, released from association with TAP, and transported to the cell surface.

The evolutionary struggle between microbes and their hosts is well illustrated by the numerous strategies that viruses have developed to block the class I MHC pathway of antigen presentation. These strategies include removing newly synthesized MHC molecules from the ER, inhibiting the transcription of MHC genes, and blocking peptide transport by TAP. By inhibiting the class I MHC pathway, viruses reduce presentation of their own antigens to CD8+ T cells and are thus able to evade the adaptive immune system. These mechanisms of immune evasion are discussed in Chapter 6.

Cross-Presentation of Internalized Antigens to CD8+ T Cells

Some dendritic cells can present ingested antigens on class I MHC molecules to CD8+ T lymphocytes. This pathway of antigen presentation violates the presumption that internalized proteins are displayed only by class II MHC molecules to CD4+ T cells. The initial response of naive CD8+ T cells, similar to CD4+

cells, requires that the antigens be presented by mature dendritic cells. However, some viruses may infect only particular cell types and not dendritic cells, and these infected cells may not travel to lymph nodes or produce all the signals needed to initiate T cell activation. How, then, are naive CD8+ T lymphocytes in lymph nodes able to respond to the intracellular antigens of infected cells? Similarly, tumors arise from many different types of cells, and how can diverse tumor antigens be presented by dendritic cells?

A subset of classical dendritic cells have the ability to ingest infected host cells, dead tumor cells, microbes, and microbial and tumor antigens and transport the ingested antigens into the cytosol, where they are processed by the proteasome. The antigenic peptides that are generated then enter the ER and bind to class I molecules, which display the antigens for recognition by CD8+ T lymphocytes (Fig. 3-16). This process is called **cross-presentation** (or cross-priming), to indicate that one type of cell, dendritic cells, can present the antigens of other, infected or dying, cells or cell fragments, and prime (or activate) naive T lymphocytes specific for these antigens. Once the CD8+ T cells have differentiated into CTLs, they kill infected host cells or tumor cells without the need for dendritic cells or signals other than recognition of antigen (see Chapter 6). The same pathway of cross-presentation is involved in initiating CD8+ T cell responses to some antigens in organ transplants (see Chapter 10).

Physiologic Significance of MHC-Associated Antigen Presentation

Many fundamental features of T cell–mediated immunity are closely linked to the peptide display function of MHC molecules:

- The restriction of T cell recognition to MHC-associated peptides ensures that T cells see and respond only to cell-associated antigens. This is because MHC molecules are cell membrane proteins and because peptide loading and subsequent expression of MHC molecules depend on intracellular biosynthetic

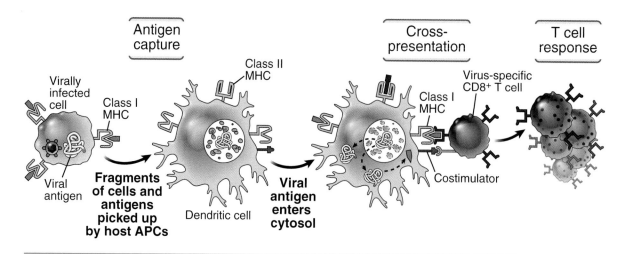

FIGURE 3-16 **Class I MHC-restricted cross-presentation of microbial antigens from infected cells by dendritic cells.** Fragments of cells infected with intracellular microbes (e.g., viruses) or antigens produced in these cells are ingested by dendritic cells, and the antigens of the infectious microbes are broken down and presented in association with class I MHC molecules of the antigen-presenting cells (APCs). T cells recognize the microbial antigens expressed on the APCs, and the T cells are activated. By convention, the term *cross-presentation* (or *cross-priming*) is applied to CD8+ T cells (cytotoxic T lymphocytes) recognizing class I MHC–associated antigens (as shown); the same cross-presenting APC may display class II MHC–associated antigens from the microbe for recognition by CD4+ helper T cells.

and assembly steps. In other words, MHC molecules can be loaded with peptides only inside cells, where intracellular and ingested antigens are present. Therefore, T lymphocytes can recognize the antigens of intracellular microbes, which require T cell–mediated effector mechanisms, as well as antigens ingested from the extracellular environment, such as those against which antibody responses are generated.

- By segregating the class I and class II pathways of antigen processing, the immune system is able to respond to extracellular and intracellular microbes in different ways that are specialized to defend against these microbes (Fig. 3-17). Many bacteria, fungi, and even extracellular viruses are typically captured and ingested by macrophages and their antigens are presented by class II molecules. Because of the specificity of CD4 for class II, class II–associated peptides are recognized by CD4+ T lymphocytes, which function as helper cells. These T cells help the macrophages to destroy ingested microbes, thereby activating an effector mechanism that can eliminate microbes that are internalized from the extracellular environment. B lymphocytes ingest protein antigens of microbes and also present processed peptides for recognition by CD4+ helper T cells. These helper cells stimulate the production of antibodies, which serve to eliminate extracellular microbes. Neither phagocytes nor antibodies are effective against intracellular viruses and other pathogens that can survive and replicate in the cytoplasm of host cells. Cytosolic antigens are processed and displayed by class I MHC molecules, which are expressed on all nucleated cells—again, as expected, because all nucleated cells can be infected with some viruses. Class I–associated peptides are recognized by CD8+ T lymphocytes, which differentiate into CTLs. The CTLs kill the infected cells and eradicate the infection, this being the most effective mechanism for eliminating cytoplasmic microbes.

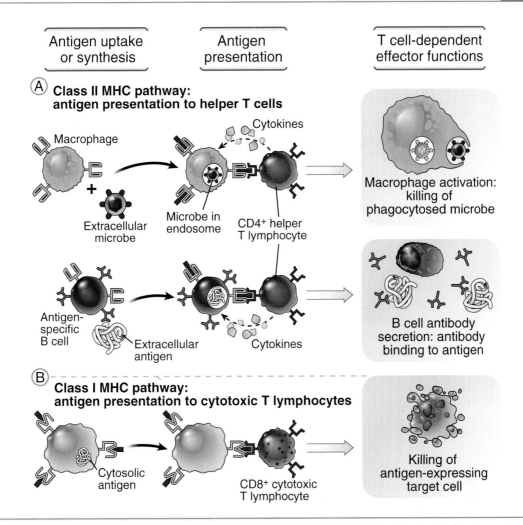

FIGURE 3-17 Role of MHC-associated antigen presentation in recognition of microbial antigens by CD4$^+$ and CD8$^+$ T cells. **A,** Protein antigens of microbes that are endocytosed from the extracellular environment by macrophages and B lymphocytes enter the class II MHC pathway of antigen processing. As a result, these proteins are recognized by CD4$^+$ helper T lymphocytes, whose functions are to activate macrophages to destroy phagocytosed microbes and activate B cells to produce antibodies against extracellular microbes and toxins. **B,** Protein antigens of microbes that live in the cytoplasm of infected cells enter the class I MHC pathway of antigen processing. As a result, these proteins are recognized by CD8$^+$ cytotoxic T lymphocytes, whose function is to kill infected cells.

Thus, the nature of the protective immune response to different microbes is optimized by linking several features of antigen presentation and T cell recognition: the pathways of processing of vesicular and cytosolic antigens, the cellular expression of class II and class I MHC molecules, the specificity of CD4 and CD8 co-receptors for class II and class I molecules, and the functions of CD4$^+$ cells as helper cells and of CD8$^+$ cells as CTLs. This function of MHC-associated antigen-processing pathways is important because the antigen receptors of T cells cannot distinguish between extracellular and intracellular microbes. In fact, as previously mentioned, the same virus can be extracellular early after infection and becomes intracellular once the infection is established. During its extracellular life, the virus is fought by antibodies and phagocytes activated by helper T cells, but once the virus has found a haven in the cytoplasm of cells, it can be eradicated only by CTL-mediated killing of the infected cells. The segregation of class I and class II antigen presentation pathways ensures the correct, specialized immune response against microbes in different locations.

The structural constraints on peptide binding to different MHC molecules, including length and anchor residues, account for the immunodominance of some peptides derived from complex protein antigens and for the inability of some individuals to respond to certain protein antigens. When any protein is proteolytically degraded in APCs, many peptides may be generated, but only those peptides able to bind to the MHC molecules in that individual can be presented for recognition by T cells. These MHC-binding peptides are the **immunodominant** peptides of the antigen. Even microbes with complex protein antigens express a limited number of immunodominant peptides. Many attempts have been made to identify these peptides in order to develop vaccines, but it is difficult to select a small number of peptides from any microbe that would be immunogenic in a large number of people, because of the enormous polymorphism of MHC molecules in the population. The polymorphism of the MHC also means that some individuals may not express MHC molecules capable of binding any peptide derived from a particular antigen. These individuals would be nonresponders to that antigen. One of the earliest observations that established the physiologic importance of the MHC was the discovery that some inbred animals did not respond to simple protein antigens and responsiveness (or lack of) mapped to genes called immune response (Ir) genes, later shown to be MHC genes.

Finally, it should be mentioned that T cells also recognize and react against small molecules and even metal ions in an MHC-restricted manner. In fact, exposure to some small molecules that are used as therapeutic drugs and to metals such as nickel and beryllium often leads to pathologic T cell reactions (so-called hypersensitivity reactions; see Chapter 11). There are several ways in which these nonpeptide antigens may be recognized by MHC-restricted CD4+ and CD8+ T cells. Some of the chemicals are thought to covalently modify self peptides or the MHC molecules themselves, creating altered molecules that are recognized as foreign. Other chemicals bind noncovalently to MHC molecules and alter the structure of the peptide-binding cleft such that the MHC molecule can display peptides that are not normally presented and these peptide-MHC complexes are seen as being foreign.

This chapter began with two questions: how do rare antigen-specific lymphocytes find antigens, and how are the appropriate immune responses generated against extracellular and intracellular microbes? Understanding the biology of APCs and the role of MHC molecules in displaying the peptides of protein antigens has provided satisfying answers to both questions, specifically for T cell–mediated immune responses.

FUNCTIONS OF ANTIGEN-PRESENTING CELLS IN ADDITION TO ANTIGEN DISPLAY

Antigen-presenting cells not only display peptides for recognition by T cells but, in response to microbes, also express additional signals for T cell activation. The two-signal hypothesis of lymphocyte activation was introduced in Chapters 1 and 2 (see Fig. 2-19), and we will return to this concept when we discuss the responses of T and B cells in Chapters 5 and 7. Recall that antigen is the necessary signal 1, and for T cells, signal 2 is provided by APCs reacting to microbes. The expression of molecules in APCs that serve as second signals for lymphocyte activation is part of the innate immune response to different microbial products. For example, many bacteria produce a substance called lipopolysaccharide (LPS, endotoxin). When the bacteria are captured by APCs for presentation of their protein antigens, LPS acts on the same APCs, through a TLR, and stimulates the expression of costimulators and the secretion of cytokines. The costimulators and cytokines act in concert with antigen recognition by the T cell to stimulate the proliferation of the T cells and their differentiation into effector and memory cells.

ANTIGEN RECOGNITION BY B CELLS AND OTHER LYMPHOCYTES

B lymphocytes use membrane-bound antibodies to recognize a wide variety of antigens, including proteins, polysaccharides, lipids, and small chemicals. These antigens may be expressed on microbial surfaces (e.g., capsular or envelope antigens) or may be in soluble form (e.g., secreted toxins). B cells differentiate in response to antigen and other signals into cells that secrete antibodies (see Chapter 7). The secreted antibodies enter the circulation and mucosal fluids and bind to the antigens, leading to their neutralization and elimination. The antigen receptors of B cells and the antibodies that are secreted usually recognize antigens in the native conformation, with no requirement for antigen processing or display by a specialized system. Macrophages in lymphatic sinuses and dendritic cells adjacent to follicles may capture antigens that enter lymph nodes and present the antigens, in intact (unprocessed) form, to B lymphocytes in the follicles.

The B cell–rich lymphoid follicles of the lymph nodes and spleen contain a population of cells called **follicular dendritic cells** (FDCs), whose function is to display antigens to activated B cells. FDCs are not bone-marrow derived, nor related to the dendritic cells that process and present antigens to T cells. The antigens that FDCs display are coated with antibodies or by complement by-products such as C3b and C3d. FDCs use receptors called Fc receptors, specific for one end of antibody molecules, to bind the antigen-antibody complexes, and receptors for complement proteins to bind antigens with these proteins attached. These antigens are seen by specific B lymphocytes during humoral immune responses, and they function to select B cells that bind the antigens with high affinity. This process is discussed in Chapter 7.

Although this chapter has focused on peptide recognition by MHC-restricted CD4$^+$ and CD8$^+$ T cells, there are other, smaller populations of T cells that recognize different types of antigens. Natural killer T cells (called NK-T cells), which are distinct from the natural killer (NK) cells described in Chapter 2, are specific for lipids displayed by class I–like CD1 molecules, and γδ T cells recognize a wide variety of molecules, some displayed by class I–like molecules and others apparently requiring no specific processing or display. The functions of these cells and the significance of their unusual specificities are poorly understood.

◼ SUMMARY

- ◼ The induction of immune responses to the protein antigens of microbes depends on a specialized system for capturing and displaying these antigens for recognition by the rare naive T cells specific for any antigen. Microbes and microbial antigens that enter the body through epithelia are captured by dendritic cells located in the epithelia and transported to regional lymph nodes or captured by dendritic cells in lymph nodes and spleen. The protein antigens of the microbes are displayed by the antigen-presenting cells (APCs) to naive T lymphocytes that recirculate through the lymphoid organs.
- ◼ Molecules encoded in the major histocompatibility complex (MHC) perform the function of displaying peptides derived from protein antigens.
- ◼ MHC genes are highly polymorphic. Their major products are class I and class II MHC molecules, which contain peptide-binding clefts, where the polymorphic residues are concentrated, and invariant regions, which bind the co-receptors CD8 and CD4, respectively.
- ◼ Proteins that are ingested by APCs from the extracellular environment are proteolytically degraded within the vesicles of the APCs, and the peptides generated bind to the clefts of newly synthesized class II MHC molecules. CD4 binds to an invariant part of class II MHC, because of which CD4$^+$ helper T cells

can only be activated by class II MHC–associated peptides derived mainly from proteins degraded in vesicles, which are typically ingested extracellular proteins.

■ Proteins that are produced in the cytosol of infected cells, or that enter the cytosol from phagosomes, are degraded by proteasomes, transported into the endoplasmic reticulum by TAP, and bind to the clefts of newly synthesized class I MHC molecules. CD8 binds class I MHC molecules, so CD8+ cytotoxic T lymphocytes can be activated only by class I MHC–associated peptides derived from proteosomal degradation of cytosolic proteins.

■ The role of MHC molecules in antigen display ensures that T cells only recognize cell-associated protein antigens and that the correct type of T cell (helper or cytotoxic) responds to the type of microbe the T cell is best able to combat.

■ Microbes activate APCs to express membrane proteins (costimulators) and to secrete cytokines that provide signals that function in concert with antigens to stimulate specific T cells. The requirement for these second signals ensures that T cells respond to microbial antigens and not to harmless, nonmicrobial substances.

■ B lymphocytes recognize proteins as well as nonprotein antigens, even in their native conformations. Follicular dendritic cells display antigens to germinal center B cells and select high-affinity B cells during humoral immune responses.

■ REVIEW QUESTIONS

1. When antigens enter through the skin, in what organs are they concentrated? What cell type(s) plays an important role in this process of antigen capture?

2. What are MHC molecules? What are human MHC molecules called? How were MHC molecules discovered, and what is their function?

3. What are the differences between the antigens that are displayed by class I and class II MHC molecules?

4. Describe the sequence of events by which class I and class II MHC molecules acquire antigens for display.

5. Which subsets of T cells recognize antigens presented by class I and class II MHC molecules? What molecules on T cells contribute to their specificity for either class I or class II MHC–associated peptide antigens?

Answers to and discussion of the Review Questions are available at https://studentconsult.inkling.com.

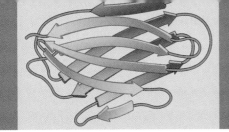

CHAPTER 4

Antigen Recognition in the Adaptive Immune System

Structure of Lymphocyte Antigen Receptors and Development of Immune Repertoires

Antigen receptors serve critical roles in the maturation of lymphocytes from progenitors and in all adaptive immune responses. In adaptive immunity, naive lymphocytes recognize antigens to initiate responses, and effector T cells and antibodies recognize antigens to perform their functions.

B and T lymphocytes express different receptors that recognize antigens: membrane-bound antibodies on B cells and T cell receptors (TCRs) on T lymphocytes. The principal function of cellular receptors in the immune system, as in other biologic systems, is to detect external stimuli (antigens, for the antigen receptors of the adaptive immune system) and trigger responses of the cells on which the receptors are expressed. To recognize a large variety of different antigens, the antigen receptors of lymphocytes must be able to bind to and distinguish between many, often closely related, chemical structures. Antigen receptors are clonally distributed, meaning that each lymphocyte clone is specific for a distinct antigen and has a

unique receptor, different from the receptors of all other clones. (Recall that a *clone* consists of a parent cell and its progeny.) The total number of distinct lymphocyte clones is very large, and this entire collection makes up the immune **repertoire**. Although each clone of B lymphocytes or T lymphocytes recognizes a different antigen, the antigen receptors transmit biochemical signals that are fundamentally the same in all lymphocytes and are unrelated to specificity. These features of lymphocyte recognition and antigen receptors raise the following questions:

- How do the antigen receptors of lymphocytes recognize extremely diverse antigens and transmit activating signals to the cells?
- What are the differences in the recognition properties of antigen receptors on B cells and T cells?
- How is the vast diversity of receptor structures in the lymphocyte repertoire generated? The diversity of antigen recognition implies the existence of many structurally different antigen receptor proteins, more than can be

79

Feature or function	Antibody (Immunoglobulin)	T cell receptor (TCR)
Forms of antigens recognized	Macromolecules (proteins, polysaccharides, lipids, nucleic acids), small chemicals	Mainly peptides displayed by MHC molecules on APCs
	Conformational and linear epitopes	Linear epitopes
Diversity	Each clone has a unique specificity; potential for >10^9 distinct specificities	Each clone has a unique specificity; potential for >10^{11} distinct specificities
Antigen recognition is mediated by:	Variable (V) regions of heavy and light chains of membrane Ig	Variable (V) regions of α and β chains of the TCR
Signaling functions are mediated by:	Proteins (Igα and Igβ) associated with membrane Ig	Proteins (CD3 and ζ) associated with the TCR
Effector functions are mediated by:	Constant (C) regions of secreted Ig	TCR does not perform effector functions

FIGURE 4-1 Properties of antibodies and T cell antigen receptors (TCRs). Antibodies (also called immunoglobulins) may be expressed as membrane receptors or secreted proteins; TCRs only function as membrane receptors. When immunoglobulin (Ig) or TCR molecules recognize antigens, signals are delivered to the lymphocytes by proteins associated with the antigen receptors. The antigen receptors and attached signaling proteins form the B cell receptor (BCR) and TCR complexes. Note that single antigen receptors are shown recognizing antigens, but signaling typically requires the binding of two or more receptors to adjacent antigen molecules. The important characteristics of these antigen-recognizing molecules are summarized. *APCs*, Antigen-presenting cells; *MHC*, major histocompatibility complex.

encoded in the inherited genome (germline). Therefore, special mechanisms must exist for generating this diversity.

In this chapter, we describe the structures of the antigen receptors of B and T lymphocytes and how these receptors recognize antigens. We also discuss how the diversity of antigen receptors is generated during the process of lymphocyte development, thus giving rise to the repertoire of mature lymphocytes. The process of antigen-induced lymphocyte activation is described in later chapters.

ANTIGEN RECEPTORS OF LYMPHOCYTES

The antigen receptors of B and T lymphocytes have several features that are important for their functions in adaptive immunity (Fig. 4-1). Although these receptors have many similarities in terms of structure and mechanisms of signaling, there are fundamental differences related to the types of antigenic structures that B cells and T cells recognize:

- **Membrane-bound antibodies, which serve as the antigen receptors of B lymphocytes, can recognize many types of chemical structures, while most T cell antigen receptors recognize only peptides bound to major histocompatibility complex (MHC) molecules. B lymphocyte antigen receptors and the antibodies that B cells secrete are able to recognize the shapes, or conformations, of macromolecules, including proteins, lipids, carbohydrates, and nucleic acids, as well as simpler, smaller chemical moieties.** This broad specificity of B cells for structurally different types of molecules enables antibodies to recognize diverse microbes and toxins in their native form. In striking contrast, most T cells see only peptides displayed on antigen-presenting cells (APCs) bound to MHC molecules. This specificity of T cells restricts their recognition to only cell-associated microbes (see Chapter 3).

- **Antigen receptor molecules consist of regions (domains) involved in antigen recognition—and therefore varying between clones of lymphocytes—and other regions required for structural integrity and effector functions—and thus relatively conserved** among all clones. The antigen-recognizing domains of the receptors are called variable (V) regions, and the conserved portions are the **constant (C) regions.** Even within each V region, most of the sequence variability is concentrated within short stretches, which are called hypervariable regions, or complementarity-determining regions (CDRs), because they form the parts of the receptor that bind antigens (i.e., they are complementary to the shapes of antigens). By concentrating sequence variation in small regions of the receptor, it is possible to maximize the variability of the antigen-binding part, while retaining the basic structure of the receptors. As discussed later, special mechanisms exist in developing lymphocytes to create genes that encode different variable regions of antigen receptor proteins in individual clones.

- **Antigen receptor chains are associated with invariant membrane proteins whose function is to deliver intracellular signals**

following antigen recognition (see Fig. 4-1). These signals, which are transmitted to the cytosol and the nucleus, may cause a lymphocyte to divide, to differentiate, or in certain circumstances to die. Thus, the two functions of lymphocyte receptors for antigen—specific antigen recognition and signal transduction—are mediated by different polypeptides. This again allows variability to be segregated in one set of molecules—the receptors themselves—while leaving the conserved function of signal transduction in other, invariant proteins. The set of associated plasma membrane antigen receptor and signaling molecules in B lymphocytes is called the **B cell receptor (BCR) complex**, and in T lymphocytes it is called the **T cell receptor (TCR) complex.** When antigen molecules bind to antigen receptors of lymphocytes, the associated signaling proteins of the receptor complexes are brought into proximity. As a result, enzymes attached to the cytoplasmic portions of the signaling proteins catalyze the phosphorylation of other proteins. Phosphorylation triggers complex signaling cascades that culminate in the transcriptional activation of many genes and the production of numerous proteins that mediate the responses of the lymphocytes. We return to the processes of T and B lymphocyte activation in Chapters 5 and 7, respectively.

- **Antibodies exist in two forms—as membrane-bound antigen receptors on B cells or as secreted proteins—but TCRs exist only as membrane receptors on T cells.** Secreted antibodies are present in the blood and mucosal secretions, where they function to defend against microbes (i.e., they are the effector molecules of humoral immunity). Antibodies are also called **immunoglobulins** (Igs), referring to immunity-conferring proteins with the characteristic slow electrophoretic mobility of globulins. Secreted antibodies recognize microbial antigens and toxins by their variable domains, the same as the membrane-bound antigen receptors of B lymphocytes. The constant regions of some secreted antibodies have the ability to bind to other molecules that participate in the elimination

of antigens: these molecules include receptors on phagocytes and proteins of the complement system. Thus, antibodies serve different functions at different stages of humoral immune responses: membrane-bound antibodies on B cells recognize antigens to initiate the responses, and secreted antibodies neutralize and eliminate microbes and their toxins in the effector phase of humoral immunity. In cell-mediated immunity, the effector function of microbe elimination is performed by T lymphocytes themselves and by other leukocytes responding to the T cells. The antigen receptors of T cells are involved only in antigen recognition and T cell activation, and these proteins are not secreted and do not mediate effector functions.

With this introduction, we describe next the antigen receptors of lymphocytes, first antibodies and then T cell receptors.

Antibodies

An antibody molecule is composed of four polypeptide chains—two identical heavy (H) chains and two identical light (L) chains—with each chain containing a variable region and a constant region (Fig. 4-2). The four chains are assembled to form a Y-shaped molecule. Each light chain is attached to one heavy chain, and the two heavy chains are attached to each other, all by disulfide bonds. A light chain is made up of one V and one C domain, and a heavy chain has one V and three or four C domains. Each domain folds into a characteristic three-dimensional shape, called the immunoglobulin (Ig) domain (Fig. 4-2, D). An Ig domain consists of two layers of β-pleated sheet held together by a disulfide bridge. The adjacent strands of each β-sheet are connected by short, protruding loops; in the V regions of Ig molecules, these loops make up the three CDRs responsible for antigen recognition. Ig domains are present in many other proteins in the immune system, as well as outside the immune system, and most of these proteins are involved in responding to stimuli from the environment and from other cells. All of these proteins are said to be members of the immunoglobulin

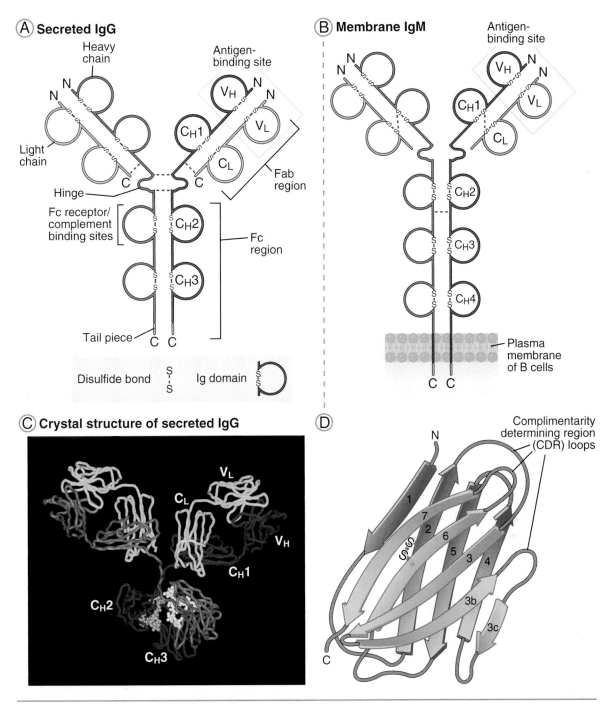

FIGURE 4-2 Structure of antibodies. Schematic diagrams of **A,** a secreted immunoglobulin G (IgG) molecule, and **B,** a molecule of a membrane-bound form of IgM, illustrating the domains of the heavy and light chains and the regions of the proteins that participate in antigen recognition and effector functions. N and C refer to the amino-terminal and carboxy-terminal ends of the polypeptide chains, respectively. **C,** The crystal structure of a secreted IgG molecule illustrates the domains and their spatial orientation; the heavy chains are colored blue and red, the light chains are green, and carbohydrates are gray. **D,** The ribbon diagram of the Ig V domain shows the basic β-pleated sheet structure and the projecting loops that form the three CDRs. *CDR*, Complementarity determining region. (**C,** Courtesy of Dr. Alex McPherson, University of California, Irvine.)

superfamily, and they may have evolved from a common ancestral gene.

The antigen-binding site of an antibody is composed of the V regions of both the heavy chain and the light chain, and the core antibody structure contains two identical antigen binding sites (see Fig. 4-2). Each variable region of the heavy chain (called V_H) or of the light chain (called V_L) contains three hypervariable regions, or CDRs. Of these three, the greatest variability is in CDR3, which is located at the junction of the V and C regions. As may be predicted from this variability, CDR3 is also the portion of the Ig molecule that contributes most to antigen binding.

Functionally distinct portions of antibody molecules were first identified based on fragments generated by proteolysis. The fragment of an antibody that contains a whole light chain (with its single V and C domains) attached to the V and first C domains of a heavy chain contains the portion of the antibody required for antigen recognition and is therefore called **Fab** (fragment, antigen-binding). The remaining heavy-chain C domains make up the **Fc** (fragment, crystalline) region; this fragment tends to crystallize in solution. In each Ig molecule, there are two identical Fab regions that bind antigen and one Fc region that is responsible for most of the biologic activity and effector functions of the antibodies. (As discussed later, some types of antibodies exist as multimers of two or five Ig molecules attached to one another.) Between the Fab and Fc regions of most antibody molecules is a flexible portion called the hinge region. The hinge allows the two antigen-binding Fab regions of each antibody molecule to move independent of each other, enabling them to simultaneously bind antigen epitopes that are separated from one another by varying distances.

The C-terminal end of the heavy chain may be anchored in the plasma membrane, as seen in B cell receptors, or it may terminate in a tail piece that lacks the membrane anchor so that the antibody is produced as a secreted protein. Light chains in the B cell receptor are not attached to cell membranes.

There are five types of heavy chains, called μ, δ, γ, ε, and α, which differ in their C regions; in humans, there are four subtypes of γ chain and two of the α chain. Antibodies that contain different heavy chains belong to different **classes,** or **isotypes,** and are named according to their heavy chains (IgM, IgD, IgG, IgE, and IgA). Each isotype has distinct physical and biologic properties and effector functions (Fig. 4-3). The antigen receptors of naive B lymphocytes, which are mature B cells that have not encountered antigen, are membrane-bound IgM and IgD. After stimulation by antigen and helper T lymphocytes, the antigen-specific B lymphocyte clone may expand and differentiate into progeny that secrete antibodies. Some of the progeny of IgM and IgD expressing B cells may secrete IgM, and other progeny of the same B cells may produce antibodies of other heavy-chain classes. This change in Ig isotype production is called **heavy-chain class** (or **isotype**) **switching;** its mechanism and importance are discussed in Chapter 7. Although heavy-chain C regions may switch during humoral immune responses, each clone of B cells maintains its specificity, because the V regions do not change.

The two types of light chains, called κ and λ, differ in their C regions. Each B cell expresses either κ or λ but not both. Each type of light chain may complex with any type of heavy chain in an antibody molecule, but unlike the heavy chains, the two types of light chains have no functional differences. The light-chain class (κ or λ) also remains fixed throughout the life of each B cell clone, regardless of whether or not heavy-chain class switching has occurred.

Binding of Antigens by Antibodies

Antibodies are capable of binding a wide variety of antigens, including macromolecules and small chemicals. The reason for this is that the antigen-binding CDR loops of antibody molecules can either come together to form clefts capable of accommodating small molecules or form more extended surfaces capable of accommodating many larger molecules, including portions of proteins (Fig. 4-4). Antibodies bind to antigens by reversible, noncovalent interactions, including hydrogen bonds, hydrophobic interactions, and charge-based interactions. The parts

Isotype of antibody	Subtypes (H chain)	Serum concentration (mg/ml)	Serum half-life (days)	Secreted form	Functions
IgA	IgA1,2 (α1 or α2)	3.5	6	Mainly dimer, also monomer, trimer Cα1 Cα2 Cα3 J chain	Mucosal immunity
IgD	None (δ)	Trace	3	Monomer	Naive B cell antigen receptor
IgE	None (ϵ)	0.05	2	Monomer Cϵ1 Cϵ2 Cϵ3 Cϵ4	Defense against helminthic parasites, immediate hypersensitivity
IgG	IgG1-4 (γ1, γ2, γ3 or γ4)	13.5	23	Monomer Cγ1 Cγ2 Cγ3	Opsonization, complement activation, antibody-dependent cell-mediated cytotoxicity, neonatal immunity, feedback inhibition of B cells
IgM	None (μ)	1.5	5	Pentamer Cμ1 Cμ3 Cμ4 Cμ2 J chain 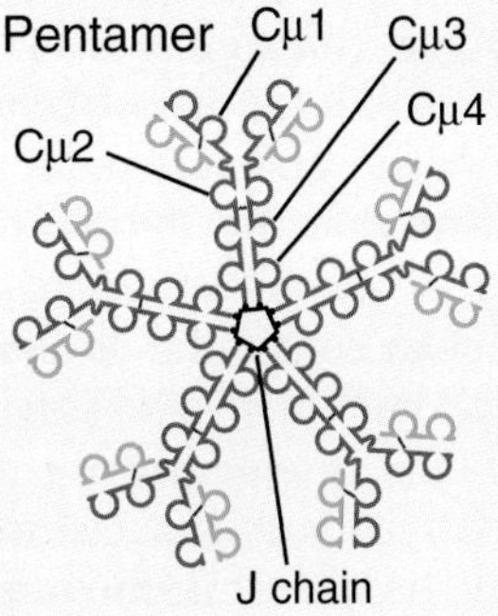	Naive B cell antigen receptor (monomeric form), complement activation

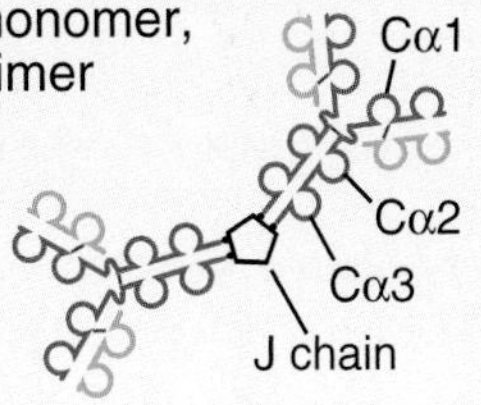

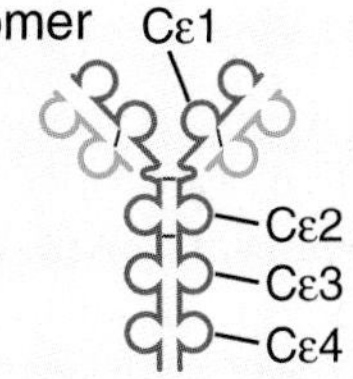

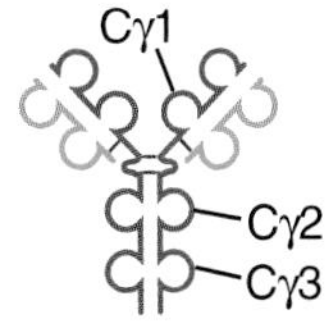

FIGURE 4-3 Features of the major isotypes (classes) of antibodies. This table summarizes some important features of the major antibody isotypes of humans. Isotypes are classified on the basis of their heavy (H) chains; each isotype may contain either κ or λ light chain. The schematic diagrams illustrate the distinct shapes of the secreted forms of these antibodies. Note that IgA consists of two subclasses, called IgA1 and IgA2, and IgG consists of four subclasses, called IgG1, IgG2, IgG3, and IgG4. (IgG subclasses are given different names in other species, for historical reasons; in mice, they are called IgG1, IgG2a, IgG2b, IgG2c, and IgG3.) The domains of the heavy chains in each isotype are labeled. The plasma concentrations are average values in normal individuals.

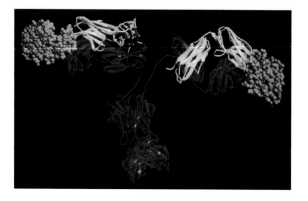

FIGURE 4-4 Binding of an antigen by an antibody. This model of a protein antigen bound to an antibody molecule shows how the antigen-binding site can accommodate soluble macromolecules in their native (folded) conformation. The heavy chains of the antibody are red, the light chains are yellow, and the antigens are blue. (Courtesy of Dr. Dan Vaughn, Cold Spring Harbor Laboratory, Cold Spring Harbor, NY.)

of antigens that are recognized by antibodies are called **epitopes,** or **determinants.** Different epitopes of protein antigens may be recognized based on the sequence of a stretch of amino acids (linear epitopes) or on the shape (conformational epitopes). Some of these epitopes are hidden within antigen molecules and are exposed as a result of a physicochemical change.

The strength with which one antigen-binding surface of an antibody binds to one epitope of an antigen is called the **affinity** of the interaction. Affinity often is expressed as the dissociation constant (K_d), which is the molar concentration of an antigen required to occupy half the available antibody molecules in a solution; the lower the K_d, the higher the affinity. Most antibodies produced in a primary immune response have a K_d in the range of 10^{-6} to 10^{-9} M, but with repeated stimulation (e.g., in a secondary immune response), the affinity increases to a K_d of 10^{-8} to 10^{-11} M. This increase in antigen-binding strength is called **affinity maturation** (see Chapter 7). Each IgG, IgD, and IgE antibody molecule has 2 antigen-binding sites. Secreted IgA is a dimer and therefore has 4 antigen-binding sites, and secreted IgM is a pentamer, with 10 antigen-binding sites. Therefore, each antibody molecule can bind 2 to 10 epitopes of an antigen,

or epitopes on 2 or more neighboring antigens. The total strength of binding is much greater than the affinity of a single antigen-antibody bond and is called the **avidity** of the interaction. Antibodies produced against one antigen may bind other, structurally similar antigens. Such binding to similar epitopes is called a **cross-reaction.**

In B lymphocytes, membrane-bound Ig molecules are noncovalently associated with two other proteins, called Igα and Igβ, and the three proteins make up the BCR complex. When the B cell receptor recognizes antigen, Igα and Igβ transmit signals to the interior of the B cell that initiate the process of B cell activation. These and other signals in humoral immune responses are discussed in Chapter 7.

Monoclonal Antibodies

The realization that one clone of B cells makes an antibody of only one specificity has been exploited to produce **monoclonal antibodies,** one of the most important technical advances in immunology, with far-reaching implications for clinical medicine and research. To produce monoclonal antibodies, B cells, which have a short life span in vitro, are obtained from an animal immunized with an antigen and fused with myeloma cells (tumors of plasma cells), which can be propagated indefinitely in tissue culture (Fig. 4-5). The myeloma cell line lacks a specific enzyme, as a result of which these cells cannot grow in the presence of a certain toxic drug; fused cells, containing both myeloma and normal B cell nuclei, however, do grow in the presence of this drug because the normal B cells provide the missing enzyme. Thus, by fusing the two cell populations and culturing them with the drug, it is possible to grow out fused cells derived from the B cells and the myeloma, which are called **hybridomas.** These hybridoma cells grow continuously, having acquired the immortal property of the myeloma tumor. From a population of hybridomas, one can select and expand individual cells that secrete the antibody of desired specificity; such antibodies, derived from a single B cell clone, are homogeneous monoclonal antibodies, meaning monoclonal antibodies against virtually any antigen can be produced.

Most monoclonal antibodies are made by fusing cells from immunized mice with mouse myelomas.

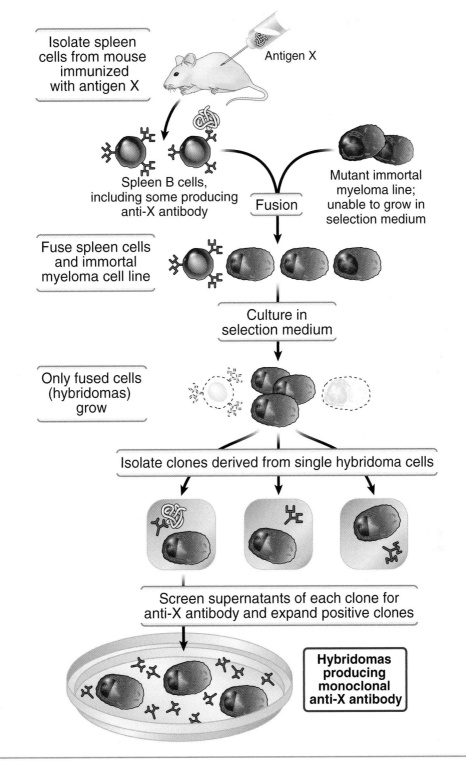

Isolate spleen cells from mouse immunized with antigen X

Antigen X

Spleen B cells, including some producing anti-X antibody

Fusion

Mutant immortal myeloma line; unable to grow in selection medium

Fuse spleen cells and immortal myeloma cell line

Culture in selection medium

Only fused cells (hybridomas) grow

Isolate clones derived from single hybridoma cells

Screen supernatants of each clone for anti-X antibody and expand positive clones

Hybridomas producing monoclonal anti-X antibody

FIGURE 4-5 Generation of hybridomas and monoclonal antibodies. In this procedure, spleen cells from a mouse that has been immunized with a known antigen are fused with an enzyme-deficient myeloma cell line that does not secrete its own immunoglobulins. The fused cells are then placed in a selection medium that permits the survival of only immortalized hybrids; the normal B cells provide the enzyme that the myeloma lacks, and unfused B cells cannot survive indefinitely. These hybrid cells are then grown as single-cell clones and tested for the secretion of antibody of the desired specificity. The clone producing this antibody is expanded and becomes a source of the monoclonal antibody.

Such mouse monoclonal antibodies cannot be injected repeatedly into human subjects, because the human immune system sees the mouse Ig as foreign and mounts an immune response against the injected antibodies. This problem has been overcome by genetic engineering approaches that retain the antigen-binding V regions of the mouse monoclonal antibody and replace the rest of the Ig with human Ig; such humanized antibodies are suitable for administration to people (although with prolonged use, even some humanized monoclonal antibodies may elicit anti-Ig antibody responses in treated individuals). More recently, monoclonal antibodies have been generated by using recombinant DNA technology to clone the DNA-encoding human antibodies of desired specificity. Another approach is to replace the Ig genes of mice with human antibody genes and then immunize these mice with an antigen to produce specific human antibodies. Monoclonal antibodies are now in widespread use as therapeutic agents for many diseases in humans (Fig. 4-6).

Inflammatory (immunological) diseases		
Target	Effect	Diseases
CD20	Depletion of B cells	B cell lymphomas, rheumatoid arthritis, multiple sclerosis, other autoimmune diseases
IgE	Blocking IgE function	Allergy-related asthma
IL-6 receptor	Blocking inflammation	Rheumatoid arthritis
TNF	Blocking inflammation	Rheumatoid arthritis, Crohn's disease, psoriasis
Cancer		
Target	Effect	Diseases
CD52	Depletion of lymphocytes	Chronic lymphocytic leukemia
CTLA-4	Activation of T cells	Melanoma
EGFR	Growth inhibition of epithelial tumors	Colorectal, lung, and head and neck cancers
HER2/Neu	Inhibition of EGF signaling; depletion of tumor cells	Breast cancer
PD-1	Activation of effector T cells	Melanoma, renal cell carcinoma, other tumors
PD-L1	Activation of effector T cells	Melanoma, renal cell carcinoma, other tumors
VEGF	Blocking tumor angiogenesis	Breast cancer, colon cancer, age-related macular degeneration
Other diseases		
Target	Effect	Diseases
Glycoprotein IIb/IIIa	Inhibition of platelet aggregation	Cardiovascular disease

FIGURE 4-6 Selected monoclonal antibodies in clinical use. The table lists some of the monoclonal antibodies that are approved for the treatment of various types of diseases or are in clinical trials for these diseases.

T Cell Receptors for Antigens

The TCR, which recognizes peptide antigens displayed by MHC molecules, is a membrane-bound heterodimeric protein composed of an α chain and a β chain, each chain containing one variable (V) region and one constant (C) region (Fig. 4-7). The V and C regions are homologous to immunoglobulin V and C regions. In the V region of each TCR chain, there are three hypervariable, or complementarity-determining, regions, each corresponding to a loop in the V domain. As in antibodies, CDR3 is the most variable among different TCRs.

Antigen Recognition by the TCR

Both the α chain and the β chain of the TCR participate in specific recognition of MHC molecules and bound peptides (Fig. 4-8). One of the remarkable features of T cell antigen recognition that has emerged from x-ray crystallographic analyses of TCRs bound to MHC-peptide complexes is that each TCR recognizes as few as one to three residues of the MHC-associated peptide.

The TCR recognizes antigen, but as with membrane Ig on B cells, it is incapable of transmitting signals to the T cell on its own. Associated with the TCR is a complex of proteins, called the CD3 and ζ proteins, which together with the TCR make up the TCR complex (see Fig. 4-1). The CD3 and ζ chains transmit some of the signals that are initiated when the TCR recognizes antigen. In addition, T cell activation requires engagement of the coreceptor molecule

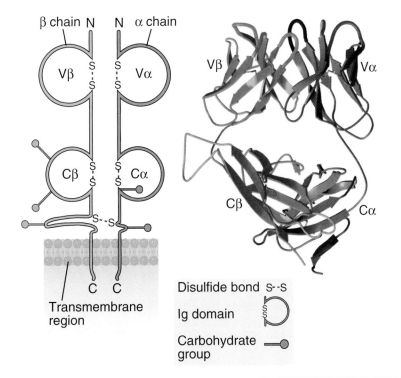

FIGURE 4-7 **Structure of the T cell antigen receptor (TCR).** The schematic diagram of the αβ TCR (left) shows the domains of a typical TCR specific for a peptide-MHC complex. The antigen-binding portion of the TCR is formed by the Vα and Vβ domains. *N* and *C* refer to the amino-terminal and carboxy-terminal ends of the polypeptides. The ribbon diagram (right) shows the structure of the extracellular portion of a TCR as revealed by x-ray crystallography. (From Bjorkman PJ: MHC restriction in three dimensions: a view of T cell receptor/ligand interactions. *Cell* 89:167-170, 1997. © Cell Press; with permission.)

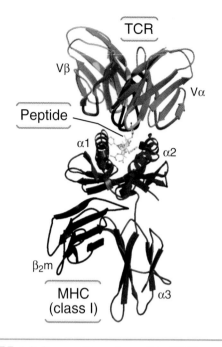

FIGURE 4-8 Recognition of peptide-MHC complex by T cell antigen receptor. This ribbon diagram is drawn from the crystal structure of the extracellular portion of a peptide-MHC complex bound to a TCR that is specific for the peptide displayed by the MHC molecule. The peptide can be seen attached to the cleft at the top of the MHC molecule, and one residue of the peptide contacts the V region of a TCR. The structure of MHC molecules and their function as peptide display proteins are described in Chapter 3. $\beta_2 m$, β_2-Microglobulin; *MHC*, major histocompatibility complex; *TCR*, T cell receptor. (From Bjorkman PJ: MHC restriction in three dimensions: a view of T cell receptor/ligand interactions. *Cell* 89:167-170, 1997. © Cell Press; with permission.)

CD4 or CD8, which recognize nonpolymorphic portions of MHC molecules and also transmit activating signals. The functions of these TCR-associated proteins and coreceptors are discussed in Chapter 5.

Antigen recognition by B and T lymphocyte receptors differs in important ways (Fig. 4-9). Antibodies can bind many different types of chemical structures, often with high affinities, which is why antibodies can bind to and neutralize many different microbes and toxins that

may be present at low concentrations in the circulation. TCRs only recognize peptide-MHC complexes and bind these with relatively low affinity, which may be why the binding of T cells to APCs has to be strengthened by additional cell surface adhesion molecules (see Chapter 5). The three-dimensional structure of the TCR is similar to that of the Fab region of an Ig molecule. Unlike in antibodies, both TCR chains are anchored in the plasma membrane; TCRs are not produced in a secreted form and do not undergo class switching or affinity maturation during the life of a T cell.

From 5% to 10% of T cells in the body express receptors composed of gamma (γ) and delta (δ) chains, which are structurally similar to the αβ TCR but have very different specificities. The γδ TCR may recognize a variety of protein and nonprotein antigens, usually not displayed by classical MHC molecules. T cells expressing γδ TCRs are abundant in epithelia. This observation suggests that γδ T cells recognize microbes usually encountered at epithelial surfaces, but neither the specificity nor the function of these T cells is well established. Another subpopulation of T cells, comprising less than 5% of all T cells, express markers of natural killer cells and are called natural killer T cells (NK-T cells). NK-T cells express αβ TCRs with limited diversity, and they recognize lipid antigens displayed by nonpolymorphic class I MHC–like molecules. The functions of NK-T cells also are not well understood.

DEVELOPMENT OF IMMUNE REPERTOIRES

Now that we have discussed the structure of antigen receptors of B and T lymphocytes and how these receptors recognize antigens, the next question is how the enormous diversity of these receptors is produced. As the clonal selection hypothesis predicted, there are many clones of lymphocytes with distinct specificities, perhaps as many as 10^9, and these clones arise before encounter with antigen. There are not enough genes in the human genome for every possible receptor to be encoded by a different gene.

Feature	Antigen-binding molecule	
	Immunoglobulin (Ig)	T cell receptor (TCR)
	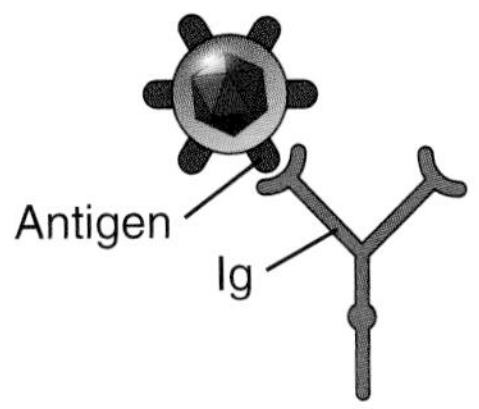 Antigen — Ig	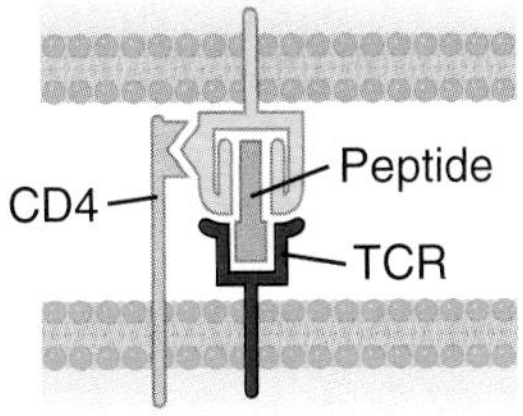 CD4 — Peptide, TCR
Antigen binding	Made up of three CDRs in V_H and three CDRs in V_L	Made up of three CDRs in $V\alpha$ and three CDRs in $V\beta$
Changes in constant regions	Heavy-chain class switching and change from membrane to secretory Ig	None
Affinity of antigen binding	K_d 10^{-7}-10^{-11} M; average affinity of Igs increases during immune responses to protein antigens	K_d 10^{-5}-10^{-7} M; No change during immune responses
On-rate and off-rate	Rapid on-rate, variable off-rate	Slow on-rate, slow off-rate

FIGURE 4-9 Features of antigen recognition by immunoglobulins and T cell antigen receptors. The important similarities and differences of Ig and TCR molecules, the antigen receptors of B and T lymphocytes, respectively.

In fact, the immune system has developed mechanisms for generating extremely diverse antigen receptors from a limited number of inherited genes, and the generation of diverse receptors is intimately linked to the process of B and T lymphocyte maturation.

The goal of lymphocyte maturation is to generate the largest possible number of cells with different antigen receptors (with one receptor on each cell) and then preserve the cells with useful receptors. The generation of very large numbers of receptors (as many as several billion) is a molecular process that cannot be influenced by what the receptors recognize, because recognition must follow receptor generation and expression. Once these

antigen receptors are expressed on developing lymphocytes, selection processes come into play that promote the survival of cells with useful receptors and eliminate cells that cannot recognize antigens in the individual or that have the potential to cause harm. We discuss each of these events next.

Lymphocyte Development

The development of lymphocytes from bone marrow stem cells involves commitment of hematopoietic progenitors to the B or T cell lineage, the proliferation of these progenitors, the rearrangement and expression of antigen receptor genes, and selection events to preserve and expand cells that

express potentially useful antigen receptors (Fig. 4-10). These steps are common to B and T lymphocytes, even though B lymphocytes mature in the bone marrow and T lymphocytes mature in the thymus. Each of the processes that occur during lymphocyte maturation plays a special role in the generation of the lymphocyte repertoire:

• **Commitment to the B cell or T cell lineage is associated with changes in common lymphoid progenitors in the bone marrow.** These changes include the activation of several lineage-specific transcription factors and increased accessibility of Ig and TCR genes to the gene recombination machinery, described later.

• **Immature lymphocytes undergo proliferation at several stages during their maturation.** Proliferation of developing lymphocytes is necessary to ensure that an adequate number of cells will be available to express useful antigen receptors and mature into functionally competent lymphocytes. Survival and proliferation of the earliest lymphocyte precursors are stimulated mainly by the growth factor interleukin-7 (IL-7), which is produced by stromal cells in the bone marrow and the thymus. IL-7 maintains and expands

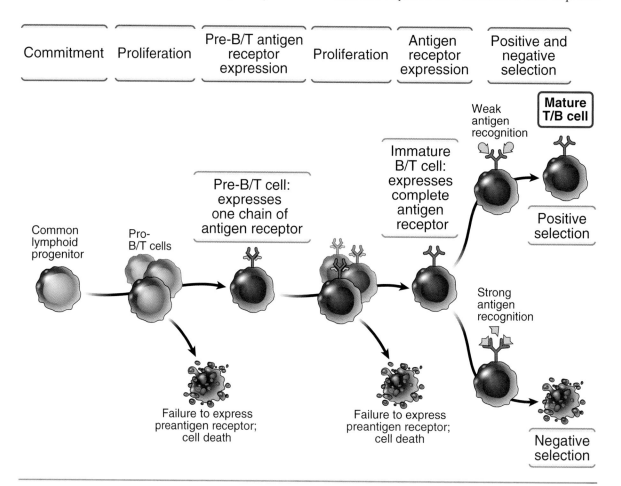

Commitment   Proliferation   Pre-B/T antigen receptor expression   Proliferation   Antigen receptor expression   Positive and negative selection

Common lymphoid progenitor

Pro-B/T cells

Pre-B/T cell: expresses one chain of antigen receptor

Immature B/T cell: expresses complete antigen receptor

Weak antigen recognition

Mature T/B cell

Positive selection

Strong antigen recognition

Negative selection

Failure to express preantigen receptor; cell death

Failure to express preantigen receptor; cell death

FIGURE 4-10 Steps in maturation of lymphocytes. During their maturation, B and T lymphocytes go through cycles of proliferation and expression of antigen receptor proteins by gene recombination. Cells that fail to express intact, functional receptors die by apoptosis, because they do not receive the necessary survival signals. At the end of the process, the cells undergo positive and negative selection. The lymphocytes shown may be B or T cells.

the number of lymphocyte progenitors (mainly T cell progenitors in humans, and both B and T cell precursors in mice) before they express antigen receptors, thus generating a large pool of cells in which diverse antigen receptors may be produced. Even greater proliferative expansion of the B and T cell lineages occurs after the developing lymphocytes have completed their first antigen receptor gene rearrangement and assembled a preantigen receptor (described later). This step is a quality control checkpoint in lymphocyte development that ensures preservation of cells with functional receptors.

- **Lymphocytes are selected at multiple steps during their maturation to preserve the useful specificities.** Selection is based on the expression of intact antigen receptor components and what they recognize. As discussed later, many attempts to generate antigen receptors fail because of errors during the gene recombination process. Therefore, checkpoints are needed at which only cells with intact, functional antigen receptors are selected to survive and proliferate. Prelymphocytes and immature lymphocytes that fail to express antigen receptors die by apoptosis (see Fig. 4-10). The gene rearrangements in the developing lymphocytes randomly generate antigen receptors with highly diverse specificities. Some of these may be incapable of recognizing antigens in the individual—for instance, if the TCR happens to be specific for an MHC molecule that is not present in the individual. In order to preserve the T cells that will be functional, immature T cells are selected to survive only if they recognize MHC molecules in the thymus. This process, called **positive selection,** ensures that cells that complete maturation will be capable of recognizing antigens displayed by the same MHC molecules on APCs (which are the only MHC molecules these cells can normally encounter). Other antigen receptors may recognize self antigens. Therefore, another selection process is needed to eliminate these potentially dangerous lymphocytes and prevent the development of autoimmune responses. The mechanisms that eliminate strongly self-reactive B and T lymphocytes constitute **negative selection.**

The processes of B and T lymphocyte maturation and selection share some important features but also differ in many respects. We start with the central event that is common to both lineages: the recombination and expression of antigen receptor genes.

Production of Diverse Antigen Receptors

The formation of functional genes that encode B and T lymphocyte antigen receptors is initiated by somatic recombination of gene segments that code for the variable regions of the receptors, and diversity is generated during this process.

Inherited Antigen Receptor Genes

Hematopoietic stem cells in the bone marrow and early lymphoid progenitors contain Ig and TCR genes in their inherited, or germline, configuration. In this configuration, Ig heavy-chain and light-chain loci and the TCR α-chain and β-chain loci each contain multiple variable region (V) gene segments, numbering about 100, and one or a few constant region (C) genes (Fig. 4-11). Between the V and C genes are groups of several short coding sequences called diversity (D) and joining (J) gene segments. (All antigen receptor gene loci contain V, J, and C genes, but only the Ig heavy-chain and TCR β-chain loci also contain D gene segments.)

Somatic Recombination and Expression of Antigen Receptor Genes

The commitment of a lymphocyte progenitor to become a B lymphocyte is associated with the recombination of randomly selected gene segments in the Ig heavy-chain locus—first one D gene segment with one J segment, followed by the rearrangement of a V segment to the fused D-J element (Fig. 4-12). Thus, the committed but still-developing B cell now has a recombined V-D-J exon in the heavy-chain locus. This gene is transcribed, and in the primary transcript, the VDJ exon is spliced to the C-region exons of the μ chain, the most 5′ C region, to form a complete μ messenger RNA (mRNA). The μ mRNA is translated

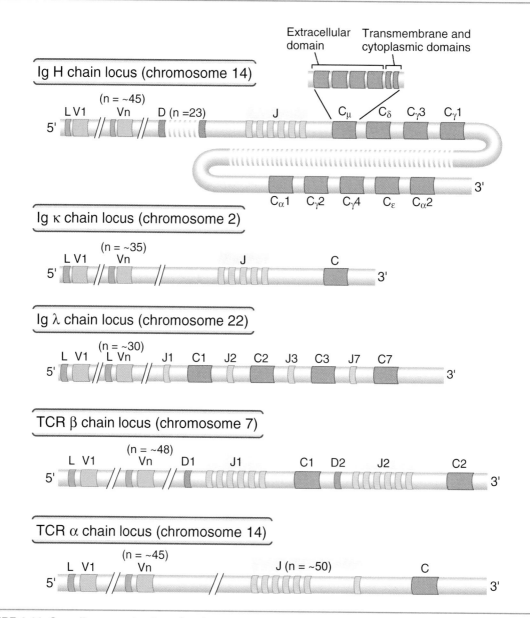

FIGURE 4-11 Germline organization of antigen receptor gene loci. In the germline, inherited antigen receptor gene loci contain coding segments (exons, shown as colored blocks of various sizes) that are separated by segments that are not expressed (introns, shown as gray sections). Each immunoglobulin heavy-chain constant (C) region and T cell receptor (TCR) C region consists of multiple exons that encode the domains of the C regions; the organization of the C_μ exons in the Ig heavy-chain locus is shown as an example. The diagrams illustrate the antigen receptor gene loci in humans; the basic organization is the same in all species, although the precise order and number of gene segments may vary. The sizes of the segments and the distances between them are not drawn to scale. D, Diversity; J, joining; L, leader sequence (a small stretch of nucleotides that encodes a peptide that guides proteins through the endoplasmic reticulum and is cleaved from the mature proteins); V, variable.

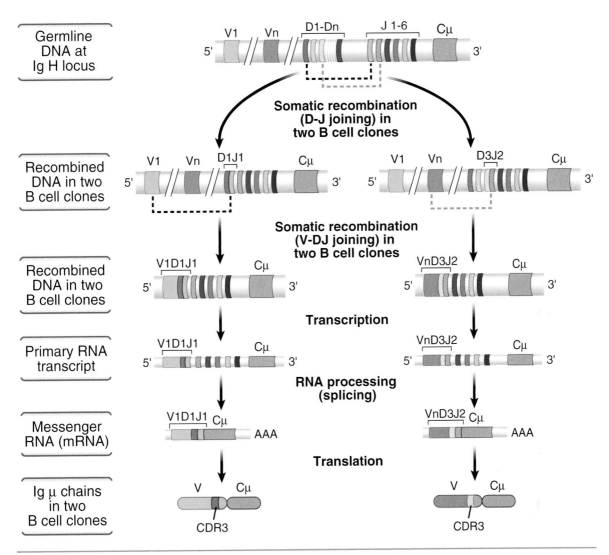

FIGURE 4-12 Recombination and expression of immunoglobulin (Ig) genes. The expression of an Ig heavy chain involves two gene recombination events (D-J joining, followed by joining of a V region to the DJ complex, with deletion and loss of intervening gene segments). The recombined gene is transcribed, and the VDJ segment is spliced onto the first heavy-chain RNA (which is μ), to give rise to the μ mRNA. The mRNA is translated to produce the μ heavy-chain protein. The recombination of other antigen receptor genes—that is, the Ig light chain and the T cell receptor (TCR) α and β chains—follows essentially the same sequence, except that in loci lacking D segments (Ig light chains and TCR α), a V gene recombines directly with a J gene segment.

to produce the μ heavy chain, which is the first Ig protein synthesized during B cell maturation. Essentially the same sequence of DNA recombination and RNA splicing leads to production of a light chain in B cells, except that the light-chain loci lack D segments, so a V region exon recombines directly with a J segment. The rearrangement of TCR α-chain and β-chain genes in T lymphocytes is similar to that of Ig L and H chains, respectively.

Mechanisms of V(D)J Recombination

The somatic recombination of V and J, or of V, D, and J, gene segments is mediated by a lymphoid-specific enzyme, the VDJ

recombinase, and additional enzymes, most of which are not lymphocyte specific and are involved in repair of double-stranded DNA breaks introduced by the recombinase. The VDJ recombinase is composed of the recombinase-activating gene 1 and 2 (RAG-1 and RAG-2) proteins. It recognizes DNA sequences that flank all antigen receptor V, D, and J gene segments. As a result of this recognition, the recombinase brings two Ig or TCR gene segments close together and cleaves the DNA at specific sites. The DNA breaks are then repaired by ligases, producing a full-length recombined V-J or V-D-J exon without the intervening DNA segments (see Fig. 4-12). The VDJ recombinase is expressed only in immature B and T lymphocytes. Although the same enzyme can mediate recombination of all Ig and TCR genes, intact Ig heavy-chain and light-chain genes are rearranged and expressed only in B cells, and TCR α and β genes are rearranged and expressed only in T cells. The lineage specificity of receptor gene rearrangement appears to be linked to the expression of lineage-specific transcription factors. In B cells, B lineage-specific transcription factors "open" the Ig gene locus at the chromatin level but not the TCR locus, whereas in developing T cells, transcriptional regulators help open up the TCR locus but not the Ig locus. The "open" loci are the ones that are accessible to the recombinase.

Generation of Ig and TCR Diversity

Diversity of antigen receptors is produced by the use of different combinations of V, D, and J gene segments in different clones of lymphocytes (called combinatorial diversity) and even more by changes in nucleotide sequences introduced at the junctions of the recombining V, D, and J gene segments (called junctional diversity) (Fig. 4-13). Combinatorial diversity is limited by the number of available V, D, and J gene segments, but junctional diversity is almost unlimited. Junctional diversity is produced by three mechanisms, which generate more sequences than are present in the germline genes:

- Exonucleases may remove nucleotides from V, D, and J gene segments at the sites of recombination.

- A lymphocyte-specific enzyme called terminal deoxyribonucleotidyl transferase (TdT) catalyzes the random addition of nucleotides that are not part of germline genes to the junctions between V and D segments and D and J segments, forming so-called N regions.

- During an intermediate stage in the process of V(D)J recombination, before breaks in the DNA are repaired, overhanging DNA sequences may be generated that are then filled in, forming P-nucleotides, introducing even more variability at the sites of recombination.

As a result of these mechanisms, the nucleotide sequence at the site of V(D)J recombination in antibody or TCR genes in one clone of lymphocytes differs from the sequence at the V(D)J site of antibody or TCR molecules made by every other clone. These junctional sequences and the D and J segments encode the amino acids of the CDR3 loop, mentioned earlier as the most variable of the CDRs and the most important for antigen recognition. Thus, junctional diversity maximizes the variability in the antigen-recognizing portions of antibodies and TCRs. In the process of creating junctional diversity, many genes may be produced with sequences that cannot code for proteins and are therefore useless. This is a price the immune system pays for generating tremendous diversity. The risk of producing nonfunctional genes also is why the process of lymphocyte maturation contains checkpoints at which only cells with useful receptors are selected to survive.

Maturation and Selection of B Lymphocytes

The maturation of B lymphocytes occurs mainly in the bone marrow (Fig. 4-14). Progenitors committed to the B cell lineage proliferate, giving rise to a large number of precursors of B cells, called **pro-B cells.** Subsequent maturation involves antigen receptor gene expression and selection.

Early Steps in B Cell Maturation. The Ig heavy-chain locus rearranges first, and only cells that are able to make an Ig μ heavy-chain protein are selected to survive and become pre-B cells. These cells begin to rearrange Ig genes, initially in the heavy-chain locus. Cells that make productive VDJ rearrangements at the Ig heavy-chain

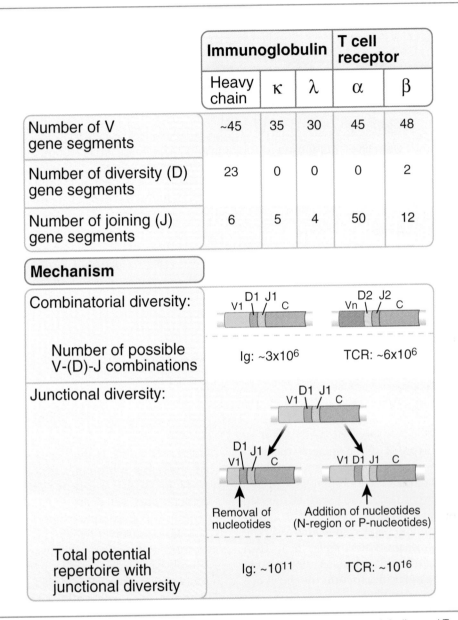

	Immunoglobulin			T cell receptor	
	Heavy chain	κ	λ	α	β
Number of V gene segments	~45	35	30	45	48
Number of diversity (D) gene segments	23	0	0	0	2
Number of joining (J) gene segments	6	5	4	50	12

Mechanism

Combinatorial diversity:

Number of possible V-(D)-J combinations   Ig: ~3×10^6 TCR: ~6×10^6

Junctional diversity:

Removal of nucleotides

Addition of nucleotides (N-region or P-nucleotides)

Total potential repertoire with junctional diversity   Ig: ~10^{11} TCR: ~10^{16}

FIGURE 4-13 Mechanisms of diversity in antigen receptors. Diversity in immunoglobulins and T cell receptors is produced by random combinations of V, D, and J gene segments, which is limited by the numbers of these segments and by removal and addition of nucleotides at the V-J or V-D-J junctions, which is almost unlimited. The numbers of gene segments refer to the average numbers of functional genes (which are known to be expressed as RNA or protein) in humans. Junctional diversity maximizes the variations in the CDR3 regions of the antigen receptor proteins, because CDR3 is the site of V-J and V-D-J recombination. The estimated contributions of these mechanisms to the potential size of the mature B and T cell repertoires are shown. Also, diversity is increased by the ability of different Ig heavy and light chains, or different TCR α and β chains, to associate in different cells, forming different receptors (not shown). Although the upper limit on the number of immunoglobulin (Ig) and T cell receptor (TCR) proteins that may be expressed is extremely large, each individual contains on the order of only 10^7 clones of B cells and T cells with distinct specificities and receptors; in other words, only a fraction of the potential repertoire may actually be expressed. (Modified from Davis MM, Bjorkman PJ: T-cell antigen receptor genes and T-cell recognition. *Nature* 334:395-402, 1988.)

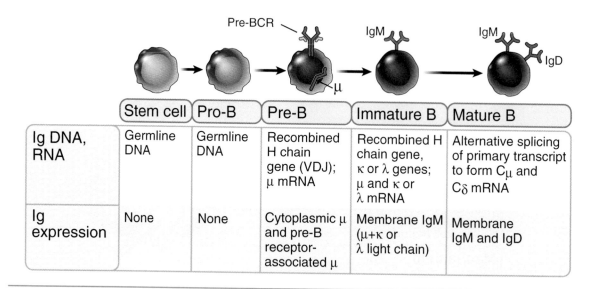

FIGURE 4-14 Steps in the maturation and selection of B lymphocytes. The maturation of B lymphocytes proceeds through sequential steps, each of which is characterized by particular changes in immunoglobulin (Ig) gene expression and in the patterns of Ig protein expression. At the pro-B cell and pre-B cell stages, failure to express functional antigen receptors (Ig heavy chain and Ig light chain, respectively) results in death of the cells by a default pathway of apoptosis. The pre-BCR consists of a membrane-associated Ig μ protein attached to two other proteins called surrogate light chains because they take the place of the light chain in a complete Ig molecule. *BCR*, B cell receptor.

locus develop into pre-B cells, defined by the presence of the Ig μ heavy-chain protein, mainly in the cytoplasm. Some of the μ protein is expressed on the cell surface in association with two other, invariant proteins, called surrogate light chains because they resemble light chains and associate with the μ heavy chain. The complex of μ chain and surrogate light chains associates with the Igα and Igβ signaling molecules to form the pre-B cell receptor (pre-BCR) complex.

Role of the Pre-BCR Complex in B Cell Maturation. The assembled pre-BCR serves essential functions in the maturation of B cells:

• Signals from the pre-BCR complex promote the survival and proliferation of B lineage cells that have made a productive rearrangement at the Ig H-chain locus. This is the first checkpoint in B cell development, and it selects and expands the pre-B cells that express a functional μ heavy chain (an essential component of the pre-BCR and BCR). Pre-B cells that make out-of-frame (nonproductive)

rearrangements at the heavy-chain locus fail to make the μ protein, cannot express a pre-BCR or receive pre-BCR signals, and die by programmed cell death (apoptosis).

• The pre-BCR complex signals to shut off recombination of Ig heavy-chain genes on the second chromosome, because of which each B cell can express an Ig heavy chain from only one of the two inherited parental alleles. This process is called **allelic exclusion,** and it helps ensure that each cell can only express a receptor of a single specificity.

• The pre-BCR triggers recombination at the Ig κ light-chain locus; the λ light chain is produced only if the rearranged κ chain locus fails to express a functional protein or if the κ chain generates a potentially harmful self-reactive receptor and has to be eliminated, by the process called receptor editing (see Chapter 9).

Whichever functional light chain is produced associates with the μ chain to form the complete membrane-associated IgM antigen receptor.

This receptor again delivers signals that promote survival, thus preserving cells that express complete antigen receptors, the second checkpoint during maturation. Signals from the antigen receptor also shut off production of the recombinase enzyme and further recombination at light chain loci. As a result, each B cell produces either one κ or one λ light chain from one of the inherited parental alleles. The presence of two sets of inherited light-chain genes simply increases the chance of completing successful gene recombination and receptor expression.

Completion of B Cell Maturation. The IgM-expressing B lymphocyte is the **immature B cell.** Its further maturation may occur in the bone marrow or after it leaves the bone marrow and enters the spleen. The final maturation step involves coexpression of IgD with IgM, which occurs because in any given B cell, the recombined heavy-chain VDJ may be spliced onto Cμ or Cδ in the primary RNA transcript, giving rise to a μ or δ mRNA, respectively. We know that the ability of B cells to respond to antigens develops together with the coexpression of IgM and IgD, but why both classes of receptor are needed is not known. The IgM⁺IgD⁺ cell is the **mature B cell,** able to respond to antigen in peripheral lymphoid tissues.

Selection of Mature B Cells. Developing B cells are positively selected mainly based on expression of complete antigen receptors, and not on the recognition specificity of these cells. (This is fundamentally different in maturing T cells, as discussed later.) The B cell repertoire is further shaped by negative selection. In this process, if an immature B cell binds an antigen in the bone marrow with high affinity, it may reactivate the VDJ recombinase enzyme, undergo additional light-chain V-J recombination, generate a different light chain, and thus change the specificity of the antigen receptor, a process called **receptor editing.** Some B cells that encounter antigens in the bone marrow may die by apoptosis, the process known as deletion. The antigens most often found in the bone marrow are self antigens that are abundantly expressed throughout the body (i.e., are ubiquitous), such as blood proteins, and membrane molecules common to all cells.

Negative selection therefore eliminates potentially dangerous cells that can recognize and react against ubiquitous self antigens.

The process of Ig gene recombination is random and cannot be inherently biased toward recognition of microbes. However, the receptors produced are able to recognize the antigens of many, varied microbes that the immune system must defend against. The repertoire of B lymphocytes is selected positively for expression of intact receptors and selected negatively against strong recognition of self antigens. What is left after these selection processes is a large collection of mature B cells, which by chance include cells that are able to recognize almost any microbial antigen that may be encountered.

Subsets of Mature B Cells. Most mature B cells are called follicular B cells because they are found within lymph node and spleen follicles. Marginal-zone B cells, which are found at the margins of splenic follicles, develop from the same progenitors (pro-B cells) as do follicular B cells. B-1 lymphocytes, a distinct population found in lymphoid organs and the peritoneal cavity, may develop earlier and from different precursors. The role of these B cell subsets in humoral immunity is described in Chapter 7.

Maturation and Selection of T Lymphocytes

T cell progenitors migrate from the bone marrow to the thymus, where the entire process of maturation occurs (Fig. 4-15). The process of T lymphocyte maturation has some unique features, primarily related to the specificity of different subsets of T cells for peptides displayed by different classes of MHC molecules.

Early Steps in T Cell Maturation. The most immature progenitors in the thymus are called **pro-T cells** or **double-negative T cells** (or double-negative thymocytes) because they do not express CD4 or CD8. These cells expand in number mainly under the influence of IL-7 produced in the thymus. TCR β gene recombination, mediated by the VDJ recombinase, occurs in some of these double-negative cells. (The γδ T cells undergo similar recombination involving TCR γ and δ loci, but they belong to a distinct lineage and are not discussed further.) If VDJ

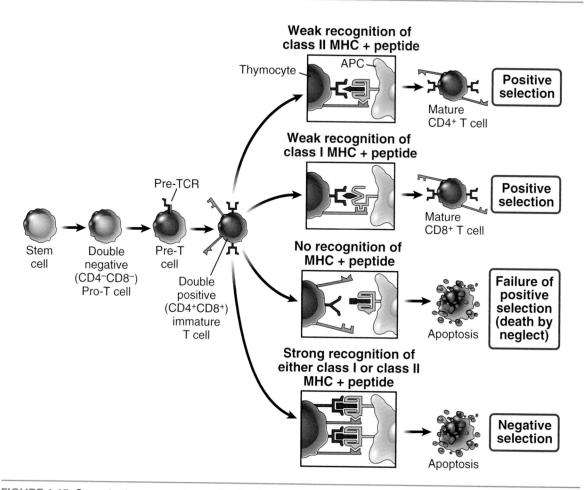

FIGURE 4-15 Steps in the maturation and selection of major histocompatibility complex (MHC)–restricted T lymphocytes. The maturation of T lymphocytes in the thymus proceeds through sequential steps often defined by the expression of the CD4 and CD8 co-receptors. The TCR β chain is first expressed at the double-negative pre-T cell stage, and the complete T cell receptor is expressed in double-positive cells. The pre-TCR consists of the TCR β chain associated with a protein called pre-Tα. Maturation culminates in the development of CD4+ and CD8+ single-positive T cells. As with B cells, failure to express antigen receptors at any stage leads to death of the cells by apoptosis.

recombination is successful in one of the two inherited loci and a TCR β-chain protein is synthesized, it is expressed on the cell surface in association with an invariant protein called pre-Tα, to form the pre-TCR complex of **pre-T cells.** If the recombination in one of the two inherited loci is not successful, recombination will take place on the other locus. If that too fails and a complete TCR β chain is not produced in a pro-T cell, the cell dies.

The pre-TCR complex delivers intracellular signals once it is assembled, similar to the signals from the pre-BCR complex in developing B cells. These signals promote survival, proliferation, and TCR α gene recombination and inhibit VDJ recombination at the second TCR β-chain locus (allelic exclusion). Failure to express the α chain and the complete TCR again results in death of the cell. The surviving cells express the complete αβ TCR and both the CD4 and CD8 coreceptors;

these cells are called **double-positive T cells** (or double-positive thymocytes).

Selection of Mature T Cells. Different clones of double-positive T cells express different αβ TCRs. If the TCR of a T cell recognizes an MHC molecule in the thymus, which must be a self MHC molecule displaying a self peptide, and if the interaction is of low or moderate affinity, this T cell is selected to survive. T cells that do not recognize an MHC molecule in the thymus die by apoptosis; these T cells would not be useful because they would be incapable of seeing MHC-displayed cell-associated antigens in that individual. This preservation of self MHC–restricted (i.e., useful) T cells is the process of **positive selection.** During this process, T cells whose TCRs recognize class I MHC–peptide complexes preserve the expression of CD8, the coreceptor that binds to class I MHC, and lose expression of CD4, the coreceptor specific for class II MHC molecules. Conversely, if a T cell recognizes class II MHC–peptide complexes, this cell maintains expression of CD4 and loses expression of CD8. Thus, what emerges are **single-positive T cells** (or single-positive thymocytes), which are either CD8+ class I MHC restricted or CD4+ class II MHC restricted. During positive selection, the T cells also become functionally segregated: the CD8+ T cells are capable of becoming CTLs on activation, and the CD4+ cells are helper cells.

Immature, double-positive T cells whose receptors strongly recognize MHC-peptide complexes in the thymus undergo apoptosis. This is the process of **negative selection,** and it serves to eliminate T lymphocytes that could react in a harmful way against self proteins that are expressed in the thymus. Some of these self proteins are present throughout the body, and others are tissue proteins that are expressed in thymic epithelial cells by special mechanisms, as discussed in Chapter 9 in the context of self-tolerance. It may seem surprising that both positive selection and negative selection are mediated by recognition of the same set of self MHC–self peptide complexes in the thymus. (Note that the thymus can contain only self MHC molecules and self peptides; microbial peptides are concentrated in peripheral lymphoid tissues and tend

not to enter the thymus.) The likely explanation for these distinct outcomes is that if the antigen receptor of a T cell recognizes a self MHC–self peptide complex with low avidity, the result is positive selection, whereas high-avidity recognition leads to negative selection. High-avidity recognition occurs if the T cell expresses a TCR that has a high affinity for that self peptide and if the self peptide is present in the thymus at a higher concentration than positively selecting peptides. If such a T cell were allowed to mature, antigen recognition could lead to harmful immune responses against the self antigen in the periphery, so the T cell must be eliminated.

As with B cells, the ability of T cells to recognize foreign antigens relies on the generation of a very diverse repertoire of clonal antigen receptors. T cells that weakly recognize self antigens in the thymus may strongly recognize and respond to foreign microbial antigens in the periphery.

▮ SUMMARY

- In the adaptive immune system, the molecules responsible for specific recognition of antigens are antibodies and T cell antigen receptors.
- Antibodies (also called immunoglobulins) may be produced as membrane receptors of B lymphocytes and as proteins secreted by antigen-stimulated B cells that have differentiated into antibody-secreting plasma cells. Secreted antibodies are the effector molecules of humoral immunity, capable of neutralizing microbes and microbial toxins and eliminating them by activating various effector mechanisms.
- T cell receptors (TCRs) are membrane receptors and are not secreted.
- The core structure of antibodies consists of two identical heavy chains and two identical light chains, forming a disulfide-linked complex. Each chain consists of a variable (V) region, which is the portion that recognizes antigen, and a constant (C) region, which provides structural stability and, in heavy chains, performs the effector functions of antibodies. The V region of one heavy chain and of one light chain together form the antigen-binding site,

and thus the core structure has two identical antigen-binding sites.

- T cell receptors consist of an α chain and a β chain. Each chain contains one V region and one C region, and both chains participate in the recognition of antigens, which for most T cells are peptides displayed by MHC molecules.
- The V regions of immunoglobulin (Ig) and TCR molecules contain hypervariable segments, also called complementarity-determining regions (CDRs), which are the regions of contact with antigens.
- The genes that encode antigen receptors consist of multiple segments separate in the germline and brought together during maturation of lymphocytes. In B cells, the Ig gene segments undergo recombination as the cells mature in the bone marrow, and in T cells, the TCR gene segments undergo recombination during maturation in the thymus.
- Receptors of different specificities are generated in part by different combinations of V, D, and J gene segments. The process of recombination introduces variability in the nucleotide sequences at the sites of recombination by adding or removing nucleotides from the junctions. The result of this introduced variability is the development of a diverse repertoire of lymphocytes, in which clones of cells with different antigen specificities express receptors that differ in sequence and recognition, and most of the differences are concentrated at the regions of gene recombination.

- During their maturation, lymphocytes are selected to survive at several checkpoints; only cells with complete functional antigen receptors are preserved and expanded. In addition, T lymphocytes are positively selected to recognize peptide antigens displayed by self MHC molecules and to ensure that the recognition of the appropriate type of MHC molecule matches the co-receptor preserved.
- Immature lymphocytes that strongly recognize self antigens are negatively selected and prevented from completing their maturation, thus eliminating cells with the potential of reacting in harmful ways against self tissues.

REVIEW QUESTIONS

1. What are the functionally distinct domains (regions) of antibody and TCR molecules? What features of the amino acid sequences in these regions are important for their functions?
2. What are the differences in the types of antigens recognized by antibodies and TCRs?
3. What mechanisms contribute to the diversity of antibody and TCR molecules? Which of these mechanisms contributes the most to the diversity?
4. What are some of the checkpoints during lymphocyte maturation that ensure survival of the useful cells?
5. What is the phenomenon of negative selection, and what is its importance?

Answers to and discussion of the Review Questions are available at https://studentconsult.inkling.com.

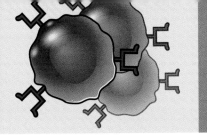

CHAPTER 5

T Cell–Mediated Immunity

Activation of T Lymphocytes by Cell-Associated Antigens

T lymphocytes perform multiple functions in defending against infections by various kinds of microbes. A major role for T lymphocytes is in **cell-mediated immunity,** which provides defense against infections by intracellular microbes. In several types of infections, microbes may find a haven inside cells, from where they must be eliminated by cell-mediated immune responses (Fig. 5-1).

• Many microbes are ingested by phagocytes as part of the early defense mechanisms of innate immunity, but some of these microbes have evolved to resist the microbicidal activities of phagocytes. Many pathogenic intracellular bacteria and protozoa are able to survive, and even replicate, in the vesicles of phagocytes. In such infections, T cells stimulate the ability of macrophages to kill the ingested microbes.

• Some microbes, notably viruses, are able to infect and replicate inside a wide variety of cells, and parts of the life cycles of the viruses take place in the cytosol. These infected cells often do not possess intrinsic mechanisms for destroying the microbes, especially in the cytosol. Even some phagocytosed microbes within macrophages can escape into the cytosol and evade the microbicidal mechanisms of the vesicular compartment. T cells kill the infected cells, thus eliminating the reservoir of infection.

In addition to cell-mediated immunity, T lymphocytes also play important roles in defense against microbes that replicate outside cells, including several types of bacteria, fungi, and helminthic parasites. Some T cells induce inflammatory responses rich in activated leukocytes that are particularly efficient at killing extracellular microbes. We discuss these T cell subsets and their functions in Chapter 6. Other populations of T cells help B cells to produce antibodies as part of humoral immune responses (see Chapter 7).

Most of the functions of T lymphocytes—activation of phagocytes, killing of infected cells, and help for B cells—require that the T

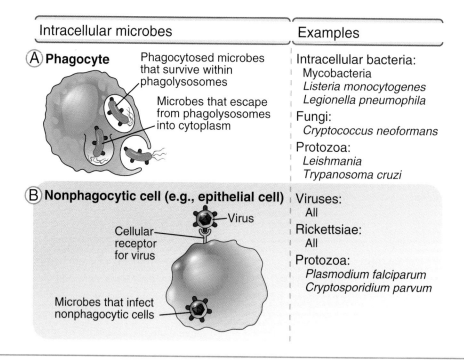

FIGURE 5-1 Types of intracellular microbes combated by T cell–mediated immunity. A, Microbes may be ingested by phagocytes and may survive within vesicles (phagolysosomes) or escape into the cytosol, where they are not susceptible to the microbicidal mechanisms of the phagocytes. **B,** Viruses may infect many cell types, including nonphagocytic cells, and replicate in the nucleus and cytosol of the infected cells. Rickettsiae and some protozoa are obligate intracellular parasites that reside in non-phagocytic cells.

lymphocytes interact with other cells, which may be phagocytes, infected host cells, or B lymphocytes. Furthermore, the initiation of T cell responses requires that the cells recognize antigens displayed by dendritic cells, which capture antigens and concentrate them in lymphoid organs. Thus, T lymphocytes work by communicating with other cells. Recall that the specificity of T cells for peptides displayed by major histocompatibility complex (MHC) molecules ensures that the T cells can see and respond only to antigens associated with other cells (see Chapters 3 and 4). This chapter discusses the way in which T lymphocytes are activated by recognition of cell-associated antigens and other stimuli. We address the following questions:

- What signals are needed to activate T lymphocytes, and what cellular receptors are used to sense and respond to these signals?
- How are the few naive T cells specific for any microbe converted into the large number of

effector T cells that have specialized functions and the ability to eliminate diverse microbes?
- What molecules are produced by T lymphocytes that mediate their communications with other cells, such as macrophages, B lymphocytes, and other leukocytes?

After describing here how T cells recognize and respond to the antigens of cell-associated microbes, in Chapter 6 we discuss how these T cells function to eliminate the microbes.

PHASES OF T CELL RESPONSES

Naive T lymphocytes recognize antigens in the peripheral (secondary) lymphoid organs, which initiates proliferation of the T cells and their differentiation into effector and memory cells, and the effector cells perform their functions when they are activated by the same antigens in peripheral tissues or lymphoid organs (Fig. 5-2). Naive T cells express antigen receptors and co-receptors

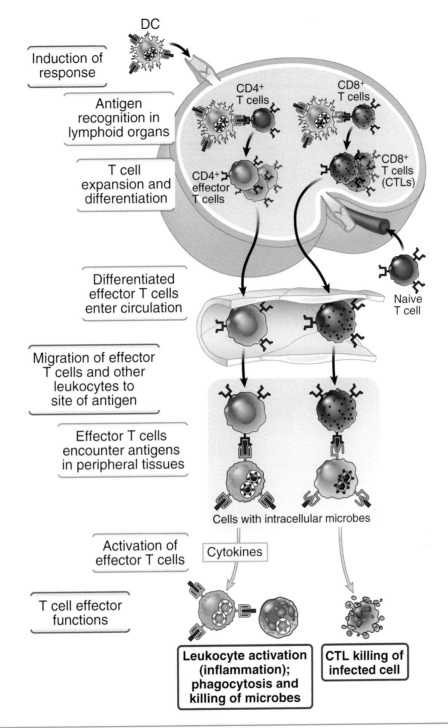

FIGURE 5-2 Induction and effector phases of cell-mediated immunity. Induction of response: Naive CD4+ T cells and CD8+ T cells recognize peptides that are derived from protein antigens and presented by dendritic cells (DCs) in peripheral lymphoid organs. The T lymphocytes are stimulated to proliferate and differentiate into effector cells, many of which enter the circulation. Some of the activated CD4+ T cells remain in the lymph node, migrate into follicles, and help B cells to produce antibodies (shown in Fig. 5-13). Migration of effector T cells and other leukocytes to site of antigen: effector T cells and other leukocytes migrate through blood vessels in peripheral tissues by binding to endothelial cells that have been activated by cytokines produced in response to infection in these tissues. T cell effector functions: CD4+ T cells recruit and activate phagocytes to destroy microbes, and CD8+ cytotoxic T lymphocytes (CTLs) kill infected cells.

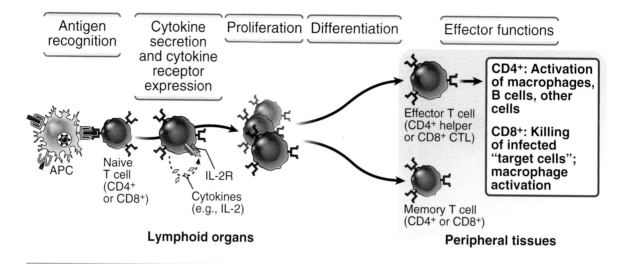

FIGURE 5-3 Steps in the activation of T lymphocytes. Naive T cells recognize major histocompatibility complex (MHC)–associated peptide antigens displayed on antigen-presenting cells and other signals (not shown). The T cells respond by producing cytokines, such as interleukin-2 (IL-2), and expressing receptors for these cytokines, leading to an autocrine pathway of cell proliferation. The result is expansion of the clone of T cells that are specific for the antigen. Some of the progeny differentiate into effector cells, which serve various functions in cell-mediated immunity, and memory cells, which survive for long periods. Other changes associated with activation, such as the expression of various surface molecules, are not shown. *APC,* Antigen-presenting cell; *CTL,* cytotoxic T lymphocyte; *IL-2R,* interleukin-2 receptor.

that function in recognizing cells harboring microbes, but these cells are incapable of performing the effector functions required for eliminating the microbes. Differentiated effector cells are capable of performing these functions, which they do in lymphoid organs and in peripheral, nonlymphoid tissues. In this chapter we focus on the responses of naive T cells to antigens. The development of effector T lymphocytes and their functions in cell-mediated immunity are described in Chapter 6, and the roles of helper T cells in antibody responses in Chapter 7.

The responses of naive T lymphocytes to cell-associated microbial antigens consist of a series of sequential steps that result in an increase in the number of antigen-specific T cells and the conversion of naive T cells to effector and memory cells (Fig. 5-3).

- One of the earliest responses is the secretion of **cytokines** and increased expression of receptors for various cytokines.
- Some cytokines stimulate the **proliferation** of the antigen-activated T cells, resulting in a rapid increase in the number of antigen-specific lymphocytes, a process called **clonal expansion.**
- The activated lymphocytes undergo the process of **differentiation,** which results in the conversion of naive T cells into a population of **effector T cells** which function to eliminate microbes.
- Many of the effector T cells leave the lymphoid organs, enter the circulation, and migrate to any site of infection, where they can eradicate the infection. Some effector T cells may remain in the lymph node, where they function to eradicate infected cells at that site or provide signals to B cells that promote antibody responses against the microbes.
- Some of the progeny of the T cells that have proliferated in response to antigen develop into **memory T cells,** which are long-lived and functionally inactive, circulate for months or years, and are ready to respond rapidly to repeated exposure to the same microbe.
- As effector T cells eliminate the infectious agent, the stimuli that triggered T cell expansion and differentiation also are eliminated. As a result,

most of the cells in the greatly expanded clone of antigen-specific lymphocytes die, returning the system to a resting state, with only memory cells remaining from the immune response.

This sequence of events is common to both CD4$^+$ and CD8$^+$ T lymphocytes, although there are important differences in the properties and effector functions of CD4$^+$ and CD8$^+$ cells, as discussed in Chapter 6.

Naive and effector T cells have different patterns of circulation and migration through tissues, which are critical for their different roles in immune responses. As discussed in previous chapters, naive T lymphocytes constantly recirculate through peripheral lymphoid organs searching for foreign protein antigens. The antigens of microbes are transported from the portals of entry of the microbes to the same regions of peripheral lymphoid organs through which naive T cells recirculate. In these organs, the antigens are processed and displayed by MHC molecules on dendritic cells, the antigen-presenting cells (APCs) that are the most efficient stimulators of naive T cells (see Chapter 3). When a T cell recognizes antigen, it is transiently arrested on the dendritic cell and it initiates an activation program. Following activation and differentiation, the cells may leave the lymphoid organ and migrate preferentially to the inflamed tissue, the original source of the antigen. The control of this directed migration is discussed later in this chapter.

With this overview, we proceed to a description of the stimuli required for T cell activation and regulation. We then describe the biochemical signals that are generated by antigen recognition and the biologic responses of the lymphocytes.

ANTIGEN RECOGNITION AND COSTIMULATION

The initiation of T cell responses requires multiple receptors on the T cells recognizing ligands on APCs (Fig. 5-4).
- The T cell receptor (TCR) recognizes MHC-associated peptide antigens.
- CD4 or CD8 coreceptors on the T cells recognize MHC molecules on the APC and help the TCR complex to deliver activating signals.

- Adhesion molecules strengthen the binding of T cells to APCs.
- Molecules called costimulators, which are expressed on APCs after encounter with microbes, bind to costimulatory receptors on the naive T cells thus promoting responses to infectious pathogens.
- Cytokines amplify the T cell response and direct it along various differentiation pathways.

The roles of these molecules in T cell responses to antigens are described next. Cytokines are discussed mainly in Chapter 6.

Recognition of MHC-Associated Peptides

The T cell receptor for antigen (the TCR) and the CD4 or CD8 coreceptor together recognize complexes of peptide antigens and MHC molecules on APCs, and this recognition provides the initiating, or first, signal for T cell activation (Fig. 5-5). The TCRs expressed on all CD4$^+$ and CD8$^+$ T cells consist of an α chain and a β chain, both of which participate in antigen recognition (see Chapter 4, Fig. 4-7). (A small subset of T cells expresses TCRs composed of γ and δ chains, which do not recognize MHC-associated peptide antigens.) The TCR of a T cell specific for a foreign (e.g., microbial) peptide recognizes the displayed peptide and simultaneously recognizes residues of the MHC molecule located around the peptide-binding cleft. Every mature MHC-restricted T cell expresses either CD4 or CD8, both of which are called coreceptors because they bind to the same MHC molecules that the TCR binds and are required for initiation of signaling from the TCR complex. At the time when the TCR is recognizing the peptide-MHC complex, CD4 or CD8 recognizes the class II or class I MHC molecule, respectively, at a site separate from the peptide-binding cleft. As discussed in Chapter 3, when protein antigens are ingested by APCs from the extracellular milieu into vesicles, these antigens are processed into peptides that are displayed by class II MHC molecules. In contrast, protein antigens present in the cytosol are processed by proteasomes into peptides displayed by class I MHC molecules. Thus, CD4$^+$ and CD8$^+$ T cells recognize antigens from different cellular

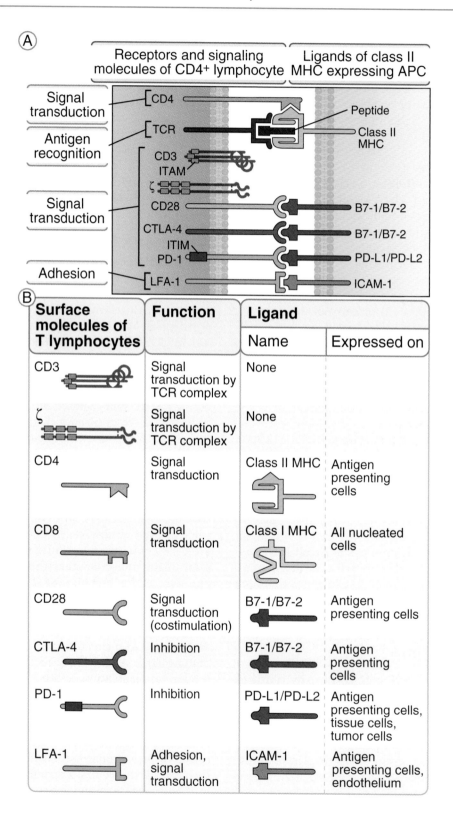

A

Receptors and signaling molecules of CD4+ lymphocyte

Ligands of class II MHC expressing APC

Signal transduction — CD4

Peptide

Antigen recognition — TCR

Class II MHC

CD3
ITAM
ζ

Signal transduction — CD28

B7-1/B7-2

CTLA-4

B7-1/B7-2

ITIM
PD-1

PD-L1/PD-L2

Adhesion — LFA-1

ICAM-1

B

Surface molecules of T lymphocytes	Function	Ligand	
		Name	Expressed on
CD3	Signal transduction by TCR complex	None	
ζ	Signal transduction by TCR complex	None	
CD4	Signal transduction	Class II MHC	Antigen presenting cells
CD8	Signal transduction	Class I MHC	All nucleated cells
CD28	Signal transduction (costimulation)	B7-1/B7-2	Antigen presenting cells
CTLA-4	Inhibition	B7-1/B7-2	Antigen presenting cells
PD-1	Inhibition	PD-L1/PD-L2	Antigen presenting cells, tissue cells, tumor cells
LFA-1	Adhesion, signal transduction	ICAM-1	Antigen presenting cells, endothelium

FIGURE 5-4 Receptors and ligands involved in T cell activation. **A,** Major surface molecules of CD4+ T cells involved in the activation of these cells and their corresponding ligands on antigen-presenting cells. CD8+ T cells use most of the same molecules, except that the TCR recognizes peptide-class I MHC complexes, and the coreceptor is CD8, which recognizes class I MHC. CD3 is composed of three polypeptide chains, δ, ε, and γ, arranged in two pairs (δε and γε); we show CD3 as three chains. Immunoreceptor tyrosine-based activation motifs (ITAMs) are the regions of signaling proteins that are phosphorylated on tyrosine residues and become docking sites for other tyrosine kinases (see Fig. 5-10). Immunoreceptor tyrosine-based inhibitory motifs (ITIMs) are the regions of signaling proteins that are sites for tyrosine phosphatases that counteract actions of ITAMs. **B,** Important properties of major surface molecules of T cells involved in functional responses. Cytokines and cytokine receptors are not listed here. The functions of most of these molecules are described in this chapter; the role of CTLA-4 and PD-1 in shutting off T cell responses is described in Chapter 9. LFA-1 is an integrin involved in leukocyte binding to endothelium and other cells. *APC,* Antigen-presenting cell; *ICAM-1,* intercellular adhesion molecule 1; *LFA-1,* leukocyte function–associated antigen 1; *MHC,* major histocompatibility complex; *PD-1,* programmed death-1; *TCR,* T cell receptor.

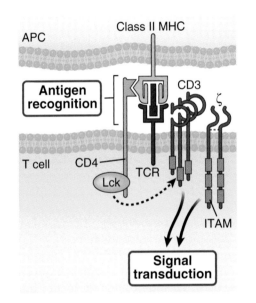

FIGURE 5-5 Antigen recognition and signal transduction during T cell activation. Different T cell molecules recognize antigen and deliver biochemical signals to the interior of the cell as a result of antigen recognition. The CD3 and ζ proteins are noncovalently attached to the T cell receptor (TCR) α and β chains by interactions between charged amino acids in the transmembrane domains of these proteins (not shown). The figure illustrates a CD4+ T cell; the same interactions are involved in the activation of CD8+ T cells, except that the coreceptor is CD8 and the TCR recognizes a peptide–class I MHC complex. *APC,* Antigen-presenting cell; *ITAM,* immunoreceptor tyrosine-based activation motifs; *MHC,* major histocompatibility complex.

compartments. The TCR and its coreceptor need to be engaged simultaneously to initiate the T cell response, and multiple TCRs likely need to be triggered for T cell activation to occur. Once these conditions are achieved, the T cell begins its activation program.

The biochemical signals that lead to T cell activation are triggered by a set of proteins linked to the TCR that are part of the TCR complex and by the CD4 or CD8 coreceptor (see Fig. 5-5). In lymphocytes, antigen recognition and subsequent signaling are performed by different sets of molecules. The TCR αβ heterodimer recognizes antigens, but it is not able to transmit biochemical signals to the interior of the cell. The TCR is noncovalently associated with a complex of transmembrane signaling molecules including three CD3 proteins and a protein called the ζ chain. The TCR, CD3, and ζ chain make up the TCR complex. Although the α and β TCRs must vary among T cell clones in order to recognize diverse antigens, the signaling functions of TCRs are the same in all clones, and therefore the CD3 and ζ proteins are invariant among different T cells. The mechanisms of signal transduction by these proteins of the TCR complex are discussed later in the chapter.

T cells can also be activated experimentally by molecules that bind to the TCRs of many or all clones of T cells, regardless of the peptide-MHC specificity of the TCR. These polyclonal activators of T cells include antibodies specific for the TCR or associated CD3 proteins, polymeric carbo-hydrate-binding proteins such as phytohemag-glutinin (PHA), and certain microbial proteins, including staphylococcal enterotoxins, which are called superantigens. Polyclonal activators often are used as experimental tools to study T cell responses, and in clinical settings to test for T cell function or to prepare metaphase spreads for karyotyping (analyzing chromosomes). Micro-bial superantigens may cause systemic inflam-matory disease by inducing excessive cytokine release from many T cells.

Role of Adhesion Molecules in T Cell Responses

Adhesion molecules on T cells recognize their ligands on APCs and stabilize the binding of the T cells to the APCs. Most TCRs bind the peptide-MHC complexes for which they are specific with low affinity. To induce a response, the binding of T cells to APCs must be stabilized for a sufficiently long period to achieve the necessary signaling threshold. This stabiliza-tion function is performed by adhesion mole-cules on the T cells that bind to ligands expressed on APCs. The most important of these adhesion molecules belong to the family of heterodimeric (two-chain) proteins called **integrins.** The major T cell integrin involved in binding to APCs is leukocyte function–associated antigen 1 (LFA-1), whose ligand on APCs is called intercellular adhesion molecule 1 (ICAM-1).

On resting naive T cells, which are cells that have not previously recognized and been acti-vated by antigen, the LFA-1 integrin is in a low-affinity state. Antigen recognition by a T cell increases the affinity of that cell's LFA-1. There-fore, once a T cell sees antigen, it increases the strength of its binding to the APC presenting that antigen, providing a positive feedback loop. Thus, integrin-mediated adhesion is critical for the ability of T cells to bind to APCs displaying microbial antigens. Integrins also play an impor-tant role in directing the migration of effector T cells and other leukocytes from the circulation to sites of infection. This process is described in Chapter 2 and later in this chapter.

Role of Costimulation in T Cell Activation

The full activation of T cells depends on the recognition of costimulators on APCs in addition to antigen (Fig. 5-6). We have previ-ously referred to costimulators as second signals for T cell activation (see Chapters 2 and 3). The name **costimulator** derives from the fact that these molecules provide stimuli to T cells that function together with stimulation by antigen.

The best-defined costimulators for T cells are two related proteins called B7-1 (CD80) and B7-2 (CD86), both of which are expressed on APCs and whose expression is increased when the APCs encounter microbes. These B7 proteins are recog-nized by a receptor called CD28, which is expressed on most T cells. Different members of the B7 and CD28 families serve to stimulate or inhibit immune responses (Fig. 5-7). The binding of CD28 on T cells to B7 on the APCs generates signals in the T cells that work together with signals gener-ated by TCR recognition of antigen presented by MHC proteins on the same APCs. CD28-mediated signaling is essential for the responses of naive T cells; in the absence of CD28:B7 interactions, antigen recognition by the TCR is insufficient for T cell activation. The requirement for costimula-tion ensures that naive T lymphocytes are acti-vated fully by microbial antigens and not by harmless foreign substances or by self antigens, because, as stated previously, microbes stimulate the expression of B7 costimulators on APCs.

A protein called ICOS (inducible costimulator), which is related to CD28 and also expressed on T cells, plays an important role in the develop-ment and function of follicular helper T cells dur-ing germinal center responses (see Chapter 7).

Another set of molecules that participate in T cell responses are CD40 ligand (CD40L, or CD154) on activated T cells and CD40 on APCs. These molecules do not directly enhance T cell activation. Instead, CD40L expressed on an antigen-stimulated T cell binds to CD40 on APCs and activates the APCs to express more B7 costimulators and to secrete cytokines (e.g., interleukin-12 (IL-12)) that enhance T cell dif-ferentiation. Thus, the CD40L-CD40 interaction promotes T cell activation by making APCs bet-ter at stimulating T cells.

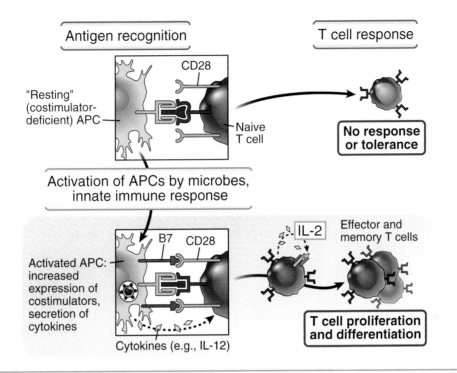

FIGURE 5-6 Role of costimulation in T cell activation. Resting antigen-presenting cells (APCs), which have not been exposed to microbes or adjuvants, may present peptide antigens, but they do not express costimulators and are unable to activate naive T cells. T cells that recognize antigen without costimulation may become unresponsive (tolerant) to subsequent exposure to antigen. Microbes, as well as cytokines produced during innate immune responses to microbes, induce the expression of costimulators, such as B7 molecules, on the APCs. The B7 costimulators are recognized by the CD28 receptor on naive T cells, providing signal 2. In conjunction with antigen recognition (signal 1), this recognition initiates T cell responses. Activated APCs also produce cytokines that stimulate the differentiation of naive T cells into effector cells. *IL,* Interleukin.

The role of costimulation in T cell activation explains an observation mentioned in earlier chapters. Protein antigens, such as those used in vaccines, fail to elicit T cell–dependent immune responses unless these antigens are administered with substances that activate APCs, especially dendritic cells. Such substances are called **adjuvants,** and they function mainly by inducing the expression of costimulators on APCs and by stimulating the APCs to secrete cytokines that activate T cells. Most adjuvants are products of microbes (e.g., killed mycobacteria, which is often used in experimental studies) or substances that mimic microbes, and they bind to pattern recognition receptors of the innate immune system, such as Toll-like receptors and NOD-like receptors (see Chapter 2). Thus, adjuvants trick the immune system into responding to purified protein antigens in a vaccine as if these proteins were parts of infectious microbes.

The increasing understanding of costimulators has led to new strategies for inhibiting harmful immune responses. Agents that block B7:CD28 interactions are used in the treatment of rheumatoid arthritis, other inflammatory diseases, and graft rejection, and antibodies that block CD40:CD40L interactions are being tested in inflammatory diseases and to treat graft rejection.

Inhibitory Receptors of T Cells

Inhibitory receptors are critical for limiting and terminating immune responses. Two important inhibitory receptors—CTLA-4 and PD-1—are structurally related to CD28 (see

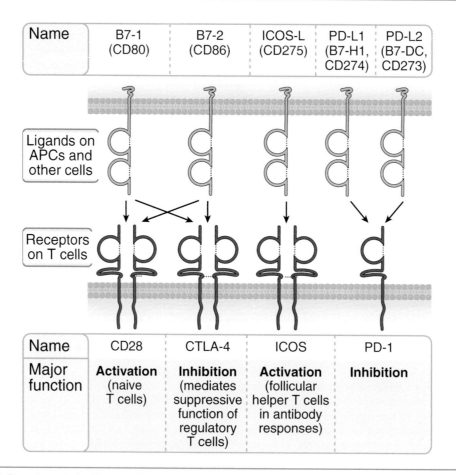

Name	B7-1 (CD80)	B7-2 (CD86)	ICOS-L (CD275)	PD-L1 (B7-H1, CD274)	PD-L2 (B7-DC, CD273)

Ligands on APCs and other cells

Receptors on T cells

Name	CD28	CTLA-4	ICOS	PD-1
Major function	**Activation** (naive T cells)	**Inhibition** (mediates suppressive function of regulatory T cells)	**Activation** (follicular helper T cells in antibody responses)	**Inhibition**

FIGURE 5-7 Proteins of the B7 and CD28 families. Ligands on APCs that are homologous to B7 bind to receptors on T cells that are homologous to CD28. Different ligand-receptor pairs serve distinct roles in immune responses. CD28 and ICOS are stimulatory receptors on T cells, and CTLA-4 and PD-1 are inhibitory receptors. Their functions are discussed in the text.

Fig. 5-7). CTLA-4, like CD28, recognizes B7-1 and B7-2 on APCs, and PD-1 recognizes different but structurally related ligands on many cell types. Both CTLA-4 and PD-1 are induced in activated T cells, and function to terminate responses of these cells. CTLA-4 also plays an important role in the suppressive function of regulatory T cells (see Chapter 9). Because these inhibitory receptors evolved to prevent immune responses against self antigens, genetic deletion or blockade of these molecules in mice and humans results in systemic autoimmune disease. CTLA-4 and PD-1 are also involved in inhibiting responses to some tumors and chronic viral infections. These discoveries are the basis for the use of antibodies that block CTLA-4 or PD-1 to enhance immune responses to tumors in patients with cancer (see Chapter 10). The function of these inhibitory receptors is discussed in more detail in Chapter 9, in the context of maintaining unresponsiveness to self antigens.

Stimuli for Activation of CD8+ T Cells

The activation of CD8+ T cells is stimulated by recognition of class I MHC–associated peptides and requires costimulation and helper T cells. The responses of CD8+ T cells may differ in several ways from responses of CD4+ T lymphocytes:

- The initiation of CD8+ T cell activation often requires cytosolic antigen from one cell (e.g.,

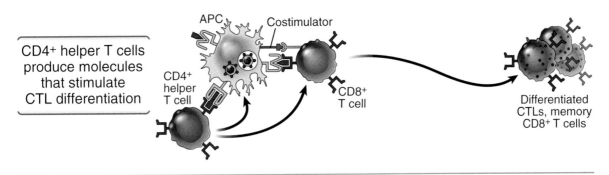

CD4+ helper T cells produce molecules that stimulate CTL differentiation

APC

Costimulator

CD4+ helper T cell

CD8+ T cell

Differentiated CTLs, memory CD8+ T cells

FIGURE 5-8 Activation of CD8+ T cells. Antigen-presenting cells (APCs), principally dendritic cells, may ingest infected cells and present microbial antigens to CD8+ T cells (cross-presentation) and to CD4+ helper T cells. Sometimes, the APC may be infected and can directly present antigens (not shown). The helper T cells then produce cytokines that stimulate the expansion and differentiation of the CD8+ T cells. Helper cells also may activate APCs to make them potent stimulators of CD8+ T cells. *CTLs*, Cytotoxic T lymphocytes.

virus-infected or tumor cells) to be cross-presented by dendritic cells (see Fig. 3-16, Chapter 3).

- The differentiation of naive CD8+ T cells into fully active cytotoxic T lymphocytes (CTLs), and, even more, into memory cells, may require the concomitant activation of CD4+ helper T cells (Fig. 5-8). When virus-infected cells are ingested by dendritic cells, the APC may present viral antigens from the cytosol in complex with class I MHC molecules and from vesicles in complex with class II MHC molecules. Thus, both CD8+ T cells and CD4+ T cells specific for viral antigens are activated near one another. The CD4+ T cells may produce cytokines or membrane molecules that help to activate the CD8+ T cells. This requirement for helper T cells in CD8+ T cell responses is the likely explanation for the defective CTL responses to many viruses in patients infected with the human immunodeficiency virus (HIV), which kills CD4+ but not CD8+ T cells. CTL responses to some viruses do not appear to require help from CD4+ T cells.

Now that we have described the stimuli required to activate naive T lymphocytes, we next consider the biochemical pathways triggered by antigen recognition and other stimuli.

BIOCHEMICAL PATHWAYS OF T CELL ACTIVATION

Following the recognition of antigens and costimulators, T cells express proteins that are involved in their proliferation, differentiation, and effector functions (Fig. 5-9). Naive T cells that have not encountered antigen have a low level of protein synthesis. Within minutes of antigen recognition, new gene transcription and protein synthesis are seen in the activated T cells. These newly expressed proteins mediate many of the subsequent responses of the T cells.

Antigen recognition activates several biochemical mechanisms that lead to T cell responses, including the activation of enzymes such as kinases, recruitment of adaptor proteins, and production of active transcription factors (Fig. 5-10). These biochemical pathways are initiated when TCR complexes and the appropriate coreceptor are brought together by binding to MHC-peptide complexes on the surface of APCs. In addition, there is an orderly movement of proteins in both the APC and T cell membranes in the region of cell-to-cell contact, such that the TCR complex, CD4/CD8 coreceptors, and CD28 coalesce to the center and the integrins move to form a peripheral ring. This redistribution of signaling and adhesion molecules is required for optimal

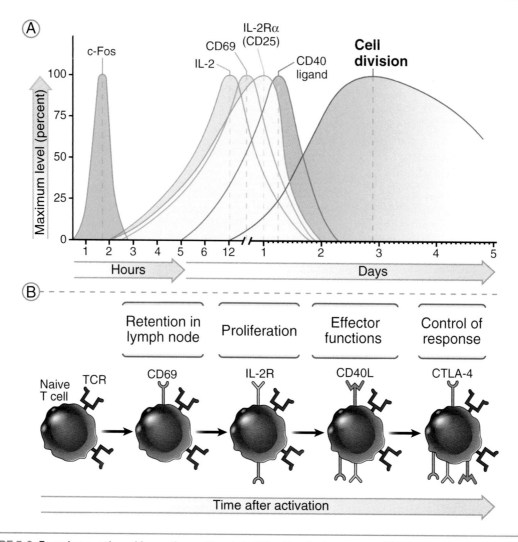

FIGURE 5-9 Proteins produced by antigen-stimulated T cells. Antigen recognition by T cells results in the synthesis and expression of a variety of proteins, examples of which are shown. The kinetics of production of these proteins **(A)** are approximations and may vary in different T cells and with different types of stimuli. The possible effects of costimulation on the patterns or kinetics of gene expression are not shown. The functions of some of the surface proteins expressed on activated T cells are shown in **B**. CD69 is a marker of T cell activation involved in cell migration; the interleukin-2 receptor (IL-2R) receives signals from the cytokine IL-2 that promotes T cell survival and proliferation; CD40 ligand is an effector molecule of T cells; CTLA-4 is an inhibitor of immune responses. c-Fos (shown in **A**) is a transcription factor. *TCR,* T cell receptor.

induction of activating signals in the T cell. The region of contact between the APC and T cell, including the redistributed membrane proteins, is called the immune synapse. Although the synapse was first described as the site of delivery of activating signals from membrane receptors to the cell's interior, it may serve other functions.

Some effector molecules and cytokines may be secreted through this region, ensuring that they do not diffuse away but are targeted to the APC. Enzymes that serve to degrade or inhibit signaling molecules are also recruited to the synapse, so it may be involved in terminating lymphocyte activation.

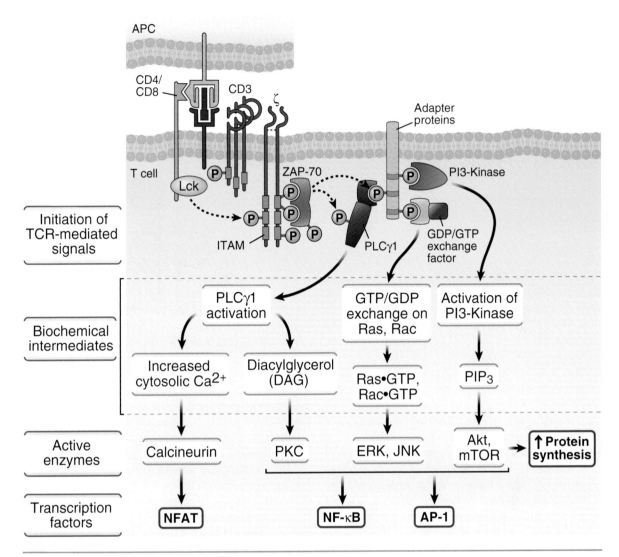

FIGURE 5-10 Signal transduction pathways in T lymphocytes. Antigen recognition by T cells induces early signaling events, which include tyrosine phosphorylation of molecules of the T cell receptor (TCR) complex and the recruitment of adaptor proteins to the site of T cell antigen recognition. These early events lead to the activation of several biochemical intermediates, which in turn activate transcription factors that stimulate transcription of genes whose products mediate the responses of the T cells. The possible effects of costimulation on these signaling pathways are not shown. These signaling pathways are illustrated as independent of one another, for simplicity, but may be interconnected in more complex networks. *AP-1*, Activating protein 1; *APC*, antigen-presenting cell; *GTP/GDP*, guanosine triphosphate/diphosphate; *ITAM*, immunoreceptor tyrosine-based activation motif; *mTOR*, mammalian target of rapamycin; *NFAT*, nuclear factor of activated T cells; *PKC*, protein kinase C; *PLCγ1*, γ1 isoform of phosphatidylinositol-specific phospholipase C; *PI-3*, phosphatidylinositol-3; *ZAP-70*, zeta-associated protein of 70 kD.

The CD4 and CD8 coreceptors facilitate signaling through a protein tyrosine kinase called Lck that is noncovalently attached to the cytoplasmic tails of these coreceptors. As discussed in Chapter 4, several transmembrane signaling proteins are associated with the TCR, including the CD3 and ζ chains. CD3 and ζ contain motifs, each with two tyrosine residues, called **immunoreceptor tyrosine-based activation motifs** (ITAMs), which are critical for signaling. Lck, which is brought near the TCR complex by the CD4 or CD8 molecules, phosphorylates tyrosine residues contained within the ITAMs of the CD3 and ζ proteins. The phosphorylated ITAMs of the ζ chain become docking sites for a tyrosine kinase called ZAP-70 (zeta-associated protein of 70 kD), which also is phosphorylated by Lck and thereby made enzymatically active. The active ZAP-70 then phosphorylates various adaptor proteins and enzymes, which assemble near the TCR complex and mediate additional signaling events.

The major signaling pathways linked to ζ-chain phosphorylation and ZAP-70 are the calcium-NFAT pathway, the Ras– and Rac–MAP kinase pathways, the PKCθ–NF-κB pathway, and the PI-3 kinase pathway:

- **Nuclear factor of activated T cells (NFAT)** is a transcription factor present in an inactive phosphorylated form in the cytoplasm of resting T cells. NFAT activation and its nuclear translocation depend on the concentration of calcium (Ca^{2+}) ions in the cytosol. This signaling pathway is initiated by ZAP-70–mediated phosphorylation and activation of an enzyme called phospholipase Cγ (PLCγ), which catalyzes the hydrolysis of a plasma membrane inositol phospholipid called phosphatidylinositol 4,5-bisphosphate (PIP2). One by-product of PLCγ-mediated PIP2 breakdown, called inositol 1,4,5-triphosphate (IP3), binds to IP3 receptors on the endoplasmic reticulum (ER) membrane and stimulates release of Ca^{2+} from the ER, thereby raising the cytosolic Ca^{2+} concentration. In response to the loss of calcium from intracellular stores, a plasma membrane calcium channel is opened, leading to the influx of extracellular Ca^{2+} into the cell, which further increases the intracellular Ca^{2+} concentration and sustains this for hours. The elevated cytoplasmic Ca^{2+} leads to activation of a phosphatase called calcineurin. This enzyme removes phosphates from cytoplasmic NFAT, enabling the transcription factor to migrate into the nucleus, where it binds to and activates the promoters of several genes, including the genes encoding the T cell growth factor IL-2 and components of the IL-2 receptor. A drug called cyclosporine inhibits calcineurin's phosphatase activity, and thus suppresses the NFAT-dependent production of cytokines by T cells. This agent is widely used as an immunosuppressive drug to prevent graft rejection; its introduction was one of the major factors in the success of organ transplantation (see Chapter 10).

- The **Ras/Rac–MAP kinase pathways** include the guanosine triphosphate (GTP)–binding Ras and Rac proteins, several adaptor proteins, and a cascade of enzymes that eventually activate one of a family of mitogen-activated protein (MAP) kinases. These pathways are initiated by ZAP-70–dependent phosphorylation and accumulation of adaptor proteins at the plasma membrane, leading to the recruitment of Ras or Rac, and their activation by exchange of bound guanosine diphosphate (GDP) with GTP. Ras•GTP and Rac•GTP, the active forms of these proteins, initiate different enzyme cascades, leading to the activation of distinct MAP kinases. The terminal MAP kinases in these pathways, called extracellular signal–regulated kinase (ERK) and c-Jun amino-terminal (N-terminal) kinase (JNK), respectively, induce the expression of a protein called c-Fos and the phosphorylation of another protein called c-Jun. c-Fos and phosphorylated c-Jun combine to form the transcription factor **activating protein 1 (AP-1)**, which enhances the transcription of several T cell genes.

- Another major pathway involved in TCR signaling consists of activation of the θ isoform of the serine-threonine kinase called protein kinase C (PKCθ), which leads to activation of the transcription factor **nuclear factor-κB (NF-κB)**.

PKC is activated by diacylglycerol, which, like IP3, is generated by PLC-mediated hydrolysis of membrane inositol lipids. PKCθ acts through adaptor proteins recruited to the TCR complex to activate NF-κB. NF-κB exists in the cytoplasm of resting T cells in an inactive form, bound to an inhibitor called IκB. TCR-induced signals downstream of PKCθ activate a kinase that phosphorylates IκB and targets it for destruction. As a result, NF-κB is released and moves to the nucleus, where it promotes the transcription of several genes.

- T cell receptor signal transduction also involves a lipid kinase called **phosphatidylinositol-3 (PI-3) kinase,** which phosphorylates the membrane phospholipid PIP2 to generate PIP3. PIP3 is required for the activation of a number of targets, including a serine-threonine kinase called Akt, or protein kinase B, which has many roles, including stimulating expression of antiapoptotic proteins and thus promoting survival of antigen-stimulated T cells. The PI-3 kinase/Akt pathway is triggered not only by the TCR but also by CD28 and IL-2 receptors. Closely linked to the Akt pathway is mTOR (mammalian target of rapamycin), a serine-threonine kinase that is involved in stimulating protein translation and promoting cell survival and growth. A drug that binds to and inactivates mTOR—rapamycin—is used to treat graft rejection.

The various transcription factors that are induced or activated in T cells, including NFAT, AP-1, and NF-κB, stimulate transcription and subsequent production of cytokines, cytokine receptors, cell cycle inducers, and effector molecules such as CD40L (see Fig. 5-9). All of these signals are initiated by antigen recognition, because binding of the TCR and coreceptors to peptide-MHC complexes is necessary to initiate signaling in T cells.

As stated earlier, recognition of costimulators, such as B7 molecules, by their receptor CD28 is essential for full T cell responses. The biochemical signals transduced by CD28 on binding to B7 costimulators are less well defined than are TCR-triggered signals. CD28 engagement likely amplifies some TCR signaling pathways that are triggered by antigen recognition (signal 1) and

also initiates a distinct set of signals that complement TCR signals.

Lymphocyte activation is also associated with a profound change in metabolic pathways. In naive (resting) T cells, low levels of glucose are taken up and used to generate energy in the form of ATP, by mitochondrial oxidative phosphorylation. Upon activation, glucose uptake increases markedly, and the cells switch to aerobic glycolysis. This process generates less ATP but facilitates the synthesis of more amino acids, lipids, and other molecules that provide building blocks for organelles and for producing new cells. As a result, it is possible for activated T cells to more efficiently manufacture the cellular constituents that are needed for their rapid increase in size and for producing daughter cells.

Having described the stimuli and biochemical pathways in T cell activation, we now discuss how T cells respond to antigens and differentiate into effector cells capable of combating microbes.

FUNCTIONAL RESPONSES OF T LYMPHOCYTES TO ANTIGEN AND COSTIMULATION

The recognition of antigen and costimulators by T cells initiates an orchestrated set of responses that culminate in the expansion of the antigen-specific clones of lymphocytes and the differentiation of the naive T cells into effector cells and memory cells (see Fig. 5-3). Many of the responses of T cells are mediated by cytokines that are secreted by the T cells and act on the T cells themselves and on many other cells involved in immune defenses. Each component of the biologic responses of T cells is discussed next.

Secretion of Cytokines and Expression of Cytokine Receptors

In response to antigen and costimulators, T lymphocytes, especially CD4+ T cells, rapidly secrete the cytokine IL-2. Cytokines are a large group of proteins that function as mediators of immunity and inflammation. We have

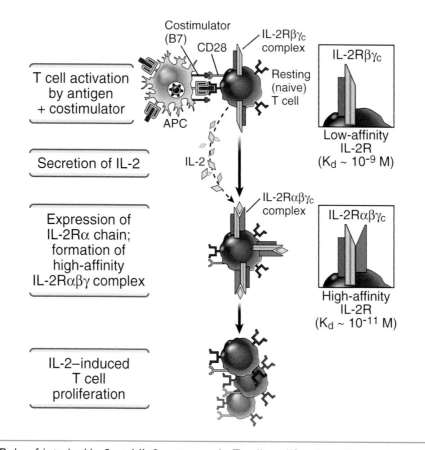

FIGURE 5-11 Role of interleukin-2 and IL-2 receptors in T cell proliferation. Naive T cells express the low-affinity IL-2 receptor (IL-2R) complex, made up of the β and γc chains (γc designates common γ chain, so called because it is a component of receptors for several cytokines). On activation by antigen recognition and costimulation, the cells produce IL-2 and express the α chain of the IL-2R (CD25), which associates with the β and γc chains to form the high-affinity IL-2 receptor. Binding of IL-2 to its receptor initiates proliferation of the T cells that recognized the antigen. *APC,* Antigen-presenting cell.

already discussed cytokines in innate immune responses, which are produced mainly by dendritic cells and macrophages (see Chapter 2). In adaptive immunity, cytokines are secreted by T cells, mainly CD4+ cells. Because most of these cytokines are produced by effector T cells and serve diverse roles in host defense, we describe them in Chapter 6 when we discuss the effector mechanisms of cell-mediated immunity.

IL-2 is produced within 1 to 2 hours after activation of CD4+ T cells. Activation also increases the expression of the high-affinity IL-2 receptor, thus rapidly enhancing the ability of the T cells to bind and respond to IL-2 (Fig. 5-11).

The receptor for IL-2 is a three-chain molecule. Naive T cells express two signaling chains but do not express the α chain (CD25) that enables the receptor to bind IL-2 with high affinity. Within hours after activation by antigens and costimulators, the T cells produce the third chain of the receptor, and now the complete IL-2 receptor is able to bind IL-2 strongly. Thus, IL-2 produced by antigen-stimulated T cells preferentially binds to and acts on the same T cells, an example of autocrine cytokine action.

The principal functions of IL-2 are to stimulate the survival and proliferation of T cells, resulting in an increase in the number

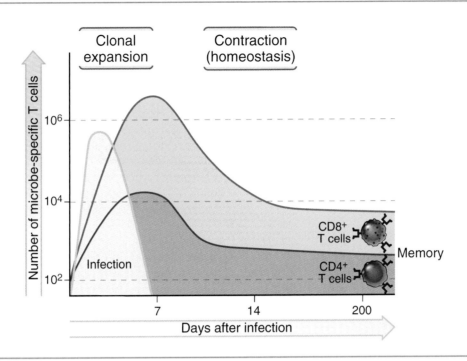

FIGURE 5-12 Expansion and decline of T cell responses. The numbers of CD4+ and CD8+ T cells specific for various antigens, and the clonal expansion and contraction during immune responses, are illustrated. The numbers are approximations based on studies of model microbial and other antigens in inbred mice; in humans, the numbers of lymphocytes are about 1000-fold greater.

of the antigen-specific T cells; because of these actions, IL-2 was originally called T cell growth factor. IL-2 also is essential for the maintenance of regulatory T cells and thus for controlling immune responses, as we discuss in Chapter 9.

CD8+ T lymphocytes that recognize antigen and costimulators do not appear to secrete large amounts of IL-2, but these lymphocytes proliferate prodigiously during immune responses. Antigen recognition and costimulation may be able to drive the proliferation of CD8+ T cells, or IL-2 may be provided by CD4+ helper T cells.

Clonal Expansion

T lymphocytes activated by antigen and costimulation begin to proliferate within 1 or 2 days, resulting in expansion of antigen-specific clones (Fig. 5-12). This expansion quickly provides a large pool of antigen-specific lymphocytes from which effector cells can be generated to combat infection.

The magnitude of clonal expansion is remarkable, especially for CD8+ T cells. Before infection, the frequency of CD8+ T cells specific for any one microbial protein antigen is about 1 in 10^5 or 1 in 10^6 lymphocytes in the body. At the peak of some viral infections, possibly within a week after the infection, as many as 10% to 20% of all the lymphocytes in the lymphoid organs may be specific for that virus. This means that the numbers of cells in antigen-specific clones have increased by more than 10,000-fold, with an estimated doubling time of about 6 hours. Several features of this clonal expansion are surprising. First, this enormous expansion of T cells specific for a microbe is not accompanied by a detectable increase in bystander cells that do not recognize that microbe. Second, even in infections with complex microbes that contain many protein antigens, a majority of the expanded clones are specific for only a few, often less than five, immunodominant peptides of that microbe.

The expansion of CD4$^+$ T cells appears to be 100-fold to 1000-fold less than that of CD8$^+$ cells. This difference may reflect differences in the functions of the two types of T cells. CD8$^+$ CTLs are effector cells that kill infected cells by direct contact, and many CTLs may be needed to kill large numbers of infected cells. By contrast, each CD4$^+$ effector cell secretes cytokines that activate many other effector cells, so a relatively small number of cytokine producers may be sufficient.

Differentiation of Naive T Cells into Effector Cells

Some of the progeny of antigen-stimulated, proliferating T cells differentiate into effector cells whose function is to eradicate infections. This process of differentiation is the result of changes in gene expression, such as the activation of genes encoding cytokines (in CD4$^+$ T cells) or cytotoxic proteins (in CD8$^+$ CTLs). It begins in concert with clonal expansion, and differentiated effector cells appear within 3 or 4 days after exposure to microbes. Effector cells of the CD4$^+$ lineage acquire the capacity to produce different sets of cytokines. The subsets of T cells that are distinguished by their cytokine profiles are named Th1, Th2, and Th17 (Fig. 5-13). Many of these cells leave the peripheral lymphoid organs and migrate to sites of infection, where their cytokines recruit other leukocytes that destroy the infectious agents. The development and functions of these effector cells are described in Chapter 6, when we discuss cell-mediated immunity. Other differentiated CD4$^+$ T cells remain in the lymphoid organs and migrate into lymphoid follicles, where they help B lymphocytes to produce antibodies (see Chapter 7). Effector cells of the CD8+ lineage acquire the ability to kill infected cells; their development and function are also described in Chapter 6.

CD4$^+$ helper T cells activate phagocytes and B lymphocytes through the action of plasma membrane proteins and by secreted cytokines (Fig. 5-14). The most important cell surface protein involved in the effector function of CD4$^+$ T cells is CD40 ligand, a member of a large family of proteins structurally related to the cytokine tumor necrosis factor (TNF). The *CD40L* gene is transcribed in CD4$^+$ T cells in response to antigen recognition and costimulation, and so CD40L is expressed on activated helper T cells (see Fig. 5-9). It binds to its receptor, CD40, which is expressed mainly on macrophages, B lymphocytes, and dendritic cells. Engagement of CD40 stimulates these cells, and thus CD40L is an important participant in the activation of macrophages and B lymphocytes by helper T cells (see Chapters 6 and 7). The interaction of CD40L on T cells with CD40 on dendritic cells increases the expression of costimulators on these APCs and the production of T cell–stimulating cytokines, thus providing a positive feedback (amplification) mechanism for APC-induced T cell activation.

Development of Memory T Lymphocytes

A fraction of antigen-activated T lymphocytes differentiates into long-lived memory cells. These cells are a pool of lymphocytes that are induced by microbes and are waiting for the infection to return. We do not know what factors determine whether the progeny of antigen-stimulated lymphocytes will differentiate into effector cells or memory cells. Memory cells have several important characteristics.

- Memory cells survive even after the infection is eradicated and antigen is no longer present. Certain cytokines, including IL-7 and IL-15, which are produced by stromal cells in tissues, may serve to keep memory cells alive and cycling slowly.
- Memory T cells may be rapidly induced to produce cytokines or kill infected cells on encountering the antigen that they recognize. These cells do not perform any effector functions until they encounter antigen, but once activated, they respond much more vigorously and rapidly than do naive lymphocytes.
- Memory T cells can be found in lymphoid organs, in various peripheral tissues, especially mucosa and skin, and in the circulation. They can be distinguished from naive and effector cells by several criteria (see Chapter 1). A subset of memory T cells, called central memory cells, populate lymphoid organs and are responsible

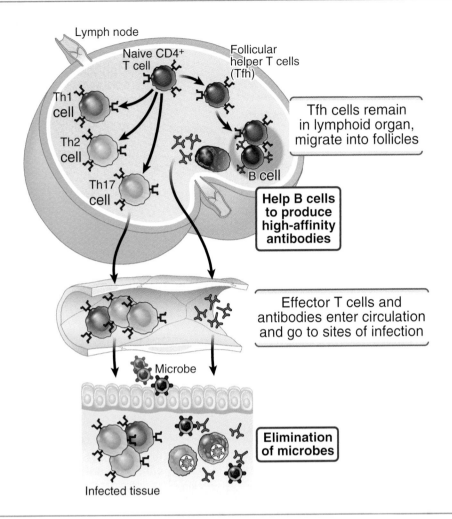

FIGURE 5-13 Development of effector CD4+ T cells When naive CD4+ T cells are activated in secondary lymphoid organs, they proliferate and differentiate into effector cells. Some of the effectors (the Th1, Th2, and Th17 populations) mostly exit the lymphoid organ and function to eradicate microbes in peripheral tissues. Other differentiated cells, called follicular helper T (Tfh) cells, remain in the lymphoid organ and help B cells to produce potent antibodies.

for rapid clonal expansion after reexposure to antigen. Another subset, called effector memory cells, localize in mucosal and other peripheral tissues and mediate rapid effector functions on reintroduction of antigen to these sites.

MIGRATION OF T LYMPHOCYTES IN CELL-MEDIATED IMMUNE REACTIONS

As we discussed at the beginning of this chapter, T cell responses are initiated primarily in

secondary lymphoid organs, and the effector phase occurs mainly in peripheral tissue sites of infection (see Fig. 5-2). Thus, **T cells at different stages of their lives have to migrate in different ways:**

• Naive T cells must migrate between blood and secondary (peripheral) lymphoid organs throughout the body, until they encounter dendritic cells within the lymphoid organ that display the antigens the T cells recognize (see Chapter 3).

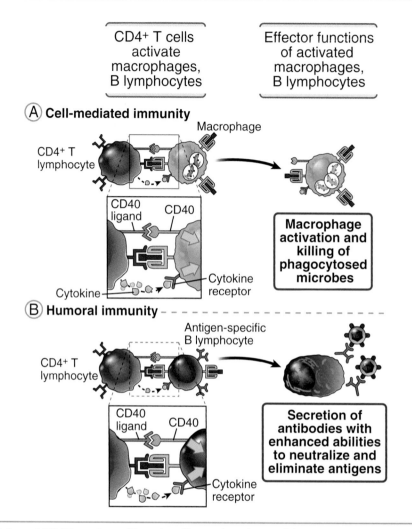

CD4⁺ T cells activate macrophages, B lymphocytes

Effector functions of activated macrophages, B lymphocytes

Ⓐ **Cell-mediated immunity**

Macrophage

CD4⁺ T lymphocyte

CD40 ligand   CD40

Cytokine

Cytokine receptor

Macrophage activation and killing of phagocytosed microbes

Ⓑ **Humoral immunity**

Antigen-specific B lymphocyte

CD4⁺ T lymphocyte

CD40 ligand   CD40

Cytokine receptor

Secretion of antibodies with enhanced abilities to neutralize and eliminate antigens

FIGURE 5-14 Roles of CD40L and cytokines in effector functions of CD4⁺ helper T cells. CD4⁺ T cells that have differentiated into effector cells express CD40L and secrete cytokines. CD40L binds to CD40 on macrophages or B lymphocytes, and cytokines bind to their receptors on the same cells. The combination of signals delivered by CD40 and cytokine receptors (arrows) activates macrophages in cell-mediated immunity **(A)** and activates B cells to produce high-affinity isotype-switched antibodies in humoral immune responses **(B)**.

- After the naive T cells are activated and differentiate into effector cells, these cells must migrate back to the sites of infection, where they function to kill microbes.

The migration of naive and effector T cells is controlled by three families of proteins—selectins, integrins, and chemokines—that regulate the migration of all leukocytes, as described in Chapter 2 (see Fig. 2-16, Chapter 2). The routes of migration of naive and effector T cells differ significantly

because of selective expression of different adhesion molecules and chemokine receptors on naive T cells versus effector T cells, together with the selective expression of endothelial adhesion molecules and chemokines in lymphoid tissues and sites of inflammation (Fig. 5-15).

Naive T cells express the adhesion molecule L-selectin (CD62L) and the chemokine receptor CCR7, which mediate the selective migration of the naive cells into

lymph nodes through specialized vessels called high endothelial venules (HEVs) (see Fig. 5-15). HEVs are located in the T cell zones of lymphoid tissues and are lined by specialized endothelial cells, which express carbohydrate ligands that bind to L-selectin. HEVs also display chemokines that are made only in lymphoid tissues and are specifically recognized by CCR7. The migration of naive T cells proceeds in a multistep sequence like that of migration of all leukocytes through blood vessels (see Chapter 2):

- Naive T cells in the blood engage in L-selectin–mediated rolling interactions with the HEV, allowing chemokines to bind to CCR7 on the T cells.
- CCR7 transduces intracellular signals that activate the integrin leukocyte function–associated antigen 1 (LFA-1) on the naive T cell, increasing the binding affinity of the integrin.
- The increased affinity of the integrin for its ligand, intercellular adhesion molecule 1 (ICAM-1) on the HEV, results in firm adhesion and arrest of the rolling T cells.
- The T cells then exit the vessel through the endothelial junctions and are retained in the T cell zone of the lymph node because of the chemokines produced there.

Thus, many naive T cells that are carried by the blood into an HEV migrate to the T cell zone of the lymph node stroma. This happens constantly in all lymph nodes and mucosal lymphoid tissues in the body. Effector T cells do not express CCR7 or L-selectin, and thus they are not drawn into lymph nodes.

The phospholipid sphingosine 1-phosphate (S1P) plays a key role in the egress of T cells from lymph nodes. The levels of S1P are higher in the blood and lymph than inside lymph nodes. S1P binds to and thereby reduces expression of its receptor, which keeps the expression of the receptor on circulating naive T cells low. When a naive T cell enters the node, it is exposed to lower concentrations of S1P, and expression of the receptor begins to increase. If the T cell does not recognize any antigen, the cell leaves the node through efferent lymphatic vessels, following the gradient of S1P into the lymph. If the T cell does encounter specific antigen and is activated, the surface expression of the S1P receptor is suppressed for several days. As a result, recently activated T cells stay in the lymph node long enough to undergo clonal expansion and differentiation. When this process is completed, S1P receptor is reexpressed on the cell surface; at the same time, the cells lose expression of L-selectin and CCR7, which previously attracted the naive T cells to the lymph nodes. Therefore, activated T cells are drawn out of the nodes into the draining lymph, which then transports the cells to the circulation. The net result of these changes is that differentiated effector T cells leave the lymph nodes and enter the circulation. The importance of the S1P pathway has been highlighted by the development of a drug (fingolimod) that binds to the S1P receptor and blocks the exit of T cells from lymph nodes. This drug is approved for the treatment of the inflammatory disease multiple sclerosis.

Effector T cells migrate to sites of infection because they express adhesion molecules and chemokine receptors that bind to ligands expressed or displayed on vascular endothelium in innate immune responses to microbes. The process of differentiation of naive T lymphocytes into effector cells is accompanied by changes in the types of adhesion molecules and chemokine receptors expressed on these cells (see Fig. 5-15). The migration of activated T cells into peripheral tissues is controlled by the same kinds of interactions involved in the migration of other leukocytes into tissues (see Chapter 2):

- Activated T cells express high levels of the glycoprotein ligands for E- and P-selectins and the integrins LFA-1 and VLA-4 (very late antigen 4). Innate immune cytokines produced at the site of infection, such as TNF and IL-1, act on the endothelial cells to increase expression of E- and P-selectins as well as ligands for integrins, especially ICAM-1 and vascular cell adhesion molecule 1 (VCAM-1), the ligand for the VLA-4 integrin.
- Effector T cells that are passing through the blood vessels at the infection site bind first to the endothelial selectins, leading to rolling interactions.

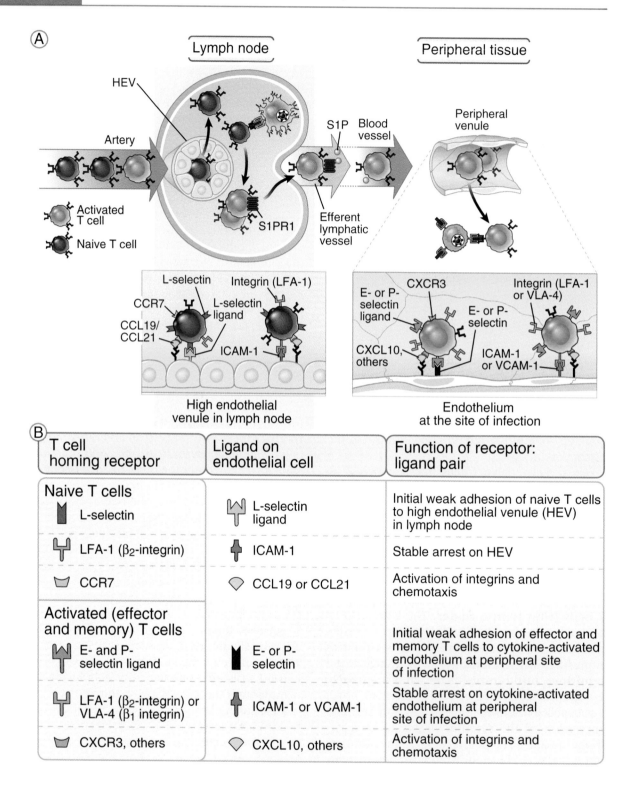

T cell homing receptor	Ligand on endothelial cell	Function of receptor: ligand pair
Naive T cells L-selectin	L-selectin ligand	Initial weak adhesion of naive T cells to high endothelial venule (HEV) in lymph node
LFA-1 (β_2-integrin)	ICAM-1	Stable arrest on HEV
CCR7	CCL19 or CCL21	Activation of integrins and chemotaxis
Activated (effector and memory) T cells E- and P-selectin ligand	E- or P-selectin	Initial weak adhesion of effector and memory T cells to cytokine-activated endothelium at peripheral site of infection
LFA-1 (β_2-integrin) or VLA-4 (β_1 integrin)	ICAM-1 or VCAM-1	Stable arrest on cytokine-activated endothelium at peripheral site of infection
CXCR3, others	CXCL10, others	Activation of integrins and chemotaxis

- Effector T cells also express receptors for chemokines that are produced by macrophages and endothelial cells at these inflammatory sites and are displayed on the surface of the endothelium. The rolling T cells recognize these chemokines, leading to increased binding affinity of the integrins for their ligands and firm adhesion of the T cells to the endothelium.
- After the effector T lymphocytes are arrested on the endothelium, they engage other adhesion molecules at the junctions between endothelial cells, crawling through these junctions into the tissue. Chemokines that were produced by macrophages and other cells in the tissues stimulate the motility of the transmigrating T cells.

The net result of these molecular interactions between the T cells and endothelial cells is that the T cells migrate out of the blood vessels to the site of infection. Naive T cells do not express ligands for E- or P-selectin and do not express receptors for chemokines produced at inflammatory sites. Therefore, naive T cells do not migrate into sites of infection or tissue injury.

The homing of effector T cells to a site of infection is independent of antigen recognition, but lymphocytes that recognize antigens are preferentially retained and activated at the site. The homing of effector T cells to sites of infection mainly depends on adhesion molecules and chemokines. Therefore, any effector T cell present in the blood, regardless of antigen specificity, can enter the site of any infection. This nonselective migration presumably maximizes the chances of effector lymphocytes entering tissues where they may encounter the microbes they recognize. The effector T cells that leave the circulation, and that specifically recognize microbial antigen presented by local tissue APCs, become reactivated and contribute to the killing of the microbe in the APC. One consequence of this reactivation is an increase in the expression of VLA integrins on the T cells. Some of these integrins specifically bind to molecules present in the extracellular matrix, such as hyaluronic acid and fibronectin. Therefore, the antigen-stimulated lymphocytes adhere firmly to the tissue matrix proteins near the antigen, which may serve to keep the cells at the inflammatory sites. This selective retention contributes to accumulation of more and more T cells specific for microbial antigens at the site of infection.

As a result of this sequence of T cell migration events, the effector phase of T cell–mediated immune responses may occur at any site of infection. In contrast with the activation of naive T cells, which requires antigen presentation and costimulation by dendritic cells, differentiated effector cells are less dependent on costimulation. Therefore, the proliferation and differentiation of naive T cells are confined to lymphoid organs, where dendritic cells (which express abundant costimulators) display antigens, but the functions of effector T cells may be reactivated by any host cell displaying microbial peptides bound to MHC molecules, not just dendritic cells.

Elucidation of the molecular interactions involved in leukocyte migration has spurred many attempts to develop agents to block the process of cell migration into tissues. Antibodies against integrins are effective in the inflammatory diseases multiple sclerosis and inflammatory bowel disease, but the clinical utility of these drugs is limited because reducing leukocyte entry into tissues, especially the central nervous system, allows the reactivation of latent viruses in occasional treated patients. A small molecule inhibitor of the S1P pathway is used for treating multiple sclerosis, as mentioned above. Small molecules that bind to and block chemokine receptors have also been developed, and some have shown efficacy in inflammatory bowel disease.

Decline of the Immune Response

Because of the remarkable expansion of antigen-specific lymphocytes at the peak of an immune response, it is predictable that once the response is over, the system must return to its steady state, called homeostasis, so that it is prepared to respond to the next infectious pathogen (see Fig. 5-12). During the response, the survival and proliferation of T cells are maintained by antigen, costimulatory signals from CD28, and cytokines such as IL-2. Once an infection is cleared and the stimuli for lymphocyte activation disappear, many of the cells that had proliferated in response to antigen are deprived of these survival signals. As a result, these cells die by apoptosis (programmed cell death). The response subsides within 1 or 2 weeks after the infection is eradicated, and the only sign that a T cell–mediated immune response had occurred is the pool of surviving memory lymphocytes.

Numerous mechanisms have evolved to overcome the challenges that T cells face in the generation of a useful cell-mediated immune response:

- Naive T cells need to find the antigen. This problem is solved by APCs that capture the antigen and concentrate it in specialized lymphoid organs in the regions through which naive T cells recirculate.
- The correct type of T lymphocytes (i.e., CD4+ helper T cells or CD8+ CTLs) must respond to antigens from the endosomal and cytosolic

compartments. This selectivity is determined by the specificity of the CD4 and CD8 coreceptors for class II and class I MHC molecules, and by the segregation of extracellular (vesicular) and intracellular (cytosolic) protein antigens for display by class II and class I MHC molecules, respectively.

- T cells should respond to microbial antigens but not to harmless proteins. This preference for microbes is maintained because T cell activation requires costimulators that are induced on APCs by microbes.
- Antigen recognition by a small number of T cells must lead to a response that is large enough to be effective. This is accomplished by robust clonal expansion after stimulation and by several amplification mechanisms induced by microbes and activated T cells themselves that enhance the response.
- The response must be optimized to combat different types of microbes. This is accomplished largely by the development of specialized subsets of effector T cells.

▌ SUMMARY

- ▪ T lymphocytes are the cells of cell-mediated immunity, the arm of the adaptive immune system that combats intracellular microbes, which may be microbes that are ingested by phagocytes and live within these cells or microbes that infect nonphagocytic cells. T lymphocytes also mediate defense against some extracellular microbes and help B lymphocytes to produce antibodies.
- ▪ The responses of T lymphocytes consist of sequential phases: recognition of cell-associated microbes by naive T cells, expansion of the antigen-specific clones by proliferation, and differentiation of some of the progeny into effector cells and memory cells.
- ▪ T cells use their antigen receptors to recognize peptide antigens displayed by MHC molecules on antigen-presenting cells (APCs), which accounts for the specificity of the ensuing response, and also recognize polymorphic residues of the MHC molecules, accounting for the MHC restriction of T cell responses.

- Antigen recognition by the T cell receptor (TCR) triggers signals that are delivered to the interior of the cells by molecules associated with the TCR (CD3 and ζ chains) and by the coreceptors CD4 and CD8, which recognize class II and class I MHC molecules, respectively.

- The binding of T cells to APCs is enhanced by adhesion molecules, notably the integrins, whose affinity for their ligands is increased by antigen recognition by the TCR.

- APCs exposed to microbes or to cytokines produced as part of the innate immune reactions to microbes express costimulators that bind to receptors on T cells and deliver necessary second signals for T cell activation.

- The biochemical signals triggered in T cells by antigen recognition and costimulation result in the activation of various transcription factors that stimulate the expression of genes encoding cytokines, cytokine receptors, and other molecules involved in T cell responses.

- In response to antigen recognition and costimulation, T cells secrete cytokines that induce proliferation of the antigen-stimulated T cells and mediate the effector functions of T cells.

- T cells proliferate following activation by antigen and costimulators, resulting in expansion of the antigen-specific clones. The survival and proliferation of activated T cells are driven by the growth factor interleukin-2.

- Some of the T cells differentiate into effector cells that are responsible for eradicating infections. CD4+ effector cells produce surface molecules, notably CD40L, and secrete various cytokines that activate other leukocytes to destroy microbes. CD8+ effector cells are able to kill infected cells.

- Other activated T cells differentiate into memory cells, which survive even after the antigen is eliminated and are capable of rapid responses to subsequent encounter with the antigen.

- Naive T cells migrate to peripheral lymphoid organs, mainly lymph nodes draining sites of microbe entry, whereas many of the effector T cells generated in lymphoid organs are able to migrate to any site of infection.

- The pathways of migration of naive and effector T cells are controlled by adhesion molecules and chemokines. The migration of T cells is independent of antigen, but cells that recognize microbial antigens in tissues are retained at these sites.

REVIEW QUESTIONS

1. What are the components of the TCR complex? Which of these components are responsible for antigen recognition and which for signal transduction?

2. What are some of the molecules in addition to the TCR that T cells use to initiate their responses to antigens, and what are the functions of these molecules?

3. What is costimulation? What is the physiologic significance of costimulation? What are some of the ligand-receptor pairs involved in costimulation?

4. Summarize the links among antigen recognition, the major biochemical signaling pathways in T cells, and the production of transcription factors.

5. What is the principal growth factor for T cells? Why do antigen-specific T cells expand more than other (bystander) T cells on exposure to an antigen?

6. What are the mechanisms by which CD4+ effector T cells activate other leukocytes?

7. What are the major properties of memory T lymphocytes?

8. Why do naive T cells migrate preferentially to lymphoid organs and differentiated effector T cells (which have been activated by antigen) migrate preferentially to tissues that are sites of infection?

Answers to and discussion of the Review Questions are available at https://studentconsult.inkling.com.

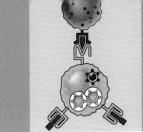

CHAPTER 6

Effector Mechanisms of T Cell–Mediated Immunity

Functions of T Cells in Host Defense

Host defense in which T lymphocytes serve as effector cells is called **cell-mediated immunity.** T cells are essential for eliminating microbes that survive and replicate inside cells and for eradicating infections by some extracellular microbes, often by recruiting other cells to clear the infectious pathogens. Cell-mediated immune responses begin with the activation of naive T cells to proliferate and to differentiate into effector cells. These effector T cells then migrate to sites of infection, and function to eliminate the microbes. In Chapter 3 we described the function of major histocompatibility complex (MHC) molecules in displaying the antigens of intracellular microbes for recognition by T lymphocytes, and in Chapter 5 we discussed the early events in the activation of naive T lymphocytes. In this chapter, we address the following questions:

- What types of effector T cells are involved in the elimination of microbes?
- How do effector T cells develop from naive T cells, and how do effector cells eradicate infections by diverse microbes?
- What are the roles of macrophages and other leukocytes in the destruction of infectious pathogens?

TYPES OF T CELL–MEDIATED IMMUNE REACTIONS

Two main types of cell-mediated immune reactions eliminate different types of microbes: CD4+ helper T cells secrete cytokines that recruit and activate other leukocytes to phagocytose (ingest) and destroy microbes, and CD8+ cytotoxic T lymphocytes (CTLs) kill any infected cell containing microbial proteins in the cytosol, eliminating cellular reservoirs of infection (Fig. 6-1). Microbial infections may occur anywhere in the body, and some infectious pathogens are able

129

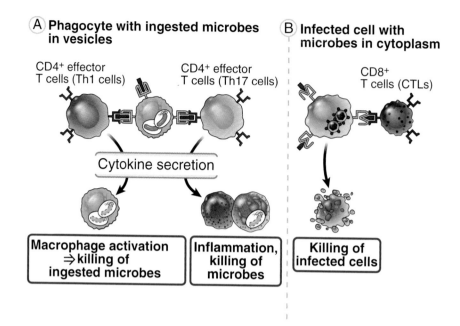

FIGURE 6-1 **Cell-mediated immunity. A,** Effector T cells of the CD4+ Th1 and Th17 subsets recognize microbial antigens and secrete cytokines that recruit leukocytes (inflammation) and activate phagocytes to kill the microbes. Effector cells of the Th2 subset (not shown) function in the eradication of infections by helminthic parasites. **B,** CD8+ cytotoxic T lymphocytes (CTLs) kill infected cells with microbes in the cytoplasm. CD8+ T cells also produce cytokines that induce inflammation and activate macrophages (not shown).

to infect and live within host cells. Pathogenic microbes that infect and survive inside host cells include (1) many bacteria, fungi, and protozoa that are ingested by phagocytes but resist the killing mechanisms of these phagocytes and thus survive in vesicles or cytosol, and (2) viruses that infect phagocytic and nonphagocytic cells and replicate in the cytosol of these cells (see Chapter 5, Fig. 5-1). The different classes of T cells recognize microbes in different cellular compartments and differ in the nature of the reactions they elicit. In general, CD4+ T cells recognize antigens of microbes in phagocytic vesicles and secrete cytokines that recruit and activate leukocytes that kill the microbes, whereas CD8+ cells recognize antigens of microbes that are present in the cytosol and destroy the infected cells.

Cell-mediated immunity against pathogens was discovered as a form of immunity to an intracellular bacterial infection that could be transferred from immune animals to naive animals by cells (now known to be T lymphocytes)

but not by serum antibodies (Fig. 6-2). It was known from the earliest studies that the specificity of cell-mediated immunity against different microbes was a function of the lymphocytes, but the elimination of the microbes was a function of activated macrophages. As already mentioned, CD4+ T cells are mainly responsible for this classical type of cell-mediated immunity, whereas CD8+ T cells can eradicate infections without a requirement for phagocytes.

T cell–mediated immune reactions consist of multiple steps (see Chapter 5, Fig. 5-2). Naive T cells are stimulated by microbial antigens in peripheral (secondary) lymphoid organs, giving rise to effector T cells whose function is to eradicate intracellular microbes. The differentiated effector T cells then migrate to the site of infection. Phagocytes at these sites that have ingested the microbes into intracellular vesicles display peptide fragments of microbial proteins bound to cell surface class II MHC molecules for recognition by CD4+ effector T cells.

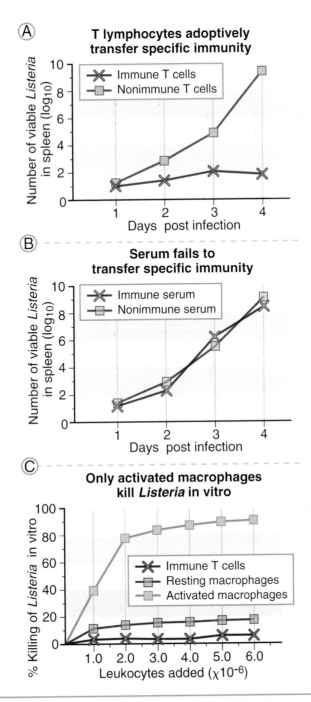

FIGURE 6-2 Cell-mediated immunity to an intracellular bacterium, _Listeria monocytogenes._ In these experiments, a sample of lymphocytes or serum (a source of antibodies) was taken from a mouse that had previously been exposed to a sublethal dose of _Listeria_ organisms (immune mouse) and transferred to a normal (naive) mouse, and the recipient of the adoptive transfer was challenged with the bacteria. The number of bacteria were measured in the spleen of the recipient mouse to determine if the transfer had conferred immunity. Protection against bacterial challenge (seen by reduced recovery of live bacteria) was induced by the transfer of immune lymphoid cells, now known to be T cells **(A)**, but not by the transfer of serum **(B)**. The bacteria were killed in vitro by activated macrophages but not by T cells **(C)**. Therefore, protection depends on antigen-specific T lymphocytes, but bacterial killing is the function of activated macrophages.

Peptide antigens derived from microbial proteins in the cytosol of infected cells are displayed by class I MHC molecules for recognition by CD8+ effector T cells. Antigen recognition activates the effector T cells to perform their task of eliminating the infectious pathogens. Thus, in cell-mediated immunity, T cells recognize protein antigens at two stages. First, naive T cells recognize antigens in lymphoid tissues and respond by proliferating and by differentiating into effector cells (see Chapter 5). Second, effector T cells recognize the same antigens anywhere in the body and respond by eliminating these microbes.

This chapter describes how CD4+ and CD8+ effector T cells develop in response to microbes and eliminate these microbes. Because CD4+ helper T lymphocytes and CD8+ CTLs employ distinct mechanisms to combat infections, we discuss the development and functions of the effector cells of these lymphocyte classes individually. We conclude by describing how the two classes of lymphocytes may cooperate to eliminate intracellular microbes.

DEVELOPMENT AND FUNCTIONS OF CD4+ EFFECTOR T LYMPHOCYTES

In Chapter 5, we introduced the concept that effector cells of the CD4+ lineage could be distinguished on the basis of the cytokines they produce. These subsets of CD4+ T cells differ in their functions and serve distinct roles in cell-mediated immunity.

Subsets of CD4+ Helper T Cells Distinguished by Cytokine Profiles

Analysis of cytokine production by helper T (Th) cells has revealed that functionally distinct subsets of CD4+ T cells exist that produce different cytokines. The existence of these subsets explains how the immune system responds differently to different microbes. For example, intracellular microbes such as mycobacteria are ingested by phagocytes but resist intracellular killing. The adaptive immune response to such microbes results in the activation of the phagocytes to kill the ingested microbes. In contrast,

the immune response to helminths is dominated by the production of immunoglobulin E (IgE) antibodies and the activation of eosinophils, which destroy the helminths. Both of these types of immune responses depend on CD4+ helper T cells, but for many years it was not clear how the CD4+ helper cells are able to stimulate such distinct immune effector mechanisms. We now know that these responses are mediated by subpopulations of CD4+ effector T cells that produce different cytokines.

CD4+ helper T cells may differentiate into three major subsets of effector cells that produce distinct sets of cytokines that perform different functions in host defense (Fig. 6-3). (A fourth subset, follicular helper T cells, which is important in humoral immune responses, is discussed in Chapter 7.) The subsets that were defined first are called Th1 cells and Th2 cells (for type 1 helper T cells and type 2 helper T cells); a third population, which was identified later, is called Th17 cells because its signature cytokine is interleukin(IL)-17. The discovery of these subpopulations has been an important milestone in understanding immune responses and provides models for studying the process of cell differentiation. However, it should be noted that many activated CD4+ T cells may produce various mixtures of cytokines and therefore cannot be readily classified into these subsets, and there may be considerable plasticity in these populations so that one subset may convert into another under some conditions.

The cytokines produced in adaptive immune responses include those made by the three major Th subsets, as well as cytokines produced by CD4+ regulatory T cells and CD8+ T cells. These cytokines of adaptive immunity share some general properties, but they each have different biologic activities and play unique roles in the effector phase or regulation of these responses (Fig. 6-4). The functions of the CD4+ T cell subsets reflect the actions of the cytokines they produce.

Each subset of CD4+ T cells develops in response to the types of microbes that subset is best at eradicating. Different microbes elicit the production of different cytokines from dendritic cells and other cells, and these

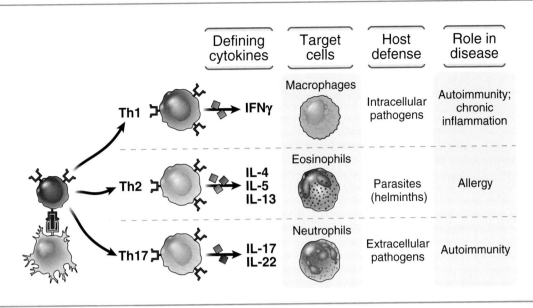

	Defining cytokines	Target cells	Host defense	Role in disease
Th1	IFNγ	Macrophages	Intracellular pathogens	Autoimmunity; chronic inflammation
Th2	IL-4 IL-5 IL-13	Eosinophils	Parasites (helminths)	Allergy
Th17	IL-17 IL-22	Neutrophils	Extracellular pathogens	Autoimmunity

FIGURE 6-3 Characteristics of subsets of CD4+ helper T lymphocytes. A naive CD4+ T cell may differentiate into subsets that produce different cytokines that recruit and activate different cell types (referred to as *target cells*) and combat different types of infections in host defense. These subsets also are involved in various kinds of inflammatory diseases. The table summarizes the major differences among Th1, Th2, and Th17 subsets of helper T cells. *IFN*, Interferon; *IL*, interleukin.

cytokines drive the differentiation of antigen-activated T cells to one or another subset. Thus, these subsets of T cells are excellent examples of the specialization of adaptive immunity, because they mediate "custom-designed" responses to combat the diversity of pathogens that may be encountered. We will see examples of such specialization when we discuss each of the major subsets, next.

Th1 Cells

The Th1 subset is induced by microbes that are ingested by and activate phagocytes, and Th1 cells stimulate phagocyte-mediated killing of ingested microbes (Fig. 6-5). The signature cytokine of Th1 cells is interferon-γ (IFN-γ), the most potent macrophage-activating cytokine known. (The name "interferon" came from the discovery of this cytokine as a protein that inhibited—or interfered with—viral infection, but IFN-γ is a much less potent antiviral cytokine than the type I IFNs [see Chapter 2]).

Th1 cells, acting through CD40-ligand and IFN-γ, increase the ability of macrophages to kill phagocytosed microbes (Fig. 6-6). Macrophages ingest and attempt to destroy microbes as part of the innate immune response (see Chapter 2). The efficiency of this process is greatly enhanced by interaction of Th1 cells with the macrophages. When the microbes are ingested into phagosomes of the macrophages, microbial peptides are presented on class II MHC molecules and are recognized by CD4+ T cells. If these T cells belong to the Th1 subset, they express CD40-ligand (CD40L, or CD154) and secrete IFN-γ. Binding of CD40L to CD40 on macrophages functions together with IFN-γ binding to its receptor on the same macrophages to trigger biochemical signaling pathways that lead to the activation of several transcription factors. These transcription factors induce the expression of genes that encode lysosomal proteases and enzymes that stimulate the synthesis of reactive oxygen species and nitric oxide, all of which are potent destroyers of microbes. The net result of CD40-mediated and IFN-γ–mediated activation is that macrophages become strongly microbicidal and can destroy most ingested

(A) General properties of T cell cytokines

Property	Significance
Produced transiently in response to antigen	Cytokine provided only when needed
Usually acts on same cell that produces the cytokine (autocrine) or nearby cells (paracrine)	Systemic effects of cytokines usually reflect severe infections or autoimmunity
Pleiotropism: each cytokine has multiple biological actions	Provides diversity of actions but may limit clinical utility of cytokines because of unwanted effects
Redundancy: multiple cytokines may share the same or similar biological activities	Blocking any one cytokine may not achieve a desired effect

(B) Biologic actions of selected T cell cytokines

Cytokine	Principal action	Cellular source(s)
IL-2	T cell proliferation; regulatory T cell survival	Activated T cells
Interferon-γ (IFN-γ)	Activation of macrophages	CD4$^+$ and CD8$^+$ T cells, natural killer (NK) cells
IL-4	B cell switching to IgE	CD4$^+$ T cells, mast cells
IL-5	Activation of eosinophils	CD4$^+$ T cells, mast cells, innate lymphoid cells
IL-17	Stimulation of acute inflammation	CD4$^+$ T cells; other cells
IL-22	Maintenance of epithelial barrier function	CD4$^+$ T cells, NK cells, innate lymphoid cells
TGF-β	Inhibition of T cell activation; differentiation of regulatory T cells	CD4$^+$ T cells; many other cell types

FIGURE 6-4 Properties of the major cytokines produced by CD4$^+$ helper T lymphocytes. A, General properties of cytokines produced during adaptive immune responses. **B,** Functions of cytokines involved in T cell–mediated immunity. Note that IL-2, which is produced by T cells early after activation and is the first identified T cell cytokine, was discussed in Chapter 5 in the context of T cell activation. Transforming growth factor β (TGF-β) functions mainly as an inhibitor of immune responses; its role is discussed in Chapter 9. The cytokines of innate immunity are shown in Figure 2-14. More information about these cytokines and their receptors is provided in Appendix II. *IgE,* Immunoglobulin E; *IL,* interleukin.

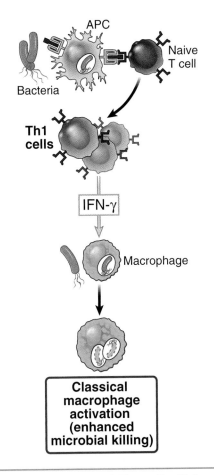

FIGURE 6-5 Functions of Th1 cells. Th1 cells produce the cytokine interferon-γ (IFN-γ), which activates macrophages to kill phagocytosed microbes (classical pathway of macrophage activation). In some species, IFN-γ stimulates the production of IgG antibodies, but follicular helper T cells may be the source of IFN-γ in this case, and a role of Th1 cytokines in isotype switching to IgG has not been established in humans. *APC*, Antigen-presenting cell.

microbes. This pathway of macrophage activation by CD40L and IFN-γ is called **classical macrophage activation**, in contrast to Th2-mediated alternative macrophage activation discussed later. Classically activated macrophages, often called M1 macrophages, also secrete cytokines that stimulate inflammation and have increased expression of MHC molecules and costimulators, which amplify the T cell response. CD8+ T cells also secrete IFN-γ

and may contribute to macrophage activation and killing of ingested microbes.

In rodents, IFN-γ produced by Th1 cells or by follicular helper T (Tfh) cells stimulates the production of IgG antibodies, which promote the phagocytosis of microbes, because these antibodies bind directly to phagocyte Fc receptors, and they activate complement, generating products that bind to phagocyte complement receptors (see Chapter 8). Thus, IFN-γ-dependent antibodies and classical macrophage activation work together in phagocyte-mediated host defense.

The critical role of Th1 cells in defense against intracellular microbes is the reason why individuals with inherited defects in the development or function of this subset are susceptible to infections with such microbes, especially normally harmless atypical (nontuberculous) mycobacteria.

Essentially the same reaction, consisting of leukocyte recruitment and activation, may be elicited by injecting a microbial protein into the skin of an individual who has been immunized against the microbe by prior infection or vaccination. This reaction is called **delayed type hypersensitivity** (DTH), and it is described in Chapter 11 when we discuss injurious immune reactions.

Development of Th1 Cells

The differentiation of CD4+ T cells to Th1 effector cells is driven by a combination of the cytokines IL-12 and IFN-γ (Fig. 6-7, *A*). In response to many bacteria (especially intracellular bacteria) and viruses, dendritic cells and macrophages produce IL-12, and NK cells produce IFN-γ. When naive T cells recognize the antigens of these microbes, the T cells are exposed to IL-12 and IFN-γ. Type I IFNs, produced in response to viral infections, also promote Th1 differentiation. These cytokines activate transcription factors (called T-bet, Stat4, and Stat1) that promote the differentiation of the T cells to the Th1 subset. IFN-γ not only activates macrophages to kill the microbes but also promotes more Th1 development and inhibits the development of Th2 and Th17 cells. Thus, IFN-γ increasingly polarizes the response to the Th1 subset.

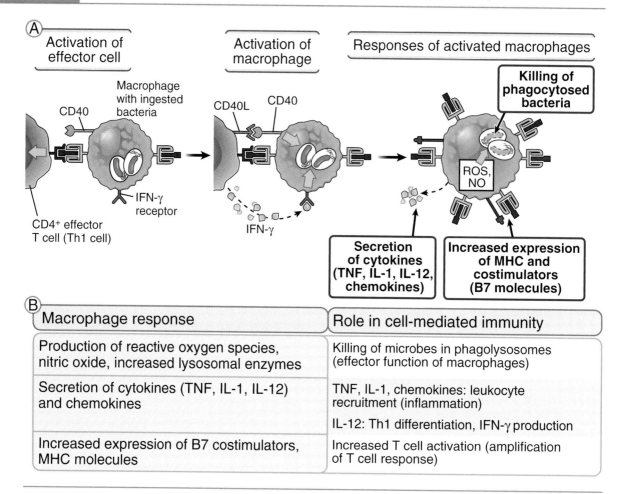

FIGURE 6-6 Activation of macrophages by Th1 lymphocytes. Effector T lymphocytes of the Th1 subset recognize the antigens of ingested microbes on macrophages. In response to this recognition, the T lymphocytes express CD40L, which engages CD40 on the macrophages, and the T cells secrete interferon-γ (IFN-γ), which binds to IFN-γ receptors on the macrophages. This combination of signals activates the macrophages to produce microbicidal substances that kill the ingested microbes. Activated macrophages also secrete tumor necrosis factor (TNF), interleukin-1 (IL-1), and chemokines, which induce inflammation, and IL-12, which promotes Th1 responses. These macrophages also express more major histocompatibility complex (MHC) molecules and costimulators, which further enhance T cell responses. **A,** Illustration shows a CD4+ T cell recognizing class II MHC–associated peptides and activating the macrophage. **B,** The figure summarizes macrophage responses and their roles in cell-mediated immunity.

Th2 Cells

Th2 cells are induced in parasitic worm infections and promote IgE-, mast cell- and eosinophil-mediated destruction of these parasites (Fig. 6-8). The signature cytokines of Th2 cells–IL-4, IL-5, and IL-13–function cooperatively in eradicating worm infections. Helminths are too large to be phagocytosed, so mechanisms other than macrophage activation are needed for their destruction. When Th2 and related Tfh cells encounter the antigens of helminths, the T cells secrete their cytokines. IL-4 produced by Tfh cells stimulates the production of IgE antibodies, which coat the helminths. Eosinophils use their Fc receptors to bind to the IgE and are activated by IL-5 produced by the Th2 cells, as well as by signals from Fc receptors. Activated eosinophils release their granule

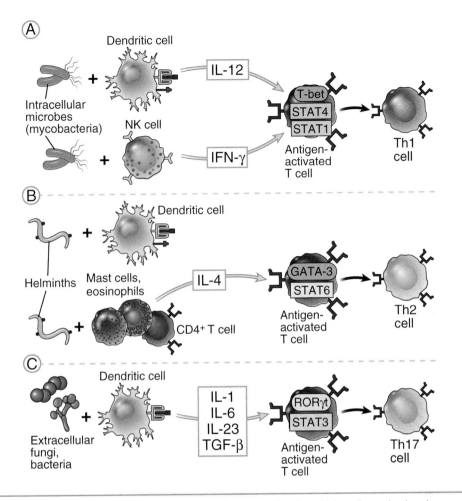

FIGURE 6-7 Development of Th1, Th2, and Th17 effector cells. Dendritic cells and other immune cells that respond to different types of microbes secrete cytokines that induce the development of antigen-activated CD4+ T cells into Th1 (**A**), Th2 (**B**), and Th17 (**C**) subsets. The transcription factors that are involved in T cell differentiation are indicated in boxes in the antigen-activated T cells.

contents, which are toxic to the parasites. IL-13 stimulates mucus secretion and intestinal peristalsis, increasing the expulsion of parasites from the intestines. IgE also coats mast cells and is responsible for the activation of mast cells; the role of this reaction in host defense is unclear.

Th2 cytokines inhibit classical macrophage activation and stimulate the alternative pathway of macrophage activation (Fig. 6-9). IL-4 and IL-13 shut down the activation of inflammatory macrophages, thus terminating these potentially damaging reactions.

These cytokines also can activate macrophages to secrete growth factors that act on fibroblasts to increase collagen synthesis and induce fibrosis. This type of macrophage response is called **alternative macrophage activation**, to distinguish it from classical activation, which enhances microbicidal functions. Alternative macrophage activation mediated by Th2 cytokines may play a role in tissue repair following injury and may contribute to fibrosis in a variety of disease states. Alternatively activated macrophages are also called M2 macrophages.

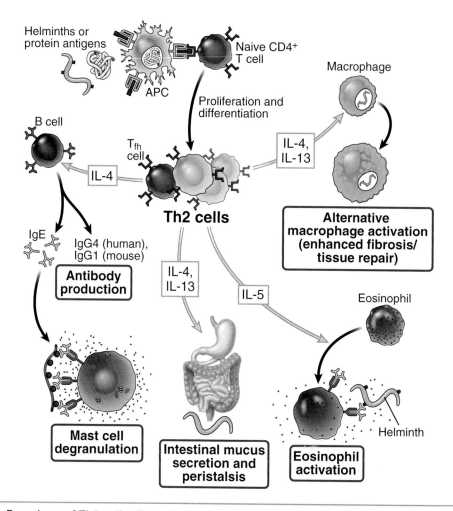

FIGURE 6-8 Functions of Th2 cells. Th2 cells produce the cytokines interleukin-4 (IL-4), IL-5, and IL-13. IL-4 (and IL-13) act on B cells to stimulate production mainly of IgE antibodies, which bind to mast cells. Help for antibody production may be provided by Tfh cells that produce Th2 cytokines and reside in lymphoid organs, and not by classical Th2 cells. IL-5 activates eosinophils, a response that is important in the destruction of helminthes. *APC*, Antigen-presenting cell; *Ig*, immunoglobulin; *IL*, interleukin.

Th2 cells are involved in allergic reactions to environmental antigens. The antigens that elicit such reactions are called allergens. They induce Th2 responses in genetically susceptible individuals, and repeat exposure to the allergens triggers mast cell and eosinophil activation. Allergies are the most common type of immune disorder; we will return to these diseases in Chapter 11 when we discuss hypersensitivity reactions. Antagonists of IL-13 are effective in the treatment of patients with severe asthma who have

strong Th2 responses, and agents that block IL-4 receptors or the cytokine IL-5 are being tested in asthma and other allergic disorders.

The relative activation of Th1 and Th2 cells in response to an infectious microbe may determine the outcome of the infection (Fig. 6-10). For example, the protozoal parasite *Leishmania major* lives inside macrophages, and its elimination requires the activation of the macrophages by *L. major*–specific Th1 cells. Most inbred strains of mice make an effective Th1 response

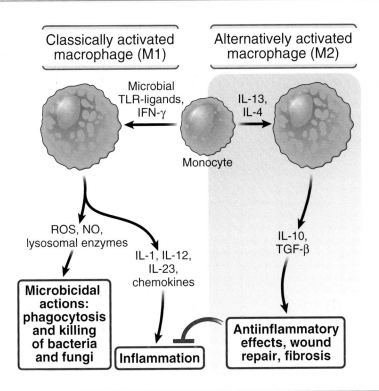

FIGURE 6-9 Classical and alternative macrophage activation. Classically activated (M1) macrophages are induced by microbial products binding to TLRs and cytokines, particularly interferon-γ (IFN-γ), and are microbicidal and proinflammatory. Alternatively activated (M2) macrophages are induced by interleukin-4 (IL-4) and IL-13 (produced by certain subsets of T lymphocytes and other leukocytes) and are important in tissue repair and fibrosis. *NO*, Nitric oxide; *ROS*, reactive oxygen species; *TGF-β*, transforming growth factor β.

to the parasite and are thus able to eradicate the infection. In some inbred mouse strains, however, the response to *L. major* is dominated by Th2 cells, and these mice succumb to the infection. *Mycobacterium leprae*, the bacterium that causes leprosy, is a pathogen for humans that also lives inside macrophages and may be eliminated by cell-mediated immune mechanisms. Some people infected with *M. leprae* are unable to eradicate the infection, which, if left untreated, will progress to a destructive form of the infection, called lepromatous leprosy. By contrast, in other patients, the bacteria induce strong cell-mediated immune responses with activated T cells and macrophages around the infection site and few surviving microbes; this form of less injurious infection is called tuberculoid leprosy. The tuberculoid form is associated with the activation of *M. leprae*–specific Th1

cells, whereas the destructive lepromatous form is associated with a defect in Th1 cell activation and sometimes a strong Th2 response. The same principle—that the T cell cytokine response to an infectious pathogen is an important determinant of the outcome of the infection—may be true for other infectious diseases.

Development of Th2 Cells

Differentiation of naive CD4⁺ T cells to Th2 cells is stimulated by IL-4, which may be produced by mast cells, other tissue cells, and T cells themselves at sites of helminth infection (see Fig. 6-7, *B*). The combination of antigen stimulation and IL-4 activates the transcription factors GATA-3 and Stat6, which together promote differentiation to the Th2 subset. These cells produce more IL-4 and thus further amplify the Th2 response.

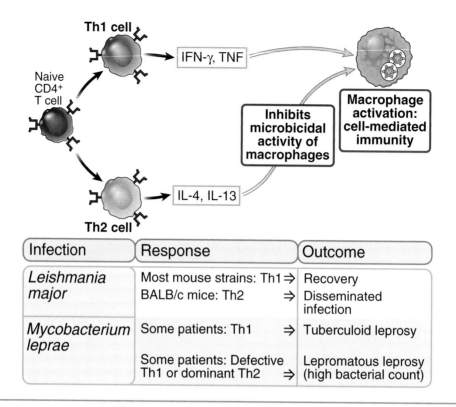

Infection	Response	Outcome
Leishmania major	Most mouse strains: Th1 ⇒ BALB/c mice: Th2 ⇒	Recovery Disseminated infection
Mycobacterium leprae	Some patients: Th1 ⇒	Tuberculoid leprosy
	Some patients: Defective Th1 or dominant Th2 ⇒	Lepromatous leprosy (high bacterial count)

FIGURE 6-10 Balance between Th1 and Th2 cell activation determines outcome of intracellular infections. Naive CD4+ T lymphocytes may differentiate into Th1 cells, which activate phagocytes to kill ingested microbes, and Th2 cells, which inhibit classical macrophage activation. The balance between these two subsets may influence the outcome of infections, as illustrated by *Leishmania* infection in mice and leprosy in humans. *IFN*, Interferon; *IL*, interleukin; *TNF*, tumor necrosis factor.

Th17 Cells

Th17 cells develop in bacterial and fungal infections and induce inflammatory reactions that destroy extracellular bacteria and fungi and may contribute to several inflammatory diseases (Fig. 6-11). The major cytokines produced by Th17 cells are IL-17 and IL-22. This T cell subset was discovered during studies of inflammatory diseases, many years after Th1 and Th2 subsets were described, and its role in host defense was established later.

The major function of Th17 cells is to stimulate the recruitment of neutrophils and, to a lesser extent, monocytes, thus inducing the inflammation that accompanies many T cell–mediated adaptive immune responses.

Recall that inflammation also is one of the principal reactions of innate immunity (see Chapter 2). Typically, when T cells stimulate inflammation, the reaction is stronger and more prolonged than when it is elicited by innate immune responses only. IL-17 secreted by Th17 cells stimulates the production of chemokines from other cells, and these chemokines are responsible for leukocyte recruitment. Th17 cells also stimulate the production of antimicrobial substances, called defensins, that function like locally produced endogenous antibiotics. IL-22 produced by Th17 cells helps to maintain the integrity of epithelial barriers and may promote repair of damaged epithelia.

These reactions of Th17 cells are critical for defense against fungal and bacterial infections.

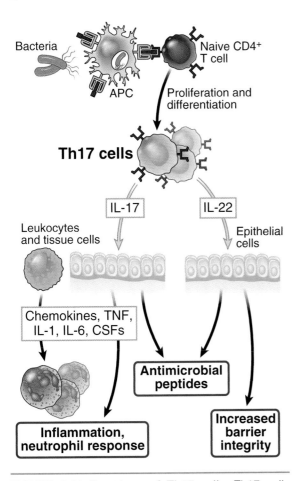

IL-17

IL-22

Leukocytes and tissue cells

Epithelial cells

Chemokines, TNF, IL-1, IL-6, CSFs

Antimicrobial peptides

Inflammation, neutrophil response

Increased barrier integrity

FIGURE 6-11 Functions of Th17 cells. Th17 cells produce the cytokine interleukin-17 (IL-17), which induces production of chemokines and other cytokines from various cells, and these recruit neutrophils (and monocytes, not shown) into the site of inflammation. Some of the cytokines made by Th17 cells, notably IL-22, function to maintain epithelial barrier function in the intestinal tract and other tissues. *APC*, Antigen-presenting cell; *CSFs*, colony-stimulating factors; *TNF*, tumor necrosis factor.

Rare individuals who have inherited defects in Th17 responses are prone to developing chronic mucocutaneous candidiasis and bacterial abscesses in the skin. Th17 cells are also implicated in numerous inflammatory diseases, and antagonists of IL-17 are very effective in the skin disease psoriasis. An antagonist that neutralizes

IL-12 and IL-23 (by binding to a protein shared by these two-chain cytokines), and thus inhibits the development of both Th1 and Th17 cells, is used for the treatment of inflammatory bowel disease and psoriasis.

Development of Th17 Cells

The development of Th17 cells from naive CD4+ cells is driven by cytokines secreted by dendritic cells (and macrophages) in response to fungi and extracellular bacteria (see Fig. 6-7, *C*). Recognition of fungal glycans and bacterial peptidoglycans and lipopeptides by innate immune receptors on dendritic cells stimulates the secretion of several cytokines, notably IL-1, IL-6, and IL-23. These act in concert to activate the transcription factors RORγt and Stat3, which induce Th17 differentiation. Another cytokine, TGF-β, also participates in this process. Interestingly, TGF-β is a powerful inhibitor of immune responses, but when present together with IL-6 or IL-1, it promotes the development of Th17 cells.

DEVELOPMENT AND FUNCTIONS OF CD8+ CYTOTOXIC T LYMPHOCYTES

Phagocytes are best at killing microbes that are confined to vesicles, and microbes that directly enter the cytoplasm (e.g., viruses) or escape from phagosomes into the cytosol (e.g., some ingested bacteria) are relatively resistant to the microbicidal mechanisms of phagocytes. Eradication of such pathogens requires another effector mechanism of T cell–mediated immunity: CD8+ cytotoxic T lymphocytes (CTLs).

CD8+ T lymphocytes activated by antigen and other signals differentiate into CTLs that are able to kill infected cells expressing the antigen. Naive CD8+ T cells can recognize antigens but are not capable of killing antigen-expressing cells. The differentiation of naive CD8+ T cells into fully active CTLs is accompanied by the synthesis of molecules involved in cell killing, giving these effector T cells the functional capacity that is the basis for their designation as cytotoxic. CD8+ T lymphocytes recognize class I MHC–associated peptides on infected cells and some tumor cells.

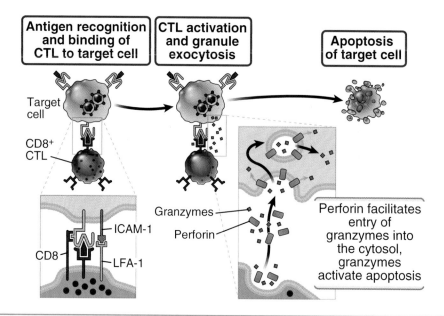

FIGURE 6-12 Mechanisms of killing of infected cells by CD8⁺ cytotoxic T lymphocytes (CTLs). CTLs recognize class I MHC–associated peptides of cytoplasmic microbes in infected cells and form tight adhesions (conjugates) with these cells. Adhesion molecules such as integrins stabilize the binding of the CTLs to infected cells (not shown). The CTLs are activated to release (exocytose) their granule contents (perforin and granzymes) toward the infected cell, referred to as the target cell. Granzymes are delivered to the cytosol of the target cell by a perforin-dependent mechanism. Granzymes then induce apoptosis. *ICAM-1,* Intercellular adhesion molecule 1; *LFA-1,* leukocyte function–associated antigen 1.

The sources of class I–associated peptides are protein antigens synthesized in the cytosol and protein antigens of phagocytosed microbes that escape from phagocytic vesicles into the cytosol (see Chapter 3). In addition, some dendritic cells may capture the antigens of infected cells and tumors, transfer these antigens into the cytosol, and thus present the ingested antigens on class I MHC molecules, by the process known as cross-presentation (see Fig. 3-16, Chapter 3). The differentiation of the naive CD8⁺ T cells into functional CTLs and memory cells requires not only antigen recognition but also costimulation and, in some situations, help from CD4⁺ T cells (see Fig. 5-7, Chapter 5).

CD8⁺ CTLs recognize class I MHC–peptide complexes on the surface of infected cells and kill these cells, thus eliminating the reservoir of infection. The T cells recognize MHC-associated peptides by their T cell receptor (TCR) and the CD8 coreceptor. (These infected cells also are called targets of CTLs, because they are attacked by the CTLs.) The TCR and CD8, as well as other signaling proteins, cluster in the CTL membrane at the site of contact with the target cell and are surrounded by the LFA-1 integrin. These molecules bind their ligands on the target cell, which firmly holds the two cells together, forming an immune synapse (see Chapter 5) into which the CTLs secrete cytotoxic proteins.

Antigen recognition by CTLs results in the activation of signal transduction pathways that lead to the exocytosis of the contents of the CTL's granules into the immune synapse between the CTL and the target cell (Fig. 6-12). Because differentiated CTLs do not require costimulation or T cell help for activation, they can be activated by and are able to kill any infected cell in any tissue. CTLs kill target cells mainly as a result of delivery of granule proteins into the target cells. Two types of granule proteins critical for killing are granzymes (granule enzymes) and perforin. **Granzyme B** cleaves and thereby activates enzymes called caspases (cysteine proteases that cleave proteins after aspartic acid residues) that are present in the cytosol of target cells and whose major function is to induce apoptosis. **Perforin** disrupts the integrity of the target cell plasma membrane and endosomal membranes, thereby facilitating the delivery of granzymes into the cytosol and the initiation of apoptosis.

Activated CTLs also express a membrane protein called Fas ligand, which binds to a death-inducing receptor, called Fas (CD95), on target cells. Engagement of Fas activates caspases and induces target cell apoptosis; this pathway does not require granule exocytosis and probably plays only a minor role in killing by CD8+ CTLs.

The net result of these effector mechanisms of CTLs is that the infected cells are killed. Cells that have undergone apoptosis are rapidly phagocytosed and eliminated. The mechanisms that induce fragmentation of target cell DNA, which is the hallmark of apoptosis, also may break down the DNA of microbes living inside the infected cells. Each CTL can kill a target cell, detach, and go on to kill additional targets.

Although we have described the effector functions of CD4+ T cells and CD8+ T cells separately, these types of T lymphocytes may function cooperatively to destroy intracellular microbes (Fig. 6-13). If microbes are phagocytosed and remain sequestered in macrophage vesicles, CD4+ T cells may be adequate to eradicate these infections by secreting IFN-γ and activating the microbicidal mechanisms of the macrophages. If the microbes are able to escape from vesicles into the cytoplasm, however, they become insusceptible to T cell–mediated macrophage activation, and their elimination requires killing of the infected cells by CD8+ CTLs.

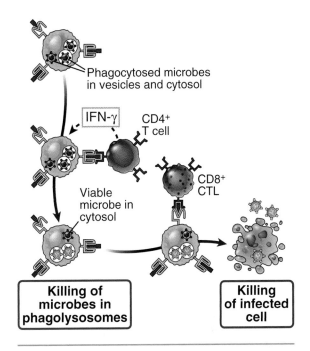

FIGURE 6-13 Cooperation between CD4+ and CD8+ T cells in eradication of intracellular infections. In a macrophage infected by an intracellular bacterium, some of the bacteria are sequestered in vesicles (phagosomes), and others may escape into the cytosol. CD4+ T cells recognize antigens derived from the vesicular microbes and activate the macrophage to kill the microbes in the vesicles. CD8+ T cells recognize antigens derived from the cytosolic bacteria and are needed to kill the infected cell, thus eliminating the reservoir of infection. *CTL*, Cytotoxic T lymphocyte; *IFN*, interferon.

RESISTANCE OF PATHOGENIC MICROBES TO CELL-MEDIATED IMMUNITY

Different microbes have developed diverse mechanisms to resist T lymphocyte–mediated host defense (Fig. 6-14). Many intracellular bacteria, such as *Mycobacterium tuberculosis, Legionella pneumophila,* and *Listeria monocytogenes,* inhibit the fusion of phagosomes with lysosomes or create pores in phagosome membranes, allowing these organisms to escape into the cytosol. Thus, these

Microbe	Mechanism	
Mycobacteria	Inhibition of phagolysosome fusion	Phagosome with ingested mycobacteria — Lysosome with enzymes. **Mycobacteria survive within phagosome**
Herpes simplex virus (HSV)	Inhibition of antigen presentation: HSV peptide interferes with TAP transporter	Cytosolic protein. **Inhibition of antigen presentation** → EBV, CMV → HSV. Proteasome, ER, TAP, CMV, CD8+ CTL
Cytomegalovirus (CMV)	Inhibition of antigen presentation: inhibition of proteasomal activity; removal of class I MHC molecules from endoplasmic reticulum (ER)	
Epstein-Barr virus (EBV)	Inhibition of antigen presentation: inhibition of proteasomal activity	
Epstein-Barr virus (EBV)	Production of IL-10, inhibition of macrophage and dendritic cell activation	EBV infected B lymphocyte, Macrophage, EBV, IL-10. **Inhibition of macrophage activation**
Pox virus	Inhibition of effector cell activation: production of soluble cytokine receptors	Pox virus, Soluble IL-1 or IFN-γ receptors, IL-1, IFN-γ. **Block cytokine activation of effector cells**

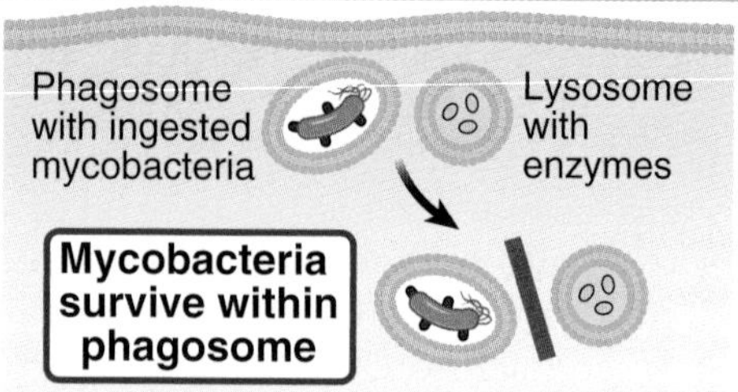

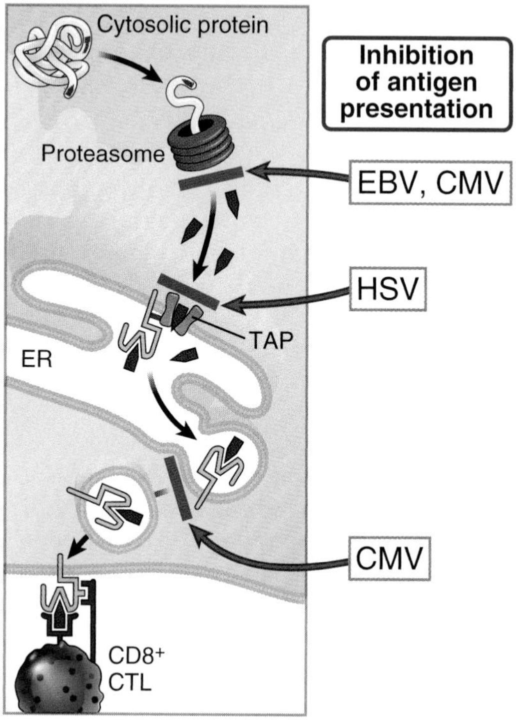

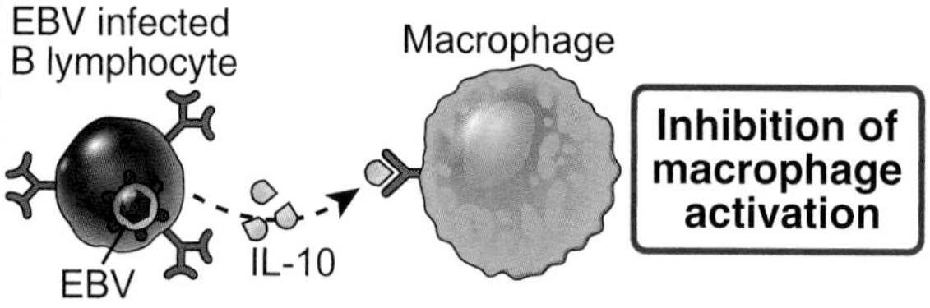

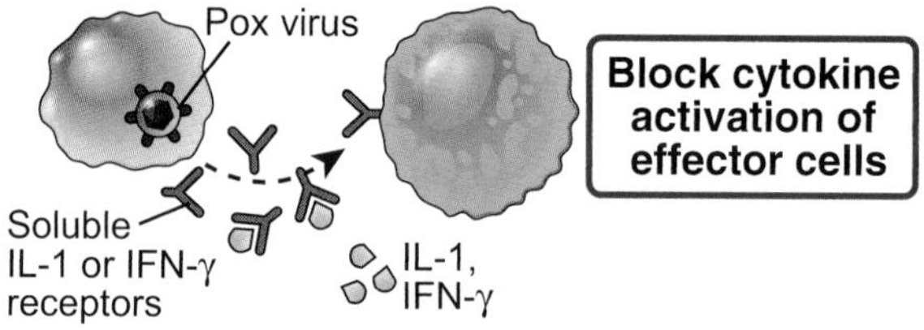

FIGURE 6-14 Evasion of cell-mediated immunity (CMI) by microbes. Select examples of different mechanisms by which bacteria and viruses resist the effector mechanisms of CMI. *CTL*, Cytotoxic T lymphocyte; *ER*, endoplasmic reticulum; *IFN*, interferon; *IL*, interleukin; *TAP*, transporter associated with antigen processing.

microbes are able to resist the microbicidal mechanisms of phagocytes and survive and even replicate inside phagocytes. Many viruses inhibit class I MHC–associated antigen presentation by inhibiting production or expression of class I molecules, by blocking transport of antigenic peptides from the cytosol into the endoplasmic reticulum (ER), and by removing newly synthesized class I molecules from the ER. All these viral mechanisms reduce the loading of class I MHC molecules by viral peptides. The result of this defective loading is reduced surface expression of class I MHC molecules, because empty class I molecules are unstable and are not expressed on the cell surface. It is interesting that natural killer (NK) cells are activated by class I–deficient cells (see Chapter 2). Thus, host defenses have evolved to combat immune evasion mechanisms of microbes: CTLs recognize class I MHC–associated viral peptides, viruses inhibit class I MHC expression, and NK cells recognize the absence of class I MHC molecules.

Other viruses produce inhibitory cytokines or soluble (decoy) cytokine receptors that bind and neutralize cytokines such as IFN-γ, reducing the amount of cytokines available to trigger cell-mediated immune reactions. Some viruses evade elimination and establish chronic infections by stimulating expression of inhibitory receptors, including PD-1 (programmed [cell] death protein 1; see Chapter 9) on CD8+ T cells, thus inhibiting the effector functions of CTLs. This phenomenon, in which the T cells mount an initial response against the virus but the response is prematurely terminated, has been called T cell exhaustion (Fig. 6-15). Still other viruses directly infect and kill immune cells, the best example being human immunodeficiency virus (HIV), which is able to survive in infected persons by killing CD4+ T cells.

The outcome of infections is influenced by the strength of host defenses and the ability of pathogens to resist these defenses. The same principle is evident when the effector mechanisms of humoral immunity are considered. One approach for tilting the balance between the host and microbes in favor of protective immunity is to vaccinate individuals to enhance cell-mediated immune responses. The principles underlying vaccination strategies are described at the end of Chapter 8, after the discussion of humoral immunity.

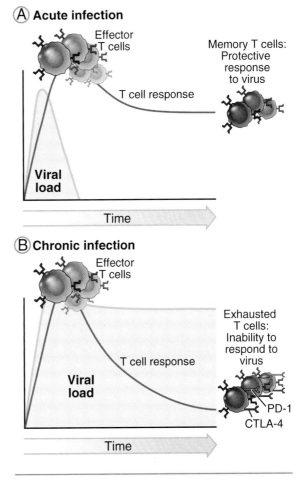

A Acute infection

Effector T cells

Memory T cells: Protective response to virus

T cell response

Viral load

Time

B Chronic infection

Effector T cells

Exhausted T cells: Inability to respond to virus

T cell response

Viral load

PD-1
CTLA-4

Time

FIGURE 6-15 T cell activation and exhaustion. **A,** In an acute viral infection, virus-specific CD8+ T cells proliferate, differentiate into effector CTLs and memory cells, and clear the virus. **B,** In some chronic viral infections, CD8+ T cells mount an initial response but begin to express inhibitory receptors (such as PD-1 and CTLA-4) and are inactivated, leading to persistence of the virus. This process is called *exhaustion* because the T cells do make a response, but this is short-lived.

SUMMARY

- Cell-mediated immunity is the arm of adaptive immunity that eradicates infections by cell-associated microbes. This form of host defense utilizes two types of T cells: CD4+ helper T cells recruit and activate phagocytes to kill ingested and some extracellular microbes, and CD8+ cytotoxic T lymphocytes (CTLs) eliminate the reservoirs of infection by killing cells harboring microbes in the cytosol.

- CD4+ T cells can differentiate into effector cells that make different cytokines and perform distinct functions.

- Effector cells of the Th1 subset recognize the antigens of microbes that have been ingested by macrophages. These T cells secrete IFN-γ and express CD40 ligand, which function cooperatively to activate macrophages.

- Classically activated macrophages produce substances, including reactive oxygen species, nitric oxide, and lysosomal enzymes, that kill ingested microbes. Macrophages also produce cytokines that induce inflammation.

- Th2 cells stimulate eosinophilic inflammation and trigger the alternative pathway of macrophage activation, and Tfh cells induced in parallel trigger IgE production. IgE and eosinophils are important in host defense against helminthic parasites.

- The balance between activation of Th1 and Th2 cells determines the outcomes of many infections, with Th1 cells promoting and Th2 cells suppressing defense against intracellular microbes.

- Th17 cells enhance neutrophil and monocyte recruitment and acute inflammation, which is essential for defense against certain extracellular bacteria and fungi.

- CD8+ T cells differentiate into CTLs that kill infected cells, mainly by inducing apoptosis of the infected cells. CD4+ and CD8+ T cells often function cooperatively to eradicate intracellular infections.

- Many pathogenic microbes have evolved mechanisms to resist cell-mediated immunity. These mechanisms include inhibiting phagolysosome fusion, escaping from the vesicles of phagocytes, inhibiting the assembly of class I MHC–peptide complexes, producing inhibitory cytokines or decoy cytokine receptors, and inactivating T cells, thus prematurely terminating T cell responses.

REVIEW QUESTIONS

1. What are the types of T lymphocyte–mediated immune reactions that eliminate microbes that are sequestered in the vesicles of phagocytes and microbes that live in the cytoplasm of infected host cells?
2. What are the major subsets of CD4+ effector T cells, how do they differ, and what are their roles in defense against different types of infectious pathogens?
3. What are the mechanisms by which T cells activate macrophages, and what are the responses of macrophages that result in the killing of ingested microbes?
4. How do CD8+ CTLs kill cells infected with viruses?
5. What are some of the mechanisms by which intracellular microbes resist the effector mechanisms of cell-mediated immunity?

Answers to and discussion of the Review Questions are available at https://studentconsult.inkling.com.

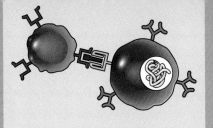

CHAPTER 7

Humoral Immune Responses

Activation of B Lymphocytes and Production of Antibodies

Humoral immunity is mediated by antibodies and is the arm of the adaptive immune response that functions to neutralize and eliminate extracellular microbes and microbial toxins. Humoral immunity is also the principal defense mechanism against microbes with capsules rich in polysaccharides and lipids, because antibodies can be produced against polysaccharides and lipids but T cells cannot respond to nonprotein antigens. Antibodies are produced by B lymphocytes and their progeny. Naive B lymphocytes recognize antigens but do not secrete antibodies, and activation of these cells stimulates their differentiation into antibody-secreting plasma cells.

This chapter describes the process and mechanisms of B cell activation and antibody production, focusing on the following questions:
- How are antigen receptor-expressing naive B lymphocytes activated and converted to antibody secreting cells?
- How is the process of B cell activation regulated so that the most useful types of antibodies are produced in response to different types of microbes?

Chapter 8 describes how the antibodies that are produced during humoral immune responses function to defend individuals against microbes and toxins.

147

PHASES AND TYPES OF HUMORAL IMMUNE RESPONSES

The activation of B lymphocytes results in the proliferation of antigen-specific cells, leading to clonal expansion, and in their differentiation into plasma cells, which actively secrete antibodies and are thus the effector cells of humoral immunity (Fig. 7-1). Naive B lymphocytes express two classes of membrane-bound antibodies, immunoglobulins M and D (IgM and IgD), that function as receptors for antigens. These naive B cells are activated by antigen binding to membrane Ig and by other signals discussed later in the chapter. The antibodies secreted in response to an antigen have the same specificity as the surface receptors on naive B cells that recognize that antigen to initiate the response. One activated B cell may generate a few thousand plasma cells, each of which can produce copious amounts of antibody molecules, in the range of

several thousand per hour. In this way, humoral immunity can keep pace with rapidly proliferating microbes. During their differentiation, some B cells may begin to produce antibodies of different heavy-chain isotypes (or classes), which mediate different effector functions and are specialized to combat different types of microbes. This process is called heavy-chain isotype (or class) switching. Repeated exposure to a protein antigen results in the production of antibodies with increasing affinity for the antigen. This process is called affinity maturation, and it leads to the production of antibodies with improved capacity to bind to and neutralize microbes and their toxins.

Antibody responses to different antigens are classified as T-dependent or T-independent, based on the requirement for T cell help (Fig. 7-2). B lymphocytes recognize and are activated by a wide variety of chemically distinct antigens, including proteins, polysaccharides, lipids, nucleic acids, and small chemicals.

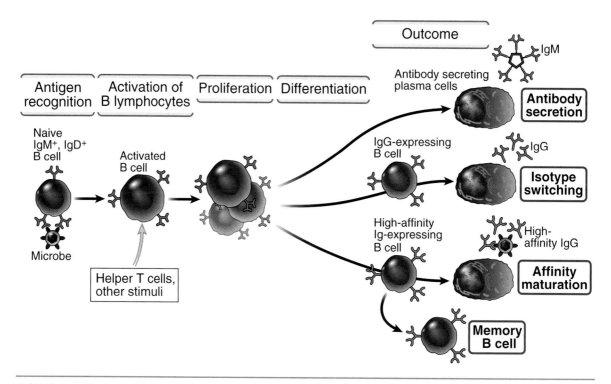

FIGURE 7-1 Phases of humoral immune responses. Naive B lymphocytes recognize antigens, and under the influence of helper T cells and other stimuli (not shown), the B cells are activated to proliferate, giving rise to clonal expansion, and to differentiate into antibody-secreting plasma cells. Some of the activated B cells undergo heavy-chain isotype switching and affinity maturation, and some become long-lived memory cells.

Protein antigens are processed and presented by antigen-presenting cells (APCs) and recognized by helper T lymphocytes, which play an important role in B cell activation and induce heavy-chain isotype switching and affinity maturation. (The designation *helper* came from the discovery that some T cells stimulate, or help, B lymphocytes to produce antibodies.) In the absence of T cell help, protein antigens elicit weak or no antibody responses. Therefore, protein antigens and the antibody responses to these antigens are called T-dependent. Polysaccharides, lipids, and other nonprotein antigens stimulate antibody production without the involvement of helper T cells. Therefore, these nonprotein antigens and the antibody responses to them are called T-independent. The antibodies produced in response to proteins show more isotype switching and affinity maturation than antibodies against T-independent antigens. Thus, the most specialized and effective antibody responses are generated under the influence of helper T cells, whereas T-independent responses are relatively simple.

Different subsets of B cells respond preferentially to protein and nonprotein antigens

(see Fig. 7-2). The majority of B cells are called **follicular B cells** because they reside in and circulate through the follicles of lymphoid organs (see Chapter 1). These follicular B cells make the bulk of T-dependent, class-switched, and high-affinity antibody responses to protein antigens and give rise to long-lived plasma cells. **Marginal-zone B cells,** which are located in the peripheral region of the splenic white pulp, respond largely to blood-borne polysaccharide and lipid antigens, and **B-1 cells** respond to nonprotein antigens in the mucosal tissues and peritoneum. Marginal-zone B cells and B-1 cells express antigen receptors of limited diversity and make predominantly T-independent IgM responses. IgM antibodies may be produced spontaneously by B-1 cells, without overt immunization. These antibodies, called **natural antibodies**, help to clear apoptotic cells and may also provide protection against some bacterial pathogens.

Antibody responses to the first exposure to an antigen, called primary responses, differ quantitatively and qualitatively from responses to subsequent exposures, called secondary responses (Fig. 7-3). The amounts of antibody produced in the primary immune

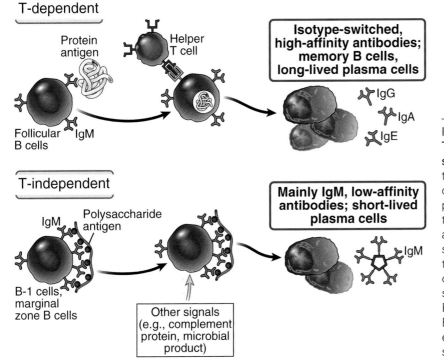

FIGURE 7-2 T-dependent and T-independent antibody responses. Antibody responses to protein antigens require T cell help, and the antibodies produced typically show isotype switching and are of high affinity. Non-protein (e.g., polysaccharide) antigens are able to activate B cells without T cell help. Most T-dependent responses are made by follicular B cells, whereas marginal zone B cells and B-1 cells play greater roles in T-independent responses. *Ig*, Immunoglobulin.

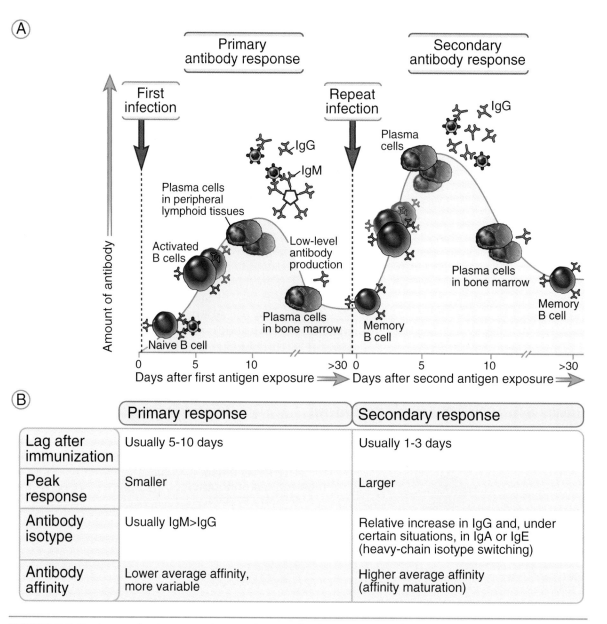

FIGURE 7-3 Features of primary and secondary antibody responses. Primary and secondary antibody responses differ in several respects, illustrated schematically in **A** and summarized in **B.** In a primary response, naive B cells in peripheral lymphoid tissues are activated to proliferate and differentiate into antibody-secreting plasma cells and memory cells. Some plasma cells may migrate to and survive in the bone marrow for long periods. In a secondary response, memory B cells are activated to produce larger amounts of antibodies, often with more heavy-chain class switching and affinity maturation. These features of secondary responses are seen mainly in responses to protein antigens, because these changes in B cells are stimulated by helper T cells, and only proteins activate T cells (not shown). The kinetics of the responses may vary with different antigens and types of immunization. *Ig,* Immunoglobulin.

response are smaller than the amounts produced in secondary responses. With protein antigens, secondary responses also show increased heavy-chain isotype switching and affinity maturation, because repeated stimulation by a protein antigen leads to an increase in the number and activity of helper T lymphocytes.

With this introduction, we now discuss B cell activation and antibody production, beginning with the responses of B cells to the initial encounter with antigen.

STIMULATION OF B LYMPHOCYTES BY ANTIGEN

Humoral immune responses are initiated when antigen-specific B lymphocytes in the spleen, lymph nodes, and mucosal lymphoid tissues recognize antigens. Some of the antigens in tissues or in the blood are transported to and concentrated in the B cell–rich follicles and marginal zones of these peripheral lymphoid organs. In lymph nodes, macrophages lining the subcapsular sinus may capture antigens and take them to the adjacent follicles, where the bound antigens are displayed to B cells. B lymphocytes specific for an antigen use their membrane-bound immunoglobulin (Ig) as receptors that recognize the antigen directly, without any need for processing. B cells are capable of recognizing the native (unprocessed) antigen, so the antibodies that are subsequently secreted (which have the same specificity as the B cell antigen receptors) are able to bind to the native microbe or microbial product.

The recognition of antigen triggers signaling pathways that initiate B cell activation. As with T lymphocytes, B cell activation also requires signals in addition to antigen recognition, and many of these second signals are produced during innate immune reactions to microbes. In the following section, we describe the biochemical mechanisms of B cell activation by antigen, followed by a discussion of the functional consequences of antigen recognition.

Antigen-Induced Signaling in B Cells

Antigen-induced clustering of membrane Ig receptors triggers biochemical signals that are transduced by receptor-associated signaling molecules (Fig. 7-4). The process of B lymphocyte activation is, in principle, similar to the activation of T cells (see Chapter 5, Fig. 5-9). In B cells, antigen receptor–mediated signal transduction requires the bringing together (cross-linking) of two or more membrane Ig molecules. Antigen receptor cross-linking occurs when two or more antigen molecules in an aggregate, or repeating epitopes of one antigen molecule, bind to adjacent membrane Ig molecules of a B cell. Polysaccharides, lipids, and other nonprotein antigens often contain multiple identical epitopes in each molecule and are therefore able to bind to numerous Ig receptors on a B cell at the same time. Even protein antigens may be expressed in an array on the surface of microbes and are thus able to cross-link multiple antigen receptors of a B cell.

Signals initiated by antigen receptor cross-linking are transduced by receptor-associated proteins. Membrane IgM and IgD, the antigen receptors of naive B lymphocytes, are membrane-bound antibodies and therefore have highly variable extracellular antigen-binding regions (see Chapter 4). However, these membrane receptors have short cytoplasmic tails, so although they recognize antigens, they do not themselves transduce signals. The receptors are noncovalently associated with two proteins, called Igα and Igβ, to form the **B cell receptor (BCR) complex,** analogous to the T cell receptor (TCR) complex of T lymphocytes. The cytoplasmic domains of Igα and Igβ each contain a conserved immunoreceptor tyrosine-based activation motif (ITAM), similar to those found in signaling subunits of many other activating receptors in the immune system (e.g., CD3 and ζ proteins of the TCR complex; see Chapter 5). When two or more antigen receptors of a B cell are clustered, the tyrosines in the ITAMs of Igα and Igβ are phosphorylated by kinases associated with the BCR complex. These phosphotyrosines recruit the Syk tyrosine kinase (equivalent to ZAP-70 in T cells), which is activated and in turn phosphorylates tyrosine residues on adaptor proteins. These phosphorylated proteins then recruit and activate a number of downstream molecules, mainly enzymes that initiate signaling cascades that activate transcription factors.

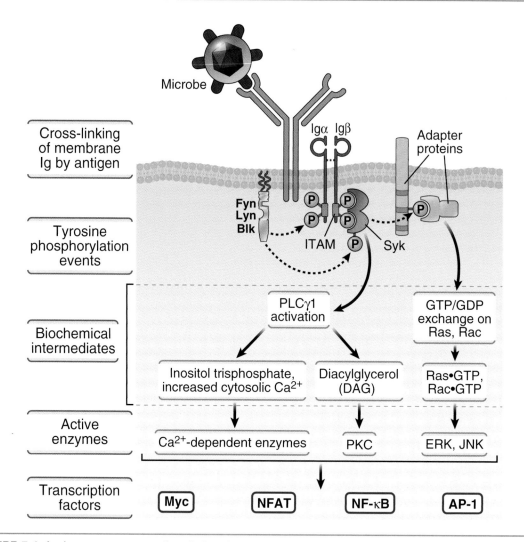

FIGURE 7-4 Antigen receptor–mediated signal transduction in B lymphocytes. Cross-linking of antigen receptors on B cells by antigen triggers biochemical signals that are transduced by the Ig-associated proteins Igα and Igβ. These signals induce early tyrosine phosphorylation events, activation of various biochemical intermediates and enzymes, and activation of transcription factors. Similar signaling events are seen in T cells after antigen recognition. Note that maximal signaling requires cross-linking of at least two Ig receptors by antigens, but only a single receptor is shown for simplicity. *AP-1,* Activating protein 1; *GDP,* guanosine diphosphate; *GTP,* guanosine triphosphate; *Ig,* immunoglobulin; *ITAM,* immunoreceptor tyrosine-based activation motif; *NFAT,* nuclear factor of activated T cells; *NF-κB,* nuclear factor κB; *PKC,* protein kinase C; *PLC,* phospholipase C.

The net result of receptor-induced signaling in B cells is the activation of transcription factors that switch on the expression of genes whose protein products are involved in B cell proliferation and differentiation. Some of the important proteins are described below.

Role of Innate Immune Signals in B Cell Activation

B lymphocytes express a receptor for a protein of the complement system that provides signals for the activation of these cells (Fig. 7-5, *A*). The complement system,

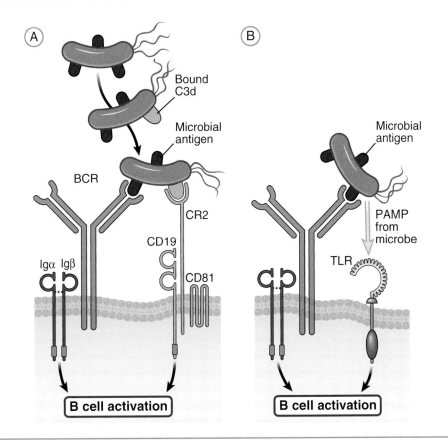

FIGURE 7-5 Role of innate immune signals in B cell activation. Signals generated during innate immune responses to microbes and some antigens cooperate with recognition of antigen by antigen receptors to initiate B cell responses. **A,** Activation of complement by microbes leads to the binding of a complement breakdown product, C3d, to the microbes. The B cell simultaneously recognizes a microbial antigen (by the immunoglobulin receptor) and bound C3d (by the CR2 receptor). CR2 is attached to a complex of proteins (CD19, CD81) that are involved in delivering activating signals to the B cell. **B,** Molecules derived from microbes (so-called pathogen-associated molecular patterns; see Chapter 2) may activate Toll-like receptors (TLRs) of B cells at the same time as microbial antigens are being recognized by the antigen receptor. *BCR,* B cell receptor.

introduced in Chapter 2, is a collection of plasma proteins that are activated by microbes and by antibodies attached to microbes and function as effector mechanisms of host defense (see Chapter 8). When the complement system is activated by a microbe, the microbe becomes coated with proteolytic fragments of the most abundant complement protein, C3. One of these fragments is called C3d. B lymphocytes express a receptor for C3d called complement receptor type 2 (CR2, or CD21). B cells that are specific for a microbe's antigens recognize the antigens by their BCRs and simultaneously recognize the bound C3d via the CR2 receptor. Engagement of CR2 greatly enhances antigen-dependent activation responses of B cells. This role of complement in humoral immune responses again illustrates that microbes or innate immune responses to microbes provide signals in addition to antigen that are necessary for lymphocyte activation. In humoral immunity, complement activation represents one way in which innate immunity facilitates B lymphocyte activation.

Microbial products also directly activate B cells by engaging innate pattern recognition receptors (see Fig. 7-5, *B*). B lymphocytes, similar to dendritic cells and other leukocytes, express numerous Toll-like receptors (TLRs; see Chapter 2). TLR engagement on the B cells by microbial products triggers activating signals that work in concert with signals from the antigen receptor. This combination of signals stimulates B cell proliferation, differentiation, and Ig secretion, thus promoting antibody responses against microbes.

Functional Consequences of B Cell Activation by Antigen

B cell activation by antigen (and other signals) initiates the proliferation and differentiation of the cells and prepares them to interact with helper T lymphocytes if the antigen is a protein (Fig. 7-6). The activated B lymphocytes enter the cell cycle and begin to proliferate. The cells may also begin to synthesize more IgM and to produce some of this IgM in a secreted form. Thus, antigen stimulation induces the early phase of the humoral immune response. This response is greatest when the antigen is multivalent, cross-links many antigen receptors, and activates complement and innate immune receptors strongly; all these features are typically seen with polysaccharides and other T-independent microbial antigens, as discussed later. Most soluble protein antigens do not contain multiple identical epitopes, are not capable of cross-linking many receptors on B cells, and by themselves, typically do not stimulate high levels of B cell proliferation and differentiation. However, protein antigens can induce signals in B lymphocytes that lead to important changes in the cells that enhance their ability to interact with helper T lymphocytes.

Activated B cells endocytose protein antigen that binds specifically to the B cell receptor, resulting in degradation of the antigen and display of peptides bound to class II MHC molecules, which can be recognized by helper T cells. Activated B cells migrate out of the follicles and toward the anatomic compartment where helper T cells are concentrated. Thus, the B cells are poised to interact with and respond to helper T cells, which were derived from naive T cells previously activated by the same antigen presented by dendritic cells.

The next section describes the interactions of helper T cells with B lymphocytes in antibody responses to T-dependent protein antigens. Responses to T-independent antigens are discussed at the end of the chapter.

FUNCTIONS OF HELPER T LYMPHOCYTES IN HUMORAL IMMUNE RESPONSES

For a protein antigen to stimulate an antibody response, B lymphocytes and helper T lymphocytes specific for that antigen must come together in lymphoid organs and interact in a way that stimulates B cell proliferation and differentiation. We know this process works efficiently because protein antigens elicit antibody responses within 3 to 7 days after antigen exposure. The efficiency of antigen-induced T-B cell interaction raises many questions. How do B cells and T cells specific for epitopes of the same antigen find one another, considering that both types of lymphocytes specific for any one antigen are rare, probably less than 1 in 100,000 of all the lymphocytes in the body? How do helper T cells specific for an antigen interact with B cells specific for an epitope of the same antigen and not with irrelevant B cells? What signals are delivered by helper T cells that stimulate not only the secretion of antibody but also the special features of the antibody response to proteins—namely, heavy-chain isotype switching and affinity maturation? As discussed next, the answers to these questions are now well understood.

The process of T-B cell interaction and T cell–dependent antibody responses is initiated by recognition of the same protein antigen by both cell types and occurs in a series of sequential steps (Fig. 7-7):

- Naive CD4$^+$ T cells are activated in the T cell zones by antigen (in the form of processed peptides bound to class II MHC molecules) presented by dendritic cells, and differentiate into functional (cytokine-producing) helper T cells.
- Naive B cells are activated in the follicles by an exposed epitope on the same protein (in its native conformation) that is transported there.

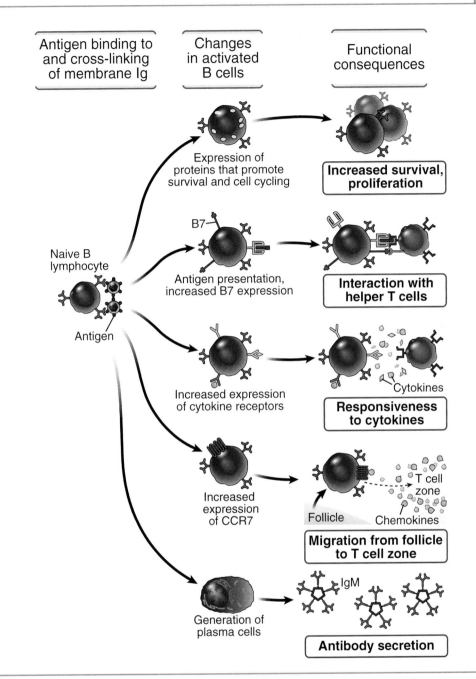

FIGURE 7-6 Functional consequences of antigen receptor-mediated B cell activation. The activation of B cells by antigen in lymphoid organs initiates the process of B cell proliferation and IgM secretion and prepares the B cell for interaction with helper T cells.

- The antigen-activated helper T cells and B cells migrate toward one another and interact at the edges of the follicles, where the initial antibody response develops.
- Some of the cells migrate back into follicles to form germinal centers, where the more specialized antibody responses are induced.

Next we describe each of these steps in detail.

Activation and Migration of Helper T Cells

Helper T cells that have been activated by dendritic cells migrate toward the B cell zone and interact with antigen-stimulated B lymphocytes in parafollicular areas of the peripheral lymphoid organs (see Fig. 7-7, *A*).

- The initial activation of T cells requires antigen recognition and costimulation, as described in Chapter 5. The antigens that stimulate CD4+ helper T cells are proteins derived from microbes that are internalized, processed in late endosomes and lysosomes, and displayed bound to class II major histocompatibility complex (MHC) molecules of APCs in the T cell–rich zones of peripheral lymphoid tissues. T cell activation is induced best by microbial protein antigens and, in the case of vaccines, by protein antigens that are administered with adjuvants, which stimulate the expression of costimulators on APCs. The CD4+ T cells differentiate into effector cells capable of producing various

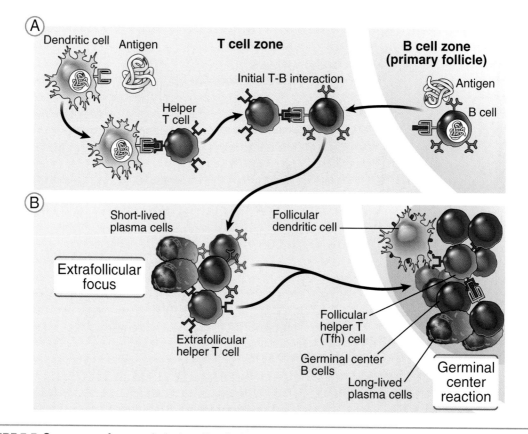

FIGURE 7-7 Sequence of events in helper T cell–dependent antibody responses. **A,** T and B lymphocytes independently recognize the antigen in different regions of peripheral lymphoid organs and are activated. The activated cells migrate toward one another and interact at the edges of lymphoid follicles. **B,** Antibody-secreting plasma cells are initially produced in the extrafollicular focus where the antigen-activated T and B cells interact. Some of the activated B and T cells migrate back into the follicle to form the germinal center, where the antibody response develops fully.

cytokines, and some of these T lymphocytes migrate toward the edges of lymphoid follicles.

- B lymphocytes are activated by antigen in the follicles, as described above, and the activated B cells begin to move out of the follicles toward the T cells.

The directed migration of activated B and T cells toward one another depends on changes in the expression of certain chemokine receptors on the activated lymphocytes. Activated T cells reduce expression of the chemokine receptor CCR7, which recognizes chemokines produced in T cell zones, and increase expression of the chemokine receptor CXCR5, which promotes migration into B cell follicles. Activated B cells undergo precisely the opposite changes, decreasing CXCR5 and increasing CCR7 expression. As a result, antigen-stimulated B and T cells migrate toward one another and meet at the edges of lymphoid follicles or in interfollicular areas. The next step in their interaction occurs here. Because antigen recognition is required for these changes, the cells that move towards one another are the ones that have been stimulated by antigen. This regulated migration is one mechanism for ensuring that rare antigen-specific lymphocytes can interact productively during immune responses to the antigen.

Protein antigens are endocytosed by the B cell and presented in a form that can be recognized by helper T cells, and this represents the next step in the process of T-dependent B cell activation.

Presentation of Antigens by B Lymphocytes to Helper T Cells

The B lymphocytes that bind protein antigens by their membrane Ig antigen receptors endocytose these antigens, process them in endosomal vesicles, and display class II MHC–associated peptides for recognition by CD4+ helper T cells (Fig. 7-8). The membrane Ig of B cells is a high-affinity receptor that enables a B cell to specifically bind a particular antigen, even when the extracellular concentration of the antigen is very low. In addition, antigen bound by membrane Ig is endocytosed efficiently and is delivered to late endosomal vesicles and lysosomes, where proteins are processed into peptides

that bind to class II MHC molecules (see Chapter 3). Therefore, B lymphocytes are efficient APCs for the antigens they specifically recognize.

Any one B cell may bind a conformational epitope of a native protein antigen, internalize and process the protein, and display multiple peptides from that protein for T cell recognition. Therefore, B cells and T cells recognize different epitopes of the same protein antigen. Because B cells efficiently present the antigen for which they have specific receptors, and helper T cells

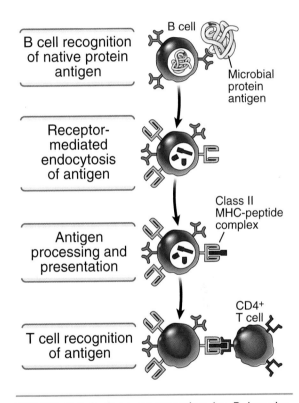

FIGURE 7-8 Antigen presentation by B lymphocytes to helper T cells. B cells specific for a protein antigen bind and internalize that antigen, process it, and present peptides attached to class II major histocompatibility complex (MHC) molecules to helper T cells. The B cells and helper T cells are specific for the same antigen, but the B cells recognize native (conformational) epitopes, and the helper T cells recognize peptide fragments of the antigen bound to class II MHC molecules. B cells also express costimulators (e.g., B7 molecules) that may play a role in T cell activation (not shown).

recognize peptides derived from the same antigen, the ensuing interaction remains antigen specific. B cells are capable of activating previously differentiated effector T cells but are inefficient at initiating the responses of naive T cells.

The idea that B cells recognize one epitope of the antigen and display different epitopes (peptides) for recognition by helper T cells was first demonstrated by studies using hapten-carrier conjugates. A hapten is a small chemical that is recognized by B cells but stimulates strong antibody responses only if it is attached to a carrier protein. In this situation the B cell binds the hapten portion, ingests the conjugate, and displays peptides derived from the carrier to helper T cells. This concept has been exploited to develop effective vaccines against microbial polysaccharides. Some bacteria have polysaccharide-rich capsules, and the polysaccharides themselves stimulate T-independent antibody responses, which are weak in infants and young children. If the polysaccharide is coupled to a carrier protein, however, effective T-dependent responses are induced against the polysaccharide because helper T cells specific for the carrier are engaged in the response. Such **conjugate vaccines** have been very useful

for inducing protective immunity against bacteria such as *Haemophilus influenzae*, especially in infants.

Mechanisms of Helper T Cell–Mediated Activation of B Lymphocytes

Activated helper T lymphocytes that recognize antigen presented by B cells use CD40 ligand (CD40L) and secreted cytokines to activate the antigen-specific B cells (Fig. 7-9). The process of helper T cell–mediated B lymphocyte activation is analogous to the process of T cell–mediated macrophage activation in cell-mediated immunity (see Chapter 6, Fig. 6-6). CD40L expressed on activated helper T cells binds to CD40 on B lymphocytes. Engagement of CD40 delivers signals to the B cells that stimulate proliferation and the synthesis and secretion of antibodies. At the same time, cytokines produced by the helper T cells bind to cytokine receptors on B lymphocytes and stimulate more B cell proliferation and Ig production. The requirement for the CD40L-CD40 interaction ensures that only T and B lymphocytes in physical contact engage in productive interactions. As described previously, the antigen-specific lymphocytes are the cells

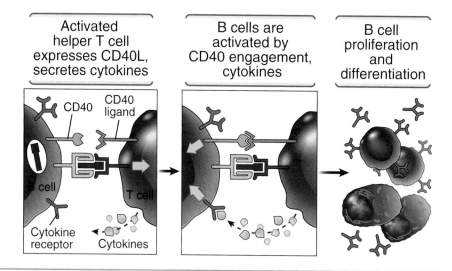

FIGURE 7-9 Mechanisms of helper T cell–mediated activation of B lymphocytes. Helper T cells recognize peptide antigens presented by B cells (and costimulators, e.g., B7 molecules, not shown) on the B cells. The helper T cells are activated to express CD40 ligand (CD40L) and secrete cytokines, both of which bind to their receptors on the same B cells and activate the B cells.

that physically interact, thus ensuring that the antigen-specific B cells are the cells that receive T cell help and are activated. Helper T cell signals also stimulate heavy-chain isotype switching and affinity maturation, which explains why these changes typically are seen in antibody responses to T-dependent protein antigens.

Extrafollicular and Germinal Center Reactions

The initial T-B interaction, which occurs at the edge of lymphoid follicles, results in the production of low levels of antibodies, which may be of switched isotypes (described next) but are generally of low affinity (see Fig. 7-7, B). The plasma cells that are generated in these extra-follicular foci are typically short-lived and produce antibodies for a few weeks, and few memory B cells are generated.

Many of the events in fully developed antibody responses occur in germinal centers that are formed in lymphoid follicles and require the participation of a specialized type of helper T cell (Fig. 7-10). Some of the activated helper T cells express high levels

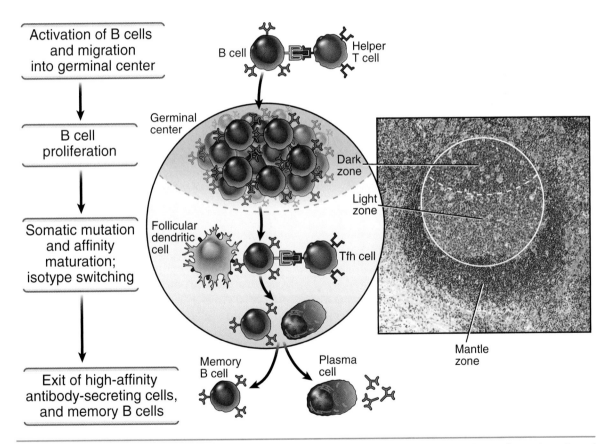

FIGURE 7-10 The germinal center reaction. B cells that have been activated by T helper cells at the edge of a primary follicle migrate into the follicle and proliferate, forming the dark zone of the germinal center. Germinal center B cells undergo extensive isotype switching and somatic mutation of Ig genes, and migrate into the light zone, where B cells with the highest affinity Ig receptors are selected to survive, and they differentiate into plasma cells or memory cells, which leave the germinal center. The right panel shows the histology of a secondary follicle with a germinal center in a lymph node. The germinal center includes a basal dark zone and an adjacent light zone. The mantle zone is the part of the follicle outside the germinal center.

of the chemokine receptor CXCR5, which draws these cells into the adjacent follicles. The CD4+ T cells that migrate into B cell–rich follicles are called **follicular helper T (Tfh) cells**. The generation and function of Tfh cells are dependent on a receptor of the CD28 family called ICOS (inducible costimulator), which binds to its ligand expressed on B cells and other cells. Inherited mutations in the *ICOS* gene are the cause of some antibody deficiencies (see Chapter 12). Tfh cells may secrete cytokines, such as interferon (IFN)-γ, interleukin (IL)-4, or IL-17, which are characteristic of Th1, Th2, and Th17 subsets; the role of these cytokines in B cell responses is described below. In addition, most Tfh cells also secrete the cytokine IL-21, which has an important but still incompletely understood role in Tfh cell function.

A few of the activated B cells from the extrafollicular focus migrate back into the lymphoid follicle and begin to divide rapidly in response to signals from Tfh cells. It is estimated that these B cells have a doubling time of approximately 6 hours, so one cell may produce several thousand progeny within a week. The region of the follicle containing these proliferating B cells is the **germinal center**, so named because it was once thought that these were the sites where new lymphocytes are generated (germinated). In the germinal center, B cells undergo extensive isotype switching and somatic mutation of Ig genes; both processes are described below. The highest-affinity B cells are the ones that are selected during the germinal center reaction to differentiate into memory B cells and long-lived plasma cells. Proliferating B cells reside in the dark zone of the germinal center (see Fig. 7-10), while selection occurs in the less dense light zone.

Heavy-Chain Isotype (Class) Switching

Helper T cells stimulate the progeny of IgM– and IgD–expressing B lymphocytes to produce antibodies of different heavy-chain isotypes (classes) (Fig. 7-11). Different antibody isotypes perform different functions, and therefore the process of isotype switching broadens the functional capabilities of humoral immune responses. For example, an important defense mechanism against the extracellular stages of most bacteria and viruses is to coat (opsonize) these microbes with antibodies and cause them to be phagocytosed by neutrophils and macrophages. This reaction is best mediated by antibody classes, such as IgG1 and IgG3 (in humans), that bind to high-affinity phagocyte Fc receptors specific for the γ heavy chain (see Chapter 8). Helminths, in contrast, are too large to be phagocytosed, and they are best eliminated by eosinophils. Therefore, defense against these parasites involves coating them with antibodies to which eosinophils bind. The antibody class that is able to do this is IgE, because eosinophils have high-affinity receptors for the Fc portion of the ε heavy chain. Thus, effective host defense requires that the immune system make different antibody isotypes in response to different types of microbes, even though all naive B lymphocytes specific for all these microbes express antigen receptors of the IgM and IgD isotypes.

Another functional consequence of isotype switching is that the IgG antibodies produced are able to bind to a specialized Fc receptor called the neonatal Fc receptor (FcRn). FcRn expressed in the placenta mediates the transfer of maternal IgG to the fetus, providing protection to the newborn, and FcRn expressed on endothelial cells and phagocytes plays a special role in protecting IgG antibodies from intracellular catabolism, thereby prolonging its half-life in the blood (see Chapter 8).

Heavy-chain isotype switching is induced by a combination of CD40L-mediated signals and cytokines. These signals act on antigen-stimulated B cells and induce switching in some of the progeny of these cells. In the absence of CD40 or CD40L, B cells secrete only IgM and fail to switch to other isotypes, indicating the essential role of this ligand-receptor pair in isotype switching. A disease called the **X-linked hyper-IgM syndrome** is caused by mutations in the CD40L gene, which is located on the X chromosome, leading to production of nonfunctional forms of CD40L. In this disease, much of the serum antibody is IgM, because of defective heavy-chain isotype switching. Patients also have defective cell-mediated immunity against intracellular microbes, because CD40L is important for T cell–mediated activation of macrophages

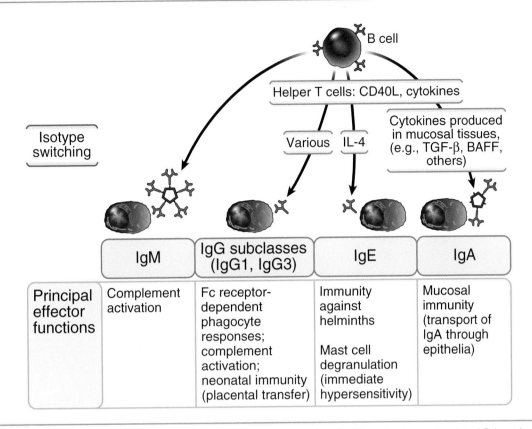

FIGURE 7-11 Immunoglobulin (Ig) heavy-chain isotype (class) switching. Antigen-stimulated B lymphocytes may differentiate into IgM antibody-secreting cells, or, under the influence of CD40 ligand (CD40L) and cytokines, some of the B cells may differentiate into cells that produce different Ig heavy-chain isotypes. The principal effector functions of some of these isotypes are listed; all isotypes may function to neutralize microbes and toxins. BAFF is a B cell–activating cytokine that may be involved in switching to IgA, especially in T-independent responses. Switching to IgG subclasses is stimulated by the cytokine interferon (IFN)-γ in mice, but in humans it is thought to be stimulated by other cytokines. *IL-4*, Interleukin-4; *TGF-β*, transforming growth factor β.

and for the amplification of T cell responses by dendritic cells (see Chapter 6).

The molecular mechanism of isotype switching, called switch recombination, takes the previously formed VDJ exon encoding the V domain of an Ig μ heavy chain and moves it adjacent to a downstream C region (Fig. 7-12). IgM-producing B cells, which have not undergone switching, contain in their Ig heavy-chain locus a rearranged *VDJ* gene adjacent to the first constant-region cluster, which is Cμ. The heavy-chain mRNA is produced by splicing a VDJ exon to Cμ exons in the initially transcribed RNA, and this mRNA is

translated to produce a μ heavy chain, which combines with a light chain to give rise to an IgM antibody. Thus, the first antibody produced by B cells is IgM. Signals from CD40 and cytokine receptors stimulate transcription through one of the constant regions that is downstream of Cμ. In the intron 5′ of each constant region (except Cδ) is a conserved nucleotide sequence called the switch region. During switch recombination, the switch region 5′ of Cμ recombines with the switch region adjacent to the transcriptionally active downstream constant region, and the intervening DNA is deleted. An enzyme called activation-induced deaminase (AID), which is induced by

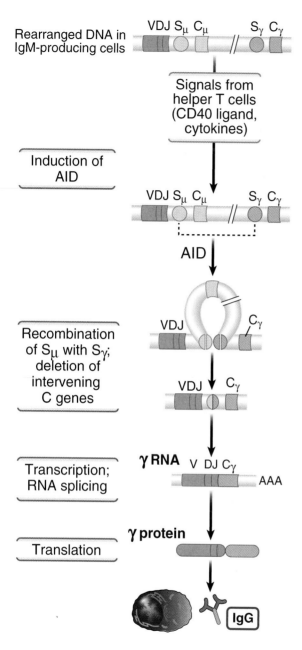

Rearranged DNA in IgM-producing cells

Signals from helper T cells (CD40 ligand, cytokines)

Induction of AID

VDJ S_μ C_μ S_γ C_γ

AID

Recombination of S_μ with S_γ; deletion of intervening C genes

VDJ C_γ

VDJ C_γ

Transcription; RNA splicing

γ RNA V DJ C_γ AAA

γ protein

Translation

IgG

FIGURE 7-12 Mechanism of immunoglobulin heavy-chain isotype switching. In an IgM-producing B cell, the rearranged VDJ heavy-chain gene is adjacent to the μ constant region genes ($C\mu$). Signals from helper T cells (CD40 ligand and cytokines) may induce recombination of switch (S) regions such that the rearranged VDJ DNA is moved close to a C gene downstream of $C\mu$, which are $C\gamma$ genes in the example shown. The enzyme activation-induced deaminase (AID), which is induced in the B cells by signals from Tfh cells, alters nucleotides in the switch regions so that they can be cleaved by other enzymes and joined to downstream switch regions. Subsequently, when the heavy chain gene is transcribed, the VDJ exon is spliced onto the exons of the downstream C gene, producing a heavy chain with a new constant region and thus a new class of Ig. Note that although the C region changes, the VDJ region, and thus the specificity of the antibody, is preserved. (Each C region gene consists of multiple exons, but only one is shown for simplicity.)

brought together and repaired, the intervening DNA is removed, and the rearranged VDJ exon that was originally close to $C\mu$ may now be brought immediately upstream of the constant region of a different isotype (e.g., IgG, IgA, IgE). The result is that the B cell begins to produce a new heavy-chain isotype (determined by the C region of the antibody) with the same specificity as that of the original B cell, because specificity is determined by the sequence of the VDJ exon, which is not altered.

Cytokines produced by follicular helper T cells determine which heavy-chain isotype is produced (see Fig. 7-11).

- The production of opsonizing IgG antibodies, which bind to phagocyte Fc receptors, is stimulated by IL-10 and other cytokines in humans and mainly by IFN-γ in mice. In antibody responses, these cytokines are produced by Tfh cells. The IgG antibodies that are produced opsonize microbes and promote their phagocytosis and intracellular killing.
- By contrast, switching to the IgE class is stimulated by IL-4 produced by Tfh cells (different from the ones that produce IFN-γ). IgE functions to eliminate helminths, acting in concert with eosinophils, which are activated by

CD40 signals, plays a key role in this process. AID converts cytosines in DNA to uracil (U). The sequential action of other enzymes results in the removal of the U's and the creation of nicks in the DNA. Such a process on both strands leads to double-stranded DNA breaks. When double-stranded DNA breaks in two switch regions are

another Th2 cytokine, IL-5. Predictably, helminths induce strong Th2 and related Tfh cell responses.

Thus, the nature of the helper T cell response to a microbe guides the subsequent antibody response, making it optimal for combating that microbe. These are excellent examples of how different components of the immune system are regulated coordinately and function together in defense against different types of microbes and how helper T cells may function as the master controllers of immune responses.

The antibody isotype produced is also influenced by the site of immune responses. For example, IgA antibody is the major isotype produced in mucosal lymphoid tissues, probably because cytokines such as transforming growth factor (TGF)-β that promote switching to IgA are made in these tissues. The B cells activated in these lymphoid tissues are also induced to express chemokine receptors and adhesion molecules that favor their migration into the sites just below mucosal epithelial barriers. IgA is the principal antibody isotype that can be actively secreted through mucosal epithelia (see Chapter 8). B-1 cells also appear to be important sources of IgA antibody in mucosal tissues, especially against nonprotein antigens.

Affinity Maturation

Affinity maturation is the process by which the affinity of antibodies produced in response to a protein antigen increases with prolonged or repeated exposure to that antigen (Fig. 7-13). Because of affinity maturation, the ability of antibodies to bind to a microbe or microbial antigen increases if the infection is persistent or recurrent. This increase in affinity is caused by point mutations in the V regions, and particularly in the antigen-binding hypervariable regions, of the genes encoding the antibodies produced. Affinity maturation is seen only in responses to helper T cell–dependent protein antigens, indicating that helper cells are critical in the process. These findings raise two intriguing questions: how do B cells undergo Ig gene mutations, and how are the high-affinity

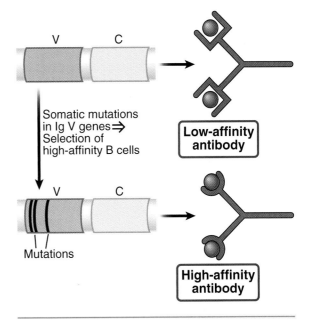

FIGURE 7-13 Affinity maturation in antibody responses. Early in the immune response, low-affinity antibodies are produced. During the germinal center reaction, somatic mutation of Ig V genes and selection of mutated B cells with high-affinity antigen receptors result in the production of antibodies with high affinity for antigen.

(i.e., most useful) B cells selected to become progressively more numerous?

Affinity maturation occurs in the germinal centers of lymphoid follicles and is the result of somatic hypermutation of Ig genes in dividing B cells, followed by the selection of high-affinity B cells by antigen (Fig. 7-14). In germinal centers the Ig genes of rapidly dividing B cells undergo numerous point mutations. The enzyme AID required for isotype switching also plays a critical role in somatic mutation. The uracils that are produced by this enzyme in Ig V-region DNA are frequently converted to thymidines during DNA replication, or they are removed and repaired by error-prone mechanisms that often lead to mutations. The frequency of Ig gene mutations is estimated to be one in 10^3 base pairs per cell per division, which is much greater than the mutation rate in most other genes. For this reason, Ig mutation in germinal center B cells is called somatic hypermutation.

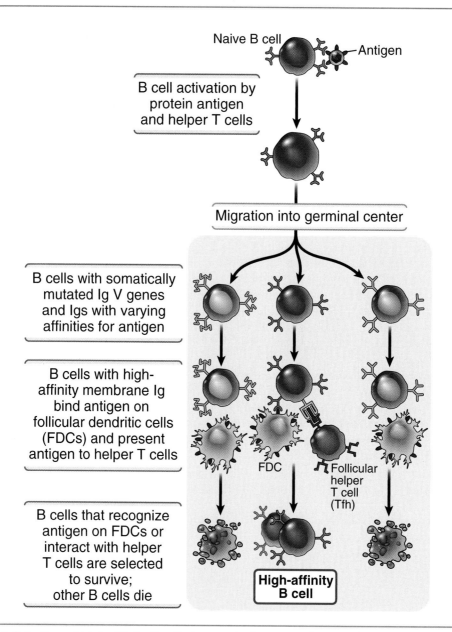

FIGURE 7-14 Selection of high-affinity B cells in germinal centers. Some activated B cells migrate into follicles to form germinal centers, where they undergo rapid proliferation and accumulate mutations in their immunoglobulin (Ig) V genes. These B cells produce antibodies with different affinities for the antigen. Follicular dendritic cells (FDCs) display the antigen, and B cells that recognize the antigen are selected to survive. FDCs display antigens by utilizing Fc receptors to bind immune complexes or by using C3 receptors to bind immune complexes with attached C3b and C3d complement proteins (not shown). B cells also bind the antigen, process it, and present it to follicular helper T (Tfh) cells in the germinal centers, and signals from the Tfh cells promote survival of the B cells. As more antibody is produced, the amount of available antigen decreases, so only the B cells that express receptors with higher affinities can bind the antigen and are selected to survive.

This extensive mutation results in the generation of different B cell clones whose Ig molecules may bind with widely varying affinities to the antigen that initiated the response. The next step in the process is the selection of B cells with the most useful antigen receptors.

Germinal center B cells undergo apoptosis unless rescued by antigen recognition and T cell help. While somatic hypermutation of Ig genes is taking place in germinal centers, the antibody secreted earlier during the immune response binds residual antigen. The antigen-antibody complexes that are formed may activate complement. These complexes are displayed by **follicular dendritic cells** (FDCs), which reside in the light zone of the germinal center and express receptors for the Fc portions of antibodies and for complement products, both of which help to display the antigen-antibody complexes. Thus, B cells that have undergone somatic hypermutation are given a chance to bind either free antigen or antigen on FDCs and to be rescued from death. These B cells can internalize the antigen, process it, and present peptides to germinal center Tfh cells, which then provide critical survival signals. High-affinity B cells efficiently bind the antigen and thus survive better than B cells that recognize the antigen weakly, akin to a process of Darwinian survival of the fittest. As the immune response to a protein antigen develops, and especially with repeated antigen exposure, the amount of antibody produced increases. As a result, the amount of available antigen decreases. The B cells that are selected to survive must be able to bind antigen at lower and lower concentrations, and therefore these are cells whose antigen receptors are of higher and higher affinity.

Generation of Plasma Cells and Memory B Cells

Activated B cells in germinal centers may differentiate into long-lived plasma cells or memory cells. The antibody-secreting cells enter the circulation and are called plasmablasts. From the blood they tend to migrate to the bone marrow or mucosal tissues, where they may survive for years as **plasma cells** and continue to produce high-affinity antibodies, even after the antigen is eliminated. It is estimated that more than half of the antibodies in the blood of a normal adult are produced by these long-lived plasma cells; thus, circulating antibodies reflect each individual's history of antigen exposure. These antibodies provide a level of immediate protection if the antigen (microbe or toxin) reenters the body.

A fraction of the activated B cells, which often are the progeny of isotype-switched high-affinity B cells, do not differentiate into active antibody secretors but instead become **memory cells.** Memory B cells do not secrete antibodies, but they circulate in the blood and reside in mucosal and other tissues. They survive for months or years in the absence of additional antigen exposure, undergo slow cycling, and are ready to respond rapidly if the antigen is reintroduced. Therefore, memory from a T-dependent antibody response can last for a lifetime.

ANTIBODY RESPONSES TO T-INDEPENDENT ANTIGENS

Polysaccharides, lipids, and other nonprotein antigens elicit antibody responses without the participation of helper T cells. Recall that these nonprotein antigens cannot bind to MHC molecules, so they cannot be seen by T cells (see Chapter 3). Many bacteria contain polysaccharide-rich capsules, and defense against such bacteria is mediated primarily by antibodies that bind to capsular polysaccharides and target the bacteria for phagocytosis. Antibody responses to T-independent antigens differ from responses to proteins, and most of these differences are attributable to the roles of helper T cells in antibody responses to proteins (Fig. 7-15). Because polysaccharide and lipid antigens often contain multivalent arrays of the same epitope, these antigens may be able to cross-link many antigen receptors on a specific B cell (see Fig. 7-2). This extensive cross-linking may activate the B cells strongly enough to stimulate their proliferation and differentiation without a requirement for T cell help. Polysaccharides also activate the complement

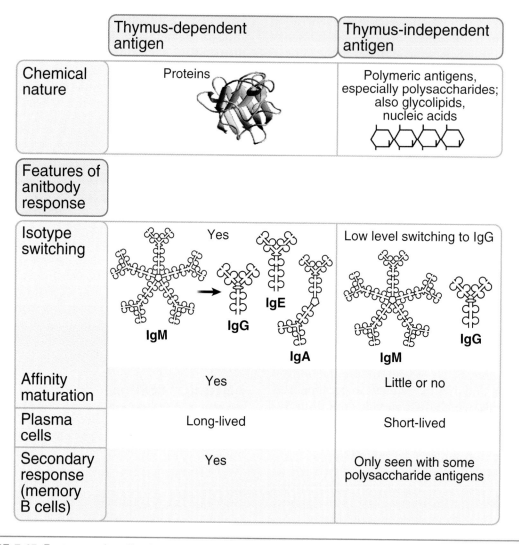

	Thymus-dependent antigen	Thymus-independent antigen
Chemical nature	Proteins	Polymeric antigens, especially polysaccharides; also glycolipids, nucleic acids
Features of anitbody response		
Isotype switching	Yes (IgM → IgG, IgE, IgA)	Low level switching to IgG (IgM → IgG)
Affinity maturation	Yes	Little or no
Plasma cells	Long-lived	Short-lived
Secondary response (memory B cells)	Yes	Only seen with some polysaccharide antigens

FIGURE 7-15 Features of antibody responses to T-dependent and T-independent antigens. T-dependent antigens (proteins) and T-independent antigens (nonproteins) induce antibody responses with different characteristics, largely reflecting the influence of helper T cells in T-dependent responses to protein antigens and the absence of T cell help in T-independent responses.

system, and many T-independent antigens engage TLRs, thus providing activating signals to the B cells that also promote B cell activation in the absence of T cell help (see Fig. 7-5). Naturally occurring protein antigens usually are not multivalent, possibly explaining why they do not induce full B cell responses themselves but depend on helper T cells to stimulate antibody production. Also, marginal-zone B cells in the spleen are the major contributors

to T-independent antibody responses to blood-borne antigens, and B-1 cells make T-independent responses to antigens in mucosal tissues and in the peritoneum.

REGULATION OF HUMORAL IMMUNE RESPONSES: ANTIBODY FEEDBACK

After B lymphocytes differentiate into antibody-secreting cells and memory cells, a fraction of

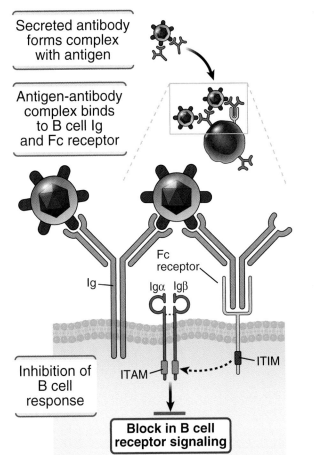

Secreted antibody forms complex with antigen

Antigen-antibody complex binds to B cell Ig and Fc receptor

Ig

Fc receptor

Igα   Igβ

Inhibition of B cell response

ITAM

ITIM

Block in B cell receptor signaling

FIGURE 7-16 **Mechanism of antibody feedback.** Secreted IgG antibodies form immune complexes (antigen-antibody complexes) with residual antigen (shown here as a virus but more commonly is a soluble antigen). The complexes interact with B cells specific for the antigen, with the membrane immunoglobulin (Ig) antigen receptors recognizing epitopes of the antigen and a certain type of Fc receptor (FcγRIIB) recognizing the bound antibody. The Fc receptors block activating signals from the antigen receptor, terminating B cell activation. The cytoplasmic domain of B cell FcγRIIB contains an ITIM that binds enzymes that inhibit antigen receptor–mediated B cell activation. *ITAM,* Immunoreceptor tyrosine-based activation motif; *ITIM,* immunoreceptor tyrosine-based inhibition motif.

these cells survive for long periods, but most of the activated B cells probably die by apoptosis. This gradual loss of the activated B cells contributes to the physiologic decline of the humoral immune response. B cells also use a special mechanism for shutting off antibody production. As IgG antibody is produced and circulates throughout the body, the antibody binds to antigen that is still available in the blood and tissues, forming immune complexes. B cells specific for the antigen may bind the antigen part of the immune complex by their Ig receptors. At the same time, the Fc tail of the attached IgG antibody may be recognized by a special type of Fc receptor expressed on B cells (as well as on many myeloid cells) called FcγRIIB (Fig. 7-16). This Fc receptor delivers inhibitory signals that shut off antigen receptor–induced signals, thereby terminating B cell responses. This process, in which antibody bound to antigen inhibits further antibody production, is called **antibody feedback.** It serves to terminate humoral immune responses once sufficient quantities of IgG antibodies have been produced. Inhibition by the FcγRIIB also functions to prevent antibody responses against self antigens, and polymorphisms in the gene encoding this receptor are associated with the autoimmune disease systemic lupus erythematosus (see Chapter 9).

■ SUMMARY

- Humoral immunity is mediated by antibodies that bind to extracellular microbes and their toxins, which are neutralized or targeted for destruction by phagocytes and the complement system.

- Humoral immune responses to nonprotein antigens are initiated by recognition of the antigens by specific membrane immunoglobulin antigen receptors of naive B cells. The binding of multivalent antigen cross-links B cell antigen receptors of specific B cells, and biochemical signals are delivered to the inside of the B cells by Ig-associated signaling proteins. These signals induce B cell clonal expansion and IgM secretion.

- Humoral immune responses to a protein antigen, called T-dependent responses, are initiated by binding of the protein to specific Ig receptors of naive B cells in lymphoid follicles. This results in the generation of signals that prepare the B cell for interaction with helper T cells. In addition, the B cells internalize and process that antigen and present class II MHC–displayed peptides to activated helper T cells also specific for the antigen. In response, the helper T cells express CD40L and secrete cytokines, which function together to stimulate high levels of B cell proliferation and differentiation. Some helper T cells, called follicular helper T cells (Tfh), migrate into germinal centers and are especially effective at stimulating isotype switching and affinity maturation.

- Heavy-chain isotype switching (or class switching) is the process by which the isotype, but not the specificity, of the antibodies produced in response to an antigen changes as the humoral response proceeds. Isotype switching is stimulated by the combination of CD40L and cytokines, both expressed by helper T cells. Different cytokines induce switching to different antibody isotypes, enabling the immune system to respond in the most effective way to different types of microbes.

- Affinity maturation is the process by which the affinity of antibodies for protein antigens increases with prolonged or repeated exposure to the antigens. The process is initiated by signals from Tfh cells, resulting in migration of the B cells into follicles and the formation of germinal centers. Here the B cells proliferate rapidly, and their Ig V genes undergo extensive somatic mutation. The antigen is displayed by follicular dendritic cells in the germinal centers. B cells that recognize the antigen with high affinity are selected to survive, giving rise to affinity maturation of the antibody response.

- The early T-dependent humoral response occurs in extrafollicular foci and generates low levels of antibodies, with little isotype switching, that are produced by short-lived plasma cells. The later response develops in germinal centers and leads to extensive isotype switching and affinity maturation, generation of long-lived plasma cells that secrete antibodies for many years, and development of long-lived memory B cells, which rapidly respond to reencounter with antigen by proliferation and secretion of high-affinity antibodies.

- Polysaccharides, lipids, and other nonprotein antigens are called T-independent antigens because they induce antibody responses without T cell help. Most T-independent antigens contain multiple identical epitopes that are able to cross-link many Ig receptors on a B cell, providing signals that stimulate B cell responses even in the absence of helper T cell activation. Antibody responses to T-independent antigens show less heavy-chain class switching and affinity maturation than typical for responses to T-dependent protein antigens.

- Secreted antibodies form immune complexes with residual antigen and shut off B cell activation by engaging an inhibitory Fc receptor on B cells.

REVIEW QUESTIONS

1. What are the signals that induce B cell responses to protein antigens and polysaccharide antigens?
2. What are the major differences between primary and secondary antibody responses to a protein antigen?
3. How do helper T cells specific for an antigen interact with B lymphocytes specific for the same antigen? Where in a lymph node do these interactions mainly occur?
4. What are the signals that induce heavy-chain isotype switching, and what is the importance of this phenomenon for host defense against different microbes?
5. What is affinity maturation? How is it induced, and how are high-affinity B cells selected to survive?
6. What are the characteristics of antibody responses to polysaccharides and lipids? What types of bacteria stimulate mostly these types of antibody responses?

Answers to and discussion of the Review Questions are available at https://studentconsult. inkling.com.

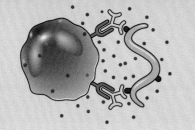

Effector Mechanisms of Humoral Immunity

Elimination of Extracellular Microbes and Toxins

Humoral immunity is the type of host defense mediated by secreted antibodies and is necessary for protection against extracellular microbes and their toxins. Antibodies prevent infections by blocking microbes from binding to and entering host cells. Antibodies also bind to microbial toxins and prevent them from damaging host cells. In addition, antibodies function to eliminate microbes, toxins, and infected cells from the body. Although antibodies are a major mechanism of adaptive immunity against extracellular microbes, they cannot reach microbes that live inside cells. However, humoral immunity is vital even for defense against microbes that live inside cells, such as viruses, because antibodies can bind to these microbes before they enter host cells or during passage from infected to uninfected cells, thus preventing spread of infection. Defects in antibody production are associated with increased susceptibility to infections by many bacteria, viruses, and parasites. Most effective vaccines work mainly by stimulating the production of antibodies.

This chapter describes how antibodies provide defense against infections, addressing the following questions:

- What are the mechanisms used by secreted antibodies to combat different types of infectious agents and their toxins?
- What is the role of the complement system in defense against microbes?
- How do antibodies combat microbes that enter through the gastrointestinal and respiratory tracts?
- How do antibodies protect the fetus and newborn from infections?

Before describing the mechanisms by which antibodies function in host defense, we summarize the features of antibody molecules that are important for these functions.

PROPERTIES OF ANTIBODIES THAT DETERMINE EFFECTOR FUNCTION

Several features of the production and structure of antibodies contribute in important ways to the functions of these molecules in host defense.

Antibodies function throughout the body and in the lumens of mucosal organs. Antibodies are produced after stimulation of B lymphocytes by antigens in peripheral lymphoid organs (lymph nodes, spleen, mucosal lymphoid tissues) and at tissue sites of inflammation. Many of the antigen-stimulated B lymphocytes differentiate into antibody-secreting plasma cells, some of which remain in lymphoid organs or inflamed tissues and others migrate to and reside in the bone marrow. Plasma cells synthesize and secrete antibodies of different heavy-chain isotypes (classes). These secreted antibodies enter the blood, from where they may reach any peripheral site of infection, and enter mucosal secretions, where they prevent infections by microbes that try to enter through epithelia. Thus, antibodies are able to perform their functions throughout the body.

Protective antibodies are produced during the first (primary) response to a microbe and in larger amounts during subsequent (secondary) responses (see Chapter 7, Fig. 7-3). Antibody production begins within the first week after infection or vaccination. The plasma cells that migrate to the bone marrow continue to produce antibodies for months or years. If the microbe again tries to infect the host, the continuously secreted antibodies provide immediate protection. Some of the antigen-stimulated B lymphocytes differentiate into memory cells, which do not secrete antibodies but are ready to respond if the antigen appears again. On encounter with the microbe, these memory cells rapidly differentiate into antibody-producing cells, providing a large burst of antibody for more effective defense against the infection. A goal of

vaccination is to stimulate the development of long-lived plasma cells and memory cells.

Antibodies use their antigen-binding (Fab) regions to bind to and block the harmful effects of microbes and toxins, and they use their Fc regions to activate diverse effector mechanisms that eliminate these microbes and toxins (Fig. 8-1). This spatial segregation of the antigen recognition and effector functions of antibody molecules was introduced in Chapter 4. Antibodies block the infectivity of microbes and the injurious effects of microbial toxins simply by binding to the microbes and toxins, using only their Fab regions to do so. Other functions of antibodies require the participation of various components of host defense, such as phagocytes and the complement system. The Fc portions of immunoglobulin (Ig) molecules, made up of the heavy-chain constant regions, contain the binding sites for Fc receptors on phagocytes and for complement proteins. The binding of antibodies to Fc and complement receptors occurs only after several Ig molecules recognize and become attached to a microbe or microbial antigen. Therefore, even the Fc-dependent functions of antibodies require antigen recognition by the Fab regions. This feature of antibodies ensures that they activate effector mechanisms only when needed—that is, when they recognize their target antigens.

Heavy-chain isotype (class) switching and affinity maturation enhance the protective functions of antibodies. Isotype switching and affinity maturation are two changes that occur in the antibodies produced by antigen-stimulated B lymphocytes, especially during responses to protein antigens (see Chapter 7). Heavy-chain isotype switching results in the production of antibodies with distinct Fc regions, capable of different effector functions (see Fig. 8-1). By switching to different antibody isotypes in response to various microbes, the humoral immune system is able to engage host mechanisms that are optimal for combating these microbes. Affinity maturation is induced by prolonged or repeated stimulation with protein antigens, and it leads to the production of antibodies with higher and higher affinities for

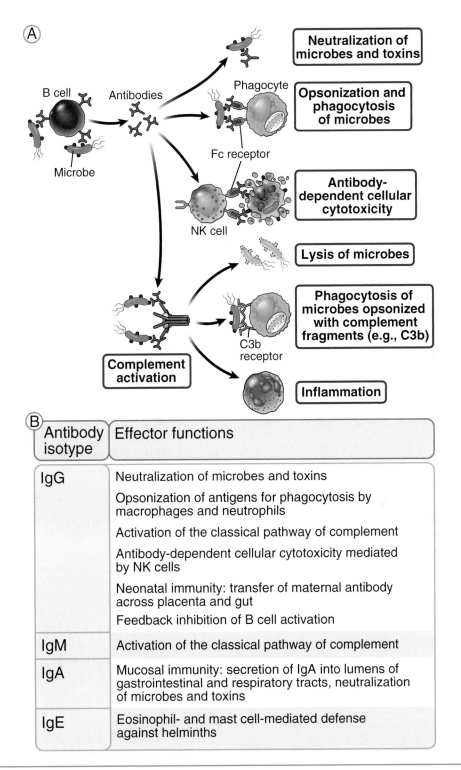

Antibody isotype	Effector functions
IgG	Neutralization of microbes and toxins
	Opsonization of antigens for phagocytosis by macrophages and neutrophils
	Activation of the classical pathway of complement
	Antibody-dependent cellular cytotoxicity mediated by NK cells
	Neonatal immunity: transfer of maternal antibody across placenta and gut
	Feedback inhibition of B cell activation
IgM	Activation of the classical pathway of complement
IgA	Mucosal immunity: secretion of IgA into lumens of gastrointestinal and respiratory tracts, neutralization of microbes and toxins
IgE	Eosinophil- and mast cell-mediated defense against helminths

FIGURE 8-1 **Effector functions of antibodies.** Antibodies are produced by the activation of B lymphocytes by antigens and other signals (not shown). Antibodies of different heavy-chain classes (isotypes) perform different effector functions, as illustrated schematically in **A** and summarized in **B**. (Some properties of antibodies are listed in Chapter 4, Figure 4-3.) *Ig,* Immunoglobulin; *NK,* natural killer.

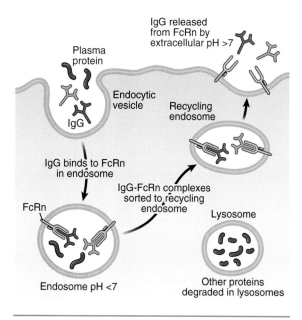

FIGURE 8-2 Neonatal Fc receptor (FcRn) contributes to the long half-life of IgG molecules. Circulating or extravascular IgG antibodies (mainly of the IgG1, IgG2 and IgG4 subclasses) are ingested by endothelial cells and phagocytes and bind the FcRn, a receptor present in the acidic environment of endosomes. In these cells, FcRn sequesters the IgG molecules in endosomal vesicles (pH ~4). The FcRn-IgG complexes recycle back to the cell surface, where they are exposed to the neutral pH (~7) of the blood, which releases the bound antibody back into the circulation or tissue fluid.

the antigen. This change increases the ability of antibodies to bind to and neutralize or eliminate microbes. The progressive increase in antibody affinity with repeated stimulation of B cells is one of the reasons for the recommended practice of giving multiple rounds of immunizations with the same antigen for generating protective immunity.

Switching to the IgG isotype prolongs the duration that an antibody remains in the blood and therefore increases the functional activity of the antibody. Most circulating proteins have half-lives of hours to days in the blood, but IgG has an unusually long half-life because of a special mechanism involving a particular Fc receptor. The neonatal Fc receptor (FcRn) is expressed in placenta, endothelium, phagocytes, and a few other cell types. In the

placenta, the FcRn transports antibodies from the mother's circulation to the fetus (discussed later). In other cell types, the FcRn protects IgG antibodies from intracellular catabolism (Fig. 8-2). FcRn is found in the endosomes of endothelial cells and phagocytes, where it binds to IgG that has been taken up by the cells. Once bound to the FcRn, the IgG is recycled back into the circulation or tissue fluids, thus avoiding lysosomal degradation. This unique mechanism for protecting a blood protein is the reason why IgG antibodies have a half-life of about 3 weeks, much longer than that of other Ig isotypes and other plasma proteins. This property of Fc regions of IgG has been exploited to increase the half-life of other proteins by coupling the proteins to an IgG Fc region (Fig. 8-3). One of several therapeutic agents based on this principle is the tumor necrosis factor (TNF) receptor–Fc fusion protein, which functions as an antagonist of TNF and is used to treat various inflammatory diseases. By coupling the extracellular domain of the receptor to the Fc portion of a human IgG molecule, the half-life of the hybrid protein becomes much greater than that of the receptor by itself.

With this introduction, we proceed to a discussion of the mechanisms used by antibodies to combat infections. Much of the chapter is devoted

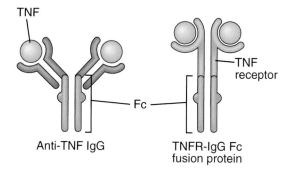

FIGURE 8-3 Antibodies and Fc-containing fusion proteins. An antibody specific for the cytokine tumor necrosis factor (TNF) (left) can bind to and block the activity of the cytokine and remain in the circulation for a long time (weeks) due to recycling by the FcRn. The extracellular domain of the TNF receptor (right) is also an antagonist of the cytokine, and coupling the soluble receptor to an IgG Fc domain results in a prolonged half-life in the blood by the same FcRn-dependent mechanism.

to effector mechanisms that are not influenced by anatomic considerations; that is, they may be active anywhere in the body. At the end of the chapter, we describe the special features of antibody functions at particular anatomic locations.

NEUTRALIZATION OF MICROBES AND MICROBIAL TOXINS

Antibodies bind to and block, or neutralize, the infectivity of microbes and the interactions of microbial toxins with host cells (Fig. 8-4). Most microbes use molecules in their envelopes or cell walls to bind to and gain entry into host cells. Antibodies may attach to these microbial surface molecules, thereby preventing the microbes from binding to and entering host cells. The most effective vaccines available today work by stimulating the production of neutralizing antibodies that block initial infection. Microbes that are able to enter host cells may replicate inside the cells and then be released and go on to infect other neighboring cells. Antibodies can neutralize the microbes during their transit from cell to cell and thus also limit the spread of infection. If an infectious

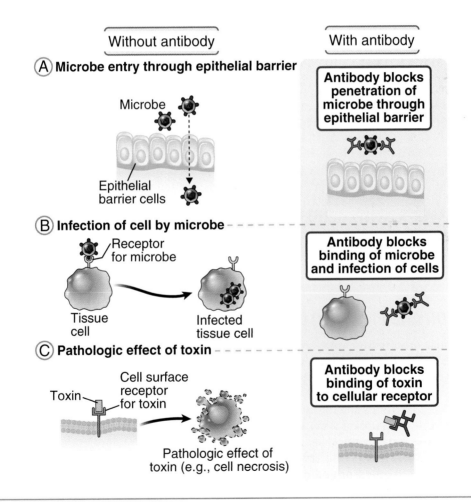

FIGURE 8-4 Neutralization of microbes and toxins by antibodies. A, Antibodies at epithelial surfaces, such as in the gastrointestinal and respiratory tracts, block the entry of ingested and inhaled microbes, respectively. **B,** Antibodies prevent the binding of microbes to cells, thereby blocking the ability of the microbes to infect host cells. **C,** Antibodies block the binding of toxins to cells, thereby inhibiting the pathologic effects of the toxins.

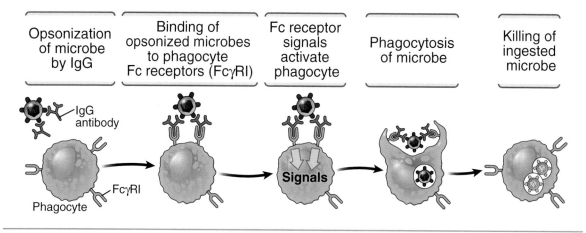

FIGURE 8-5 Antibody-mediated opsonization and phagocytosis of microbes. Antibodies of certain IgG subclasses bind to microbes and are then recognized by Fc receptors on phagocytes. Signals from the Fc receptors promote the phagocytosis of the opsonized microbes and activate the phagocytes to destroy these microbes.

microbe does colonize the host, its harmful effects may be caused by endotoxins or exotoxins, which often bind to specific receptors on host cells in order to mediate their effects. Antibodies prevent binding of the toxins to host cells and thus block their harmful effects. Emil von Behring and Shibasaburo Kitasato's demonstration of this type of protection mediated by the administration of antibodies against diphtheria toxin was the first formal demonstration of therapeutic immunity against a microbe or its toxin, then called serum therapy, and the basis for awarding Behring the first Nobel Prize in Physiology or Medicine in 1901.

OPSONIZATION AND PHAGOCYTOSIS

Antibodies coat microbes and promote their ingestion by phagocytes (Fig. 8-5). The process of coating particles for subsequent phagocytosis is called **opsonization,** and the molecules that coat microbes and enhance their phagocytosis are called **opsonins.** When several antibody molecules bind to a microbe, an array of Fc regions is formed projecting away from the microbial surface. If the antibodies belong to certain isotypes (IgG1 and IgG3 in humans), their Fc regions bind to a high-affinity receptor for the Fc regions of γ heavy chains, called FcγRI (CD64), which is expressed on neutrophils and

macrophages (Fig. 8-6). The phagocyte extends its plasma membrane around the attached microbe and ingests the microbe into a vesicle called a phagosome, which fuses with lysosomes. The binding of antibody Fc tails to FcγRI also activates the phagocytes, because the FcγRI contains a signaling chain that triggers numerous biochemical pathways in the phagocytes. Large amounts of reactive oxygen species, nitric oxide, and proteolytic enzymes are produced in the lysosomes of the activated neutrophils and macrophages, all of which contribute to the destruction of the ingested microbe.

Antibody-mediated phagocytosis is the major mechanism of defense against encapsulated bacteria, such as pneumococci. The polysaccharide-rich capsules of these bacteria protect the organisms from phagocytosis in the absence of antibody, but opsonization by antibody promotes phagocytosis and destruction of the bacteria. The spleen contains large numbers of phagocytes and is an important site of phagocytic clearance of opsonized bacteria. This is why patients who have undergone splenectomy for traumatic rupture of the organ are susceptible to disseminated infections by encapsulated bacteria.

One of the Fcγ receptors, FcγRIIB, does not mediate effector functions of antibodies but rather shuts down antibody production and reduces inflammation. The role of

Fc Receptor	Affinity for Ig	Cell distribution	Function
FcγRI (CD64)	High (K_d ~10^{-9} M); binds IgG1 and IgG3; can bind monomeric IgG	Macrophages, neutrophils; eosinophils	Phagocytosis; activation of phagocytes
FcγRIIA (CD32)	Low (K_d ~0.6–2.5x10^{-6} M)	Macrophages, neutrophils; eosinophils, platelets	Phagocytosis; cell activation (inefficient)
FcγRIIB (CD32)	Low (K_d ~0.6–2.5x10^{-6} M)	B lymphocytes, DCs, mast cells, neutrophils, macrophages	Feedback inhibition of B cells, attenuation of inflammation
FcγRIIIA (CD16)	Low (K_d ~0.6–2.5x10^{-6} M)	NK cells	Antibody-dependent cellular cytotoxicity (ADCC)
FcεRI	High (K_d ~10^{-10} M); binds monomeric IgE	Mast cells, basophils, eosinophils	Activation (degranulation) of mast cells and basophils

FIGURE 8-6 **Fc receptors.** The cellular distribution and functions of different types of human Fc receptors. *DCs,* Dendritic cells; *Ig,* immunoglobulin; *NK,* natural killer.

FcγRIIB in feedback inhibition of B cell activation was discussed in Chapter 7 (see Fig. 7-16). FcγRIIB also inhibits activation of macrophages and dendritic cells and may thus serve an anti-inflammatory function as well. Pooled IgG from healthy donors is given intravenously to treat various inflammatory diseases. This preparation is called **intravenous immune globulin (IVIG)**, and its beneficial effect in these diseases is partly mediated by its binding to FcγRIIB on various cells.

ANTIBODY-DEPENDENT CELLULAR CYTOTOXICITY

Natural killer (NK) cells and other leukocytes may bind to antibody-coated cells and destroy these cells (Fig. 8-7). NK cells express an Fcγ receptor called FcγRIII (CD16), which is one of several kinds of NK cell–activating receptors (see Chapter 2). FcγRIII binds to arrays of IgG antibodies attached to the surface of a cell, generating signals that cause the NK cell to discharge its granule proteins, which kill the opsonized cell. This process is called **antibody-dependent**

cellular cytotoxicity (ADCC). Cells infected with enveloped viruses typically express viral glycoproteins on their surface that can be recognized by specific antibodies, and this may facilitate ADCC-mediated destruction of the infected cells. ADCC is also one of the mechanisms by which therapeutic antibodies used to treat cancers eliminate tumor cells.

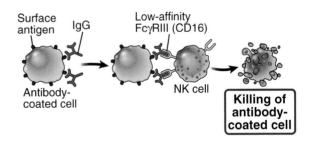

FIGURE 8-7 Antibody-dependent cellular cytotoxicity (ADCC). Antibodies of certain immunoglobulin G (IgG) subclasses (IgG1 and IgG3) bind to cells (e.g., infected cells), and their Fc regions are recognized by an Fcγ receptor on natural killer (NK) cells. The NK cells are activated and kill the antibody-coated cells.

IMMUNOGLOBULIN E– AND EOSINOPHIL/MAST CELL–MEDIATED REACTIONS

Immunoglobulin E (IgE) antibodies activate mast cell and eosinophil–mediated reactions that provide defense against helminthic parasites and are involved in allergic diseases. Most helminths are too large to be phagocytosed, and their thick integument makes them resistant to many of the microbicidal substances produced by neutrophils and macrophages. The humoral immune response to helminths is dominated by IgE antibodies. IgE binds to the worms and promotes the attachment of eosinophils through the high-affinity Fc receptor for IgE, FcεRI, which is expressed on eosinophils and mast cells. Engagement of FcεRI, together with the cytokine interleukin-5 (IL-5) produced by Th2 helper T cells reacting against the helminths, leads to activation of the eosinophils, which release their granule contents, including proteins that can kill the worms (Fig. 8-8). IgE antibodies also bind to and activate mast cells, which secrete cytokines, including chemokines, that attract more leukocytes that function to destroy the helminths.

This IgE-mediated reaction illustrates how Ig isotype switching optimizes host defense. B cells respond to helminths by switching to IgE, which is useful against helminths, but B cells respond to most bacteria and viruses by switching to IgG antibodies, which promote phagocytosis by FcγRI.

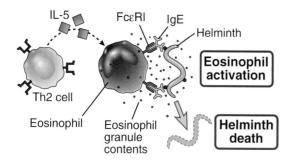

FIGURE 8-8 IgE- and eosinophil-mediated killing of helminths. IgE antibody binds to helminths and recruits and activates eosinophils via FcεRI, leading to degranulation of the cells and release of toxic mediators. IL-5 secreted by Th2 cells enhances the ability of eosinophils to kill the parasites.

As discussed in Chapters 6 and 7, these patterns of isotype switching are determined by the cytokines produced by helper T cells responding to the different types of microbes.

IgE antibodies also are involved in allergic diseases (see Chapter 11).

THE COMPLEMENT SYSTEM

The complement system is a collection of circulating and cell membrane proteins that play important roles in host defense against microbes and in antibody-mediated tissue injury. The term *complement* refers to the ability of these proteins to assist, or complement, the activity of antibodies in destroying (lysing) cells, including microbes. The complement system may be activated by microbes in the absence of antibody, as part of the innate immune response to infection, and by antibodies attached to microbes, as part of adaptive immunity (see Chapter 2, Fig. 2-12).

The activation of the complement system involves sequential proteolytic cleavage of complement proteins, leading to the generation of effector molecules that participate in eliminating microbes in different ways. This cascade of complement protein activation, like all enzymatic cascades, is capable of achieving tremendous amplification, because even a small number of activated complement molecules produced early in the cascade may generate a large number of effector molecules. Activated complement proteins become covalently attached to the cell surfaces where the activation occurs, ensuring that complement effector functions are limited to the correct sites. Normal host cells possess several regulatory mechanisms that inhibit the activation of complement and the deposition of activated complement proteins, thus preventing complement-mediated damage to healthy cells.

Pathways of Complement Activation

There are three major pathways of complement activation: the alternative and lectin pathways are initiated by microbes in the absence of antibody, and the classical pathway is initiated by certain isotypes of antibodies attached to antigens (Fig. 8-9). The alternative and lectin pathways function in

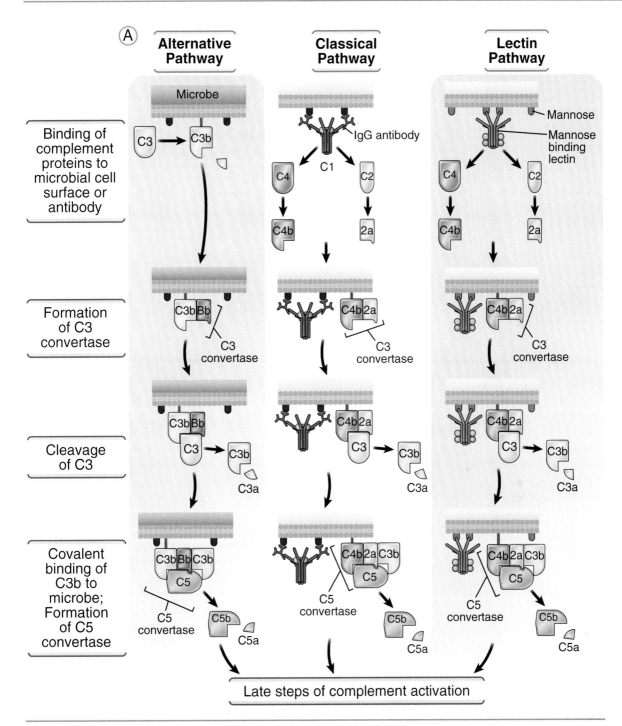

FIGURE 8-9 Early steps of complement activation. A, The steps in the activation of the alternative, classical, and lectin pathways. Although the sequence of events is similar, the three pathways differ in their requirement for antibody and the proteins used. Note that C5 is cleaved by the C5 convertase but is not a component of the enzyme.

Continued

B

Protein	Serum conc. (ug/mL)	Function
C3	640-1660	C3b binds to the surface of microbes, where it functions as an opsonin and as a component of C3 and C5 convertases C3a stimulates inflammation
Factor B	200	Bb is a serine protease and the active enzyme of C3 and C5 convertases
Factor D	1-2	Plasma serine protease that cleaves Factor B when it is bound to C3b

C

Protein	Serum conc. (ug/mL)	Function
C1 ($C1q_2r_2s_2$)		Initiates the classical pathway; C1q binds to Fc portion of antibody; C1r and C1s are proteases that lead to C4 and C2 activation
C4	150-450	C4b covalently binds to surfaces of microbes or cells where antibody is bound and complement is activated C4b binds to C2 for cleavage by C1s C4a stimulates inflammation
C2	20	C2a is a serine protease functioning as an active enzyme of C3 and C5 convertases
Mannose binding lectin (MBL)	0.8-1	Initiates the lectin pathway; MBL binds to terminal mannose residues of microbial carbohydrates. A MBL-associated protease activates C4 and C2, as in the classical pathway.

FIGURE 8-9—cont'd **B,** The important properties of the proteins involved in the early steps of the alternative pathway of complement activation. **C,** The important properties of the proteins involved in the early steps of the classical and lectin pathways. Note that C3, which is listed among the alternative pathway proteins **(B),** also is the central component of the classical and lectin pathways.

innate immune responses and were introduced in Chapter 2. Several proteins in each pathway interact in a precise sequence. The most abundant complement protein in the plasma, C3, plays a central role in all three pathways. C3 is spontaneously hydrolyzed in plasma at a low level, but its products are unstable, rapidly broken down, and lost. The early steps of all three pathways function to generate a large number of activated C3 molecules bound to the microbe or cell where complement is activated.

- The **alternative pathway** of complement activation is triggered when a breakdown product of C3 hydrolysis, called C3b, is deposited on the surface of a microbe. Here, the C3b forms stable covalent bonds with microbial proteins or polysaccharides and is thus protected from further degradation. The microbe-bound C3b binds another protein called Factor B, which is then broken down by a plasma protease called Factor D to generate the Bb fragment. This fragment remains attached to C3b, and the C3bBb complex functions as an enzyme, called the alternative pathway C3 convertase, to break down more C3. The C3 convertase is stabilized by properdin, a positive regulator of the complement system. As a result of this enzymatic activity, many more C3b and C3bBb molecules are produced and become attached to the microbe. Some of the C3bBb molecules bind an additional C3b molecule, and the resulting C3bBb3b complexes function as C5 convertases, to break down the complement protein C5 and initiate the late steps of complement activation.

- The **classical pathway** of complement activation is triggered when IgM or certain subclasses of IgG (IgG1, IgG2, and IgG3 in humans) bind to antigens (e.g., on a microbial cell surface). As a result of this binding, adjacent Fc regions of the antibodies become accessible to and bind the C1 complement protein (which is made up of a binding component called C1q and two proteases called C1r and C1s). The attached C1 becomes enzymatically active, resulting in the binding and sequential cleavage of two proteins, C4 and C2. One of the C4 fragments that is generated, C4b, becomes covalently attached to the antibody or to the microbial surface where the antibody is bound, and then binds C2, which is cleaved by active C1 to yield the C4b2a complex. This complex is the classical pathway C3 convertase, which functions to break down C3, and the C3b that is generated again becomes attached to the microbe. Some of the C3b binds to the C4b2a complex, and the resultant C4b2a3b complex functions as a C5 convertase, which cleaves the C5 complement protein.
- The **lectin pathway** of complement activation is initiated not by antibodies but by the attachment of plasma mannose-binding lectin (MBL) to microbes. Serine proteases structurally related to C1s of the classical pathway are associated with MBL and serve

to activate C4. The subsequent steps are essentially the same as in the classical pathway.

The net result of these early steps of complement activation is that microbes acquire a coat of covalently attached C3b. Note that the alternative and lectin pathways are effector mechanisms of innate immunity, whereas the classical pathway is a mechanism of adaptive humoral immunity. These pathways differ in their initiation, but once triggered, their late steps are the same.

The late steps of complement activation are initiated by the binding of C5 to the C5 convertase and subsequent proteolysis of C5, generating C5b (Fig. 8-10). The remaining components, C6, C7, C8, and C9, bind sequentially to a complex nucleated by C5b. The final protein in the pathway, C9, polymerizes to form a pore in the cell membrane through which water and ions can enter, causing death of the microbe. The C5-9 complex is called the **membrane attack complex** (MAC), and its formation is the end result of complement activation.

Functions of the Complement System

The complement system plays an important role in the elimination of microbes during innate and adaptive immune responses. The main effector functions of the complement system are illustrated in Figure 8-11.

- *Opsonization.* Microbes coated with C3b are phagocytosed by virtue of C3b being recognized by complement receptor type 1 (CR1, or CD35), which is expressed on phagocytes. Thus, C3b functions as an opsonin. Opsonization is probably the most important function of complement in defense against microbes.
- *Cell lysis.* The MAC can induce osmotic lysis of cells, including microbes. MAC-induced lysis is effective only against microbes that have thin cell walls and little or no glycocalyx, such as the *Neisseria* species of bacteria.
- *Inflammation.* The small peptide fragments C3a and C5a, which are produced by proteolysis of C3 and C5, are chemotactic for neutrophils, stimulate the release of inflammatory mediators from various leukocytes, and act on endothelial cells to enhance movement of leukocytes and plasma proteins into tissues. In this way,

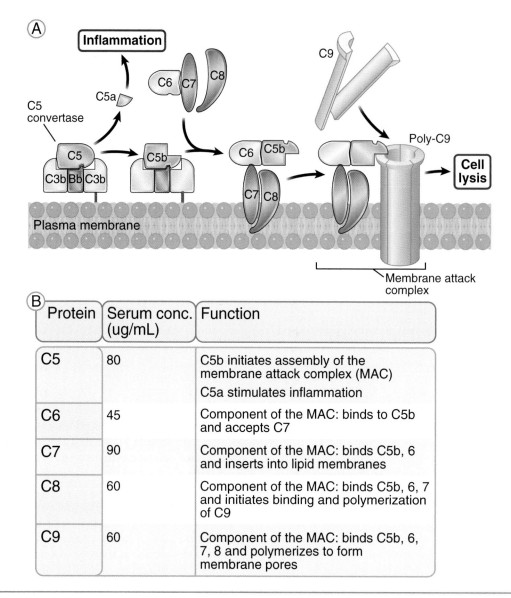

FIGURE 8-10 Late steps of complement activation. **A,** The late steps of complement activation start after the formation of the C5 convertase and are identical in the alternative and classical pathways. Products generated in the late steps induce inflammation (C5a) and cell lysis (membrane attack complex). **B,** Properties of the proteins in the late steps of complement activation.

complement fragments induce inflammatory reactions that also serve to eliminate microbes.

In addition to its antimicrobial effector functions, the complement system stimulates B cell responses and antibody production. When C3 is activated by a microbe by the alternative pathway, one of its breakdown products, C3d, is recognized by complement receptor type 2 (CR2) on B lymphocytes. Signals delivered by this receptor enhance B cell responses against the microbe. This process is described in Chapter 7 (see Fig. 7-5, *A*) and is an example of an innate immune response to a microbe (complement activation) enhancing an adaptive immune

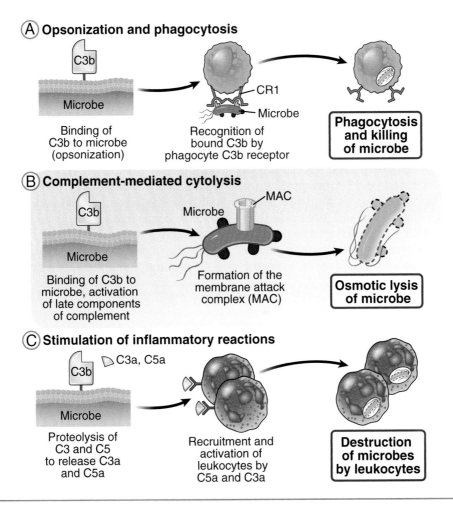

FIGURE 8-11 The functions of complement. A, C3b opsonizes microbes and is recognized by the type 1 complement receptor (CR1) of phagocytes, resulting in ingestion and intracellular killing of the opsonized microbes. Thus, C3b is an opsonin. CR1 also recognizes C4b, which may serve the same function. Other complement products, such as the inactivated form of C3b (iC3b), also bind to microbes and are recognized by other receptors on phagocytes (e.g., type 3 complement receptor, a member of integrin family of proteins). **B,** Membrane attack complex creates pores in cell membranes and induces osmotic lysis of the cells. **C,** Small peptides released during complement activation bind to receptors on neutrophils and other leukocytes and stimulate inflammatory reactions. The peptides that serve this function are mainly C5a (which is released by proteolysis of C5, not shown) and C3a.

response to the same microbe (B cell activation and antibody production). Complement proteins bound to antigen-antibody complexes are recognized by follicular dendritic cells in germinal centers, allowing the antigens to be displayed for further B cell activation and selection of high-affinity B cells. This complement-dependent antigen display is another way in which the complement system promotes antibody production.

Inherited deficiencies of complement proteins result in immune deficiencies and, in some cases, increased incidence of autoimmune disease. Deficiency of C3 results in increased susceptibility to bacterial infections that may be fatal early in life. Deficiencies of the early proteins of the classical pathway, C2 and C4, may have no clinical consequence, may result in increased susceptibility to infections, or are associated with an increased incidence of systemic lupus erythematosus, an immune complex-mediated autoimmune disease. The increased incidence of lupus may be because the classical pathway functions to eliminate immune complexes from the circulation, and these complexes accumulate in individuals lacking C2 and C4. In addition, complement deficiencies may lead to defective signaling in B cells and a failure of B cell tolerance (see Chapter 9). Deficiencies of C9 and MAC formation result in increased susceptibility to *Neisseria* infections. Some individuals inherit polymorphisms in the gene encoding MBL, leading to production of a protein that is functionally defective; such defects are associated with increased

susceptibility to infections. Inherited deficiency of the alternative pathway protein properdin also causes increased susceptibility to bacterial infection.

Regulation of Complement Activation

Mammalian cells express regulatory proteins that inhibit complement activation, thus preventing complement-mediated damage to host cells (Fig. 8-12). Many such regulatory proteins have been described, and defects in these proteins are associated with clinical syndromes caused by uncontrolled complement activation.

- A regulatory protein called C1 inhibitor (C1 INH) stops complement activation early, at

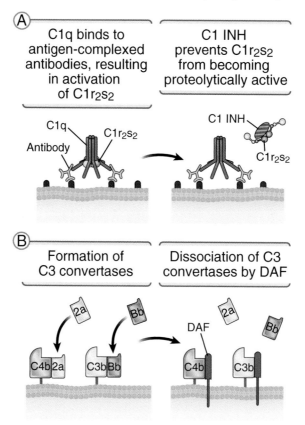

FIGURE 8-12 Regulation of complement activation. A, C1 inhibitor (C1 INH) prevents the assembly of the C1 complex, which consists of C1q, C1r, and C1s proteins, thereby blocking complement activation by the classical pathway. **B,** The lipid-linked cell surface protein decay-accelerating factor (DAF) and the type 1 complement receptor (CR1) interfere with the formation of the C3 convertase by removing Bb (in alternative pathway) or C4b (in classical pathway; not shown). Membrane cofactor protein (MCP, or CD46) and CR1 serve as cofactors for cleavage of C3b by a plasma enzyme called factor I, thus destroying any C3b that may be formed.

C | **Plasma proteins**

Protein	Plasma concentration	Function
C1 inhibitor (C1 INH)	200 µg/ml	Inhibits C1r and C1s serine protease activity
Factor I	35 µg/ml	Proteolytically cleaves C3b and C4b
Factor H	480 mg/ml	Causes dissociation of alternative pathway C3 convertase subunits Cofactor for Factor I–mediated cleavage of C3b
C4 binding protein (C4BP)	300 µg/ml	Causes dissociation of classical pathway C3 convertase subunits Cofactor for Factor I–mediated cleavage of C4b

Membrane proteins

Protein	Distribution	Function
Membrane cofactor protein (MCP, CD46)	Leukocytes, epithelial cells, endothelial cells	Cofactor for Factor I–mediated cleavage of C3b and C4b
Decay accelerating factor (DAF)	Blood cells, endothelial cells, epithelial cells	Blocks formation of C3 convertase
CD59	Blood cells, endothelial cells, epithelial cells	Blocks C9 binding and prevents formation of the MAC
Type 1 complement receptor (CR1, CD35)	Mononuclear phagocytes, neutrophils, B and T cells, erythrocytes, eosinophils, FDCs	Causes dissociation of C3 convertase subunits Cofactor for Factor I–mediated cleavage of C3b and C4b

FIGURE 8-12—cont'd **C,** The major regulatory proteins of the complement system and their functions. *FDCs,* Follicular dendritic cells; *MAC,* membrane attack complex.

the stage of C1 activation. Deficiency of C1 INH is the cause of a disease called **hereditary angioedema,** in which excessive C1 activation and the production of vasoactive proteins lead to leakage of fluid (edema) in the larynx and many other tissues.

- Decay-accelerating factor (DAF) is a glycolipid-linked cell surface protein that disrupts the binding of Bb to C3b and the binding of C4b to C2a, thus blocking C3 convertase formation and terminating complement activation by both the alternative and the classical pathways. A disease called **paroxysmal nocturnal hemoglobinuria** results from the acquired deficiency in hematopoietic stem cells of an enzyme that synthesizes the glycolipid anchor for several cell surface proteins, including the complement regulatory proteins DAF and CD59. In these patients, unregulated complement activation occurs on erythrocytes, leading to their lysis.

- A plasma enzyme called Factor I cleaves C3b into inactive fragments, with membrane cofactor protein (MCP) and the plasma protein Factor H serving as cofactors in this enzymatic process. Deficiency of the regulatory proteins Factors H and I results in increased complement activation and reduced levels of C3 because of its consumption, causing increased susceptibility to infection. Mutations in Factor H that compromise its binding to cells are associated with a rare genetic disease called atypical hemolytic uremic syndrome, in which there are clotting, vascular, and renal abnormalities. Certain genetic variants of Factor H are linked to an eye disease called age-related macular degeneration.

The presence of these regulatory proteins is an adaptation of mammals. Microbes lack the regulatory proteins and therefore the complement system can be activated on microbial surfaces much more effectively than on normal host cells. Even in mammalian cells, the regulation can be overwhelmed by too much complement activation. For instance, mammalian cells can become targets of complement if they are coated with large amounts of antibodies, as in some hypersensitivity diseases (see Chapter 11).

FUNCTIONS OF ANTIBODIES AT SPECIAL ANATOMIC SITES

The effector mechanisms of humoral immunity described so far may be active at any site in the body to which antibodies gain access. As mentioned previously, antibodies are produced in peripheral lymphoid organs and bone marrow and readily enter the blood, from which they may go anywhere. Antibodies also serve vital protective functions at two special anatomic sites: the mucosal organs and the fetus. There are special mechanisms for transporting antibodies across epithelia and across the placenta.

Mucosal Immunity

Immunoglobulin A (IgA) is produced in mucosal lymphoid tissues, transported across epithelia, and binds to and neutralizes microbes in the lumens of the mucosal organs (Fig. 8-13). Microbes often are inhaled or ingested, and antibodies that are secreted into the lumens of the respiratory or gastrointestinal tract bind to these microbes and prevent them from colonizing the host. This type of immunity is called mucosal immunity (or secretory immunity). The principal class of antibody produced in mucosal tissues is IgA. In fact, because of the vast surface area of the intestines, IgA accounts for about two-thirds of the approximately 3 grams of antibody produced daily by a healthy adult. The propensity of B cells in mucosal epithelial tissues to produce IgA is because the cytokines that induce switching to this isotype, including transforming growth factor β (TGF-β), are produced at high levels in mucosa-associated lymphoid tissues. In addition, IgA-producing B cells that are generated in regional lymph nodes or spleen tend to home to mucosal tissues in response to chemokines produced in these tissues. Also, some of the IgA is produced by a subset of B cells, called B-1 cells, which also have a propensity to migrate to mucosal tissues; these cells secrete IgA in response to nonprotein antigens, without T cell help.

Intestinal mucosal B cells are located in the lamina propria, beneath the epithelial barrier, and IgA is produced in this region. To bind and neutralize microbial pathogens in the lumen

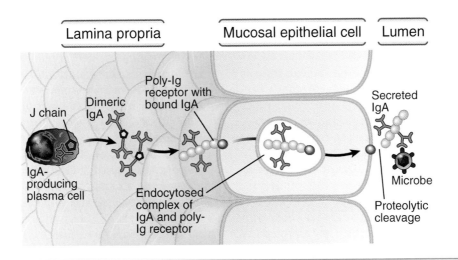

FIGURE 8-13 Transport of IgA through epithelium. In the mucosa of the gastrointestinal and respiratory tracts, IgA is produced by plasma cells in the lamina propria and is actively transported through epithelial cells by an IgA-specific Fc receptor, called the poly-Ig receptor because it recognizes IgM as well. On the luminal surface, the IgA with a portion of the bound receptor is released. Here the antibody recognizes ingested or inhaled microbes and blocks their entry through the epithelium.

before they invade, the IgA must be transported across the epithelial barrier into the lumen. Transport through the epithelium is carried out by a special Fc receptor, the poly-Ig receptor, which is expressed on the basal surface of the epithelial cells. This receptor binds IgA, endocytoses it into vesicles, and transports it to the luminal surface. Here the receptor is cleaved by a protease, and the IgA is released into the lumen still carrying a portion of the bound poly-Ig receptor (the secretory component). The attached secretory component protects the antibody from degradation by proteases in the gut. The antibody can then recognize microbes in the lumen and block their binding to and entry through the epithelium. IgA-mediated mucosal immunity is the mechanism of protection from poliovirus infection that is induced by oral immunization with the attenuated virus.

The gut contains a large number of commensal bacteria that are essential for basic functions such as absorption of food and, therefore, have to be tolerated by the immune system. IgA antibodies are produced mainly against potentially harmful and pro-inflammatory bacteria, thus blocking their entry through the gut

epithelium. Harmless commensals are tolerated by the immune system of the gut, by mechanisms that are discussed in Chapter 9.

Neonatal Immunity

Maternal antibodies are transported across the placenta to the fetus and across the gut epithelium of neonates, protecting the newborn from infections. Newborn mammals have incompletely developed immune systems and are unable to mount effective immune responses against many microbes. During their early life, they are protected from infections by antibodies acquired from their mothers. This is an example of naturally occurring passive immunity. Neonates acquire maternal IgG antibodies by two routes. During pregnancy, maternal IgG binds to the neonatal Fc receptor (FcRn) expressed in the placenta, and is actively transported into the fetal circulation. After birth, infants ingest maternal antibodies from their mothers' colostrum and milk. Ingested IgA antibodies provide mucosal immune protection to the neonate. Thus, neonates acquire the antibody profiles of their mothers and are protected from infectious microbes to which the mothers were exposed or vaccinated.

EVASION OF HUMORAL IMMUNITY BY MICROBES

Microbes have evolved numerous mechanisms to evade humoral immunity (Fig. 8-14). Many bacteria and viruses mutate their antigenic surface molecules so that they can no longer be recognized by antibodies produced in response to the original microbe. Antigenic variation typically is seen in viruses, such as influenza virus, human immunodeficiency virus (HIV), and rhinovirus. HIV mutates its genome at a high rate, and therefore different strains contain many variant forms of the major antigenic surface glycoprotein of HIV, called gp120. As a result, antibodies against exposed determinants on gp120 in any one HIV subtype may not protect against other virus subtypes that appear in infected individuals. This is one reason why gp120 vaccines are not effective in protecting people from HIV infection.

Bacteria such as *Escherichia coli* vary the antigens contained in their pili and thus evade antibody-mediated defense. The trypanosome parasite, which causes sleeping sickness, expresses new surface glycoproteins whenever it encounters antibodies against the original glycoprotein. As a result, infection with this protozoan parasite is characterized by waves of parasitemia, each wave consisting of an antigenically new parasite that is not recognized by antibodies produced against the parasites in the preceding wave. Other microbes inhibit complement activation, or resist opsonization and phagocytosis by concealing surface antigens under a hyaluronic acid capsule.

VACCINATION

Now that we have discussed the mechanisms of host defense against microbes, including cell-mediated

Mechanism of immune evasion	Example(s)	
Antigenic variation	Many viruses (e.g., influenza, HIV) Bacteria (e.g., *Neisseria gonorrhoeae*, *E. coli*)	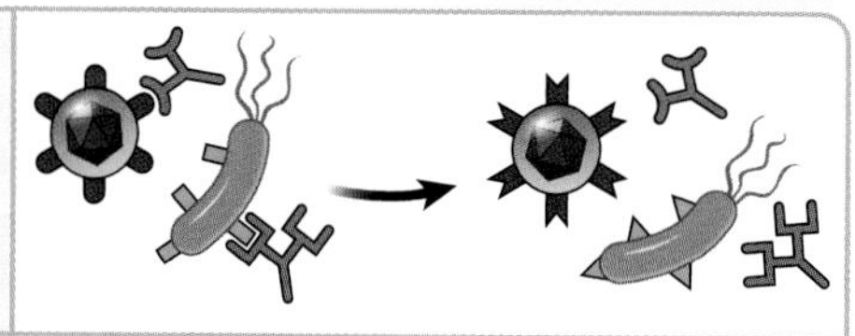
Inhibition of complement activation	Many bacteria	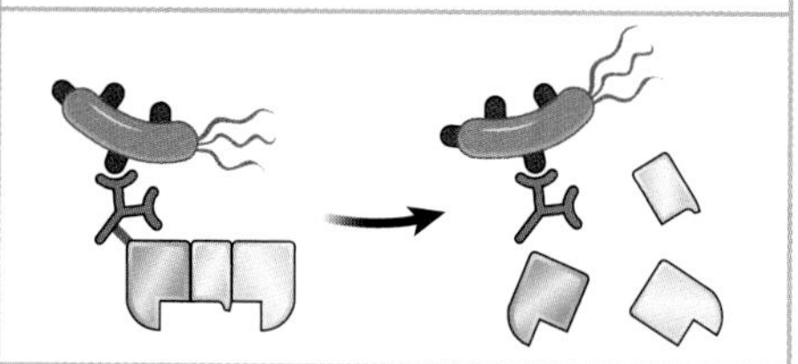
Blocking by hyaluronic acid capsule	Streptococcus	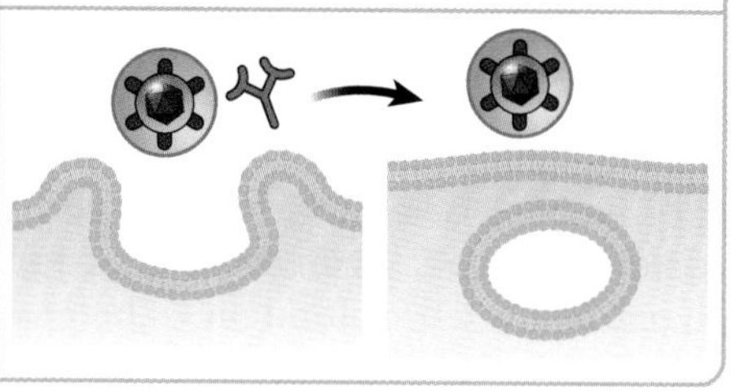

FIGURE 8-14 Evasion of humoral immunity by microbes. This figure shows some of the mechanisms by which microbes evade humoral immunity, with illustrative examples. *HIV*, Human immunodeficiency virus.

immunity in Chapter 6 and humoral immunity in this chapter, it is important to consider how these adaptive immune responses can be induced with prophylactic vaccines.

Vaccination is the process of stimulating protective adaptive immune responses against microbes by exposure to nonpathogenic forms or components of the microbes. The development of vaccines against infections has been one of the great successes of immunology. The only human disease to be intentionally eradicated from the earth is smallpox, and this was achieved by a worldwide program of vaccination. Polio is likely to be the second such disease, and as mentioned in Chapter 1, many other diseases have been largely controlled by vaccination (see Fig. 1-2).

Several types of vaccines are in use and being developed (Fig. 8-15).

- Some of the most effective vaccines are composed of attenuated microbes, which are treated to abolish their infectivity and pathogenicity while retaining their antigenicity. Immunization with these attenuated microbes stimulates the production of neutralizing antibodies against microbial antigens that protect vaccinated individuals from subsequent infections. For some infections, such as polio, the vaccines are given orally to stimulate mucosal IgA responses that protect individuals from natural infection, which occurs by the oral route.
- Vaccines composed of microbial proteins and polysaccharides, called subunit vaccines, work

Type of vaccine	Examples	Form of protection
Live attenuated, or killed, bacteria	BCG, cholera	Antibody response
Live attenuated viruses	Polio, rabies	Antibody response; cell-mediated immune response
Subunit (antigen) vaccines	Tetanus toxoid, diphtheria toxoid	Antibody response
Conjugate vaccines	*Haemophilus influenzae* infection	Helper T cell–dependent antibody response to polysaccharide antigens
Synthetic vaccines	Hepatitis virus (recombinant proteins)	Antibody response
Viral vectors	Clinical trials of HIV antigens in canary pox vector	Cell-mediated and humoral immune responses
DNA vaccines	Clinical trials ongoing for several infections	Cell-mediated and humoral immune responses

FIGURE 8-15 Vaccination strategies. A summary of different types of vaccines in use or tried, as well as the nature of the protective immune responses induced by these vaccines. *BCG*, Bacille Calmette-Guérin; *HIV*, human immunodeficiency virus.

in the same way. Some microbial polysaccharide antigens (which cannot stimulate T cell help) are chemically coupled to proteins so that helper T cells are activated and high-affinity antibodies are produced against the polysaccharides. These are called conjugate vaccines, and they are excellent examples of the practical application of our knowledge of helper T cell–B cell interactions (see Chapter 7). Immunization with inactivated microbial toxins and with microbial proteins synthesized in the laboratory stimulates antibodies that bind to and neutralize the native toxins and the microbes, respectively.

One of the continuing challenges in vaccination is to develop vaccines that stimulate cell-mediated immunity against intracellular microbes. Injected or orally administered antigens are extracellular antigens, and they induce mainly antibody responses. Many newer approaches are being tried to stimulate cell-mediated immunity by vaccination. One of these approaches is to incorporate microbial antigens into viral vectors, which will infect host cells and produce the antigens inside the cells. Another technique is to immunize individuals with DNA encoding a microbial antigen in a bacterial plasmid. The plasmid is ingested by host APCs, and the antigen is produced inside the cells. Yet another approach is to link protein antigens to monoclonal antibodies that direct the antigens into dendritic cells that are particularly efficient at cross-presentation and may thus induce CTL activation. Many of these strategies have been successfully tested in animal models, but few have shown clinical efficacy to date.

SUMMARY

- Humoral immunity is the type of adaptive immunity that is mediated by antibodies. Antibodies prevent infections by blocking the ability of microbes to invade host cells, and they eliminate microbes by activating several effector mechanisms.
- In antibody molecules, the antigen-binding (Fab) regions are spatially separate from the effector (Fc) regions. The ability of antibodies to neutralize microbes and toxins is entirely a function of the antigen-binding regions. Even Fc-dependent effector functions are activated only after antibodies bind antigens.
- Antibodies are produced in lymphoid tissues and bone marrow, but they enter the circulation and are able to reach any site of infection. Heavy-chain isotype switching and affinity maturation enhance the protective functions of antibodies.
- Antibodies neutralize the infectivity of microbes and the pathogenicity of microbial toxins by binding to and interfering with the ability of these microbes and toxins to attach to host cells.
- Antibodies coat (opsonize) microbes and promote their phagocytosis by binding to Fc receptors on phagocytes. The binding of antibody Fc regions to Fc receptors also stimulates the microbicidal activities of phagocytes.
- The complement system is a collection of circulating and cell surface proteins that play important roles in host defense. The complement system may be activated on microbial surfaces without antibodies (alternative and lectin pathways, mechanisms of innate immunity) and after the binding of antibodies to antigens (classical pathway, a mechanism of adaptive humoral immunity).
- Complement proteins are sequentially cleaved, and active components, in particular C4b and C3b, become covalently attached to the surfaces on which complement is activated. The late steps of complement activation lead to the formation of the cytolytic membrane attack complex.
- Different products of complement activation promote phagocytosis of microbes, induce cell lysis, and stimulate inflammation. Mammals express cell surface and circulating regulatory proteins that prevent inappropriate complement activation on host cells.
- IgA antibody is produced in the lamina propria of mucosal organs and is actively transported by a special Fc receptor across the epithelium into the lumen, where it blocks the ability of microbes to invade the epithelium.
- Neonates acquire IgG antibodies from their mothers through the placenta, using the

neonatal Fc receptor to capture and transport the maternal antibodies. Infants also acquire IgA antibodies from the mother's colostrum and milk by ingestion.

■ Microbes have developed strategies to resist or evade humoral immunity, such as varying their antigens and becoming resistant to complement and phagocytosis.

■ Most vaccines in current use work by stimulating the production of neutralizing antibodies. Many approaches are being tested to develop vaccines that can stimulate protective cell-mediated immune responses.

REVIEW QUESTIONS

1. What regions of antibody molecules are involved in the functions of antibodies?

2. How do heavy-chain isotype (class) switching and affinity maturation improve the ability of antibodies to combat infectious pathogens?

3. In what situations does the ability of antibodies to neutralize microbes protect the host from infections?

4. How do antibodies assist in the elimination of microbes by phagocytes?

5. How is the complement system activated?

6. Why is the complement system effective against microbes but does not react against host cells and tissues?

7. What are the functions of the complement system, and what components of complement mediate these functions?

8. How do antibodies prevent infections by ingested and inhaled microbes?

9. How are neonates protected from infection before their immune system has reached maturity?

Answers to and discussion of the Review Questions are available at https://studentconsult.inkling.com.

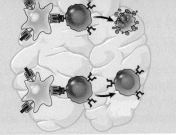

CHAPTER 9

Immunological Tolerance and Autoimmunity

Self–Nonself Discrimination in the Immune System and Its Failure

One of the remarkable properties of the normal immune system is that it can react to an enormous variety of microbes but does not react against the individual's own (self) antigens. This unresponsiveness to self antigens, also called **immunological tolerance,** is maintained despite the fact that the molecular mechanisms by which lymphocyte receptor specificities are generated are not biased to exclude receptors for self antigens. In other words, lymphocytes with the ability to recognize self antigens are constantly being generated during the normal process of lymphocyte maturation. Furthermore, many self antigens have ready access to the immune system, so unresponsiveness to these antigens cannot be maintained simply by concealing them from lymphocytes. It follows that there must exist mechanisms that prevent immune responses to self antigens. These mechanisms are responsible for one of the cardinal features of the immune system—namely, its ability to discriminate between self and nonself (usually microbial) antigens. If these mechanisms fail, the immune system may attack the individual's own cells and tissues. Such reactions are called **autoimmunity,** and the diseases they cause are called autoimmune diseases. In addition to tolerating the presence of self antigens, the immune system has to coexist with many commensal microbes that live within their human hosts, often in a state of symbiosis, and the immune system of a pregnant female has to accept the presence of a fetus that expresses antigens derived from the father. Unresponsiveness to commensal microbes and the fetus is maintained by many of the same mechanisms involved in unresponsiveness to self.

In this chapter we address the following questions:

- How does the immune system maintain unresponsiveness to self antigens?
- What are the factors that may contribute to the loss of self-tolerance and the development of autoimmunity?
- How does the immune system maintain unresponsiveness to commensal microbes and the fetus?

This chapter begins with a discussion of the important principles and features of self-tolerance. Then we discuss the different mechanisms that maintain tolerance to self antigens as well as commensal microbes and the fetus, and how mechanisms of tolerance may fail, resulting in autoimmunity.

IMMUNOLOGICAL TOLERANCE: SIGNIFICANCE AND MECHANISMS

Immunological tolerance is a lack of response to antigens that is induced by exposure of lymphocytes to these antigens. When lymphocytes with receptors for a particular antigen encounter this antigen, any of several outcomes is possible. The lymphocytes may be activated to proliferate and to differentiate into effector and memory cells, leading to a productive immune response; antigens that elicit such a response are said to be **immunogenic.** The lymphocytes may be functionally inactivated or killed, resulting in tolerance; antigens that induce tolerance are said to be **tolerogenic.** In some situations, the antigen-specific lymphocytes may not react in any way; this phenomenon has been called immunological ignorance, implying that the lymphocytes simply ignore the presence of the antigen. Normally, microbes are immunogenic and self antigens are tolerogenic.

The choice between lymphocyte activation and tolerance is determined largely by the nature of the antigen and the additional signals present when the antigen is displayed to the immune system. In fact, the same antigen may be administered in different ways to induce an immune response or tolerance. This experimental observation has been exploited to analyze what factors determine whether activation or tolerance develops as a consequence of encounter with an antigen.

The phenomenon of immunological tolerance is important for several reasons. First, as we stated at the outset, self antigens normally induce tolerance, and failure of self-tolerance is the underlying cause of autoimmune diseases. Second, if we learn how to induce tolerance in lymphocytes specific for a particular antigen, we may be able to use this knowledge to prevent or control unwanted immune reactions. Strategies for inducing tolerance are being tested to treat allergic and autoimmune diseases and to prevent the rejection of organ transplants. The same strategies may be valuable in gene therapy to prevent immune responses against the products of newly expressed genes or vectors and even for stem cell transplantation if the stem cell donor is genetically different from the recipient.

Immunological tolerance to different self antigens may be induced when developing lymphocytes encounter these antigens in the generative (central) lymphoid organs, a process called central tolerance, or when mature lymphocytes encounter self antigens in peripheral (secondary) lymphoid organs or peripheral tissues, called peripheral tolerance (Fig. 9-1). Central tolerance is a mechanism of tolerance only to self antigens that are present in the generative lymphoid organs—namely, the bone marrow and thymus. Tolerance to self antigens that are not present in these organs must be induced and maintained by peripheral mechanisms. We have only limited knowledge of how many and which self antigens induce central or peripheral tolerance or are ignored by the immune system.

With this brief background, we proceed to a discussion of the mechanisms of immunological

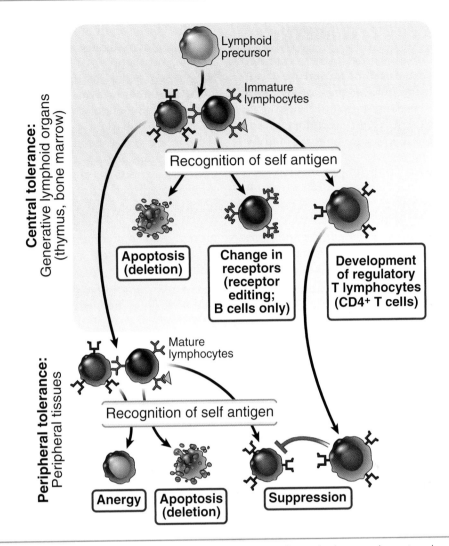

Central tolerance: Generative lymphoid organs (thymus, bone marrow)

Peripheral tolerance: Peripheral tissues

Lymphoid precursor

Immature lymphocytes

Recognition of self antigen

Apoptosis (deletion)

Change in receptors (receptor editing; B cells only)

Development of regulatory T lymphocytes (CD4+ T cells)

Mature lymphocytes

Recognition of self antigen

Anergy

Apoptosis (deletion)

Suppression

FIGURE 9-1 Central and peripheral tolerance to self antigens. Central tolerance: Immature lymphocytes specific for self antigens may encounter these antigens in the generative (central) lymphoid organs and are deleted; B lymphocytes change their specificity (receptor editing); and some T lymphocytes develop into regulatory T cells. Some self-reactive lymphocytes may complete their maturation and enter peripheral tissues. Peripheral tolerance: Mature self-reactive lymphocytes may be inactivated or deleted by encounter with self antigens in peripheral tissues or suppressed by regulatory T cells.

tolerance and how the failure of each mechanism may result in autoimmunity. Tolerance in T cells, particularly CD4+ helper T lymphocytes, is discussed first because many of the mechanisms of self-tolerance were defined by studies of these cells. In addition, CD4+ helper T cells orchestrate virtually all immune responses to protein antigens, so tolerance in these cells may be enough to prevent both cell-mediated and humoral immune responses against self proteins. Conversely, failure of tolerance in helper T cells may result in autoimmunity manifested by T cell–mediated attack against self antigens or by the production of autoantibodies against self proteins.

CENTRAL T LYMPHOCYTE TOLERANCE

The principal mechanisms of central tolerance in T cells are death of immature T cells and the generation of CD4$^+$ regulatory T cells (Fig. 9-2). The lymphocytes that develop in the thymus consist of cells with receptors capable of recognizing many antigens, both self and foreign. If a lymphocyte that has not completed its maturation interacts strongly with a self antigen, displayed as a peptide bound to a self major histocompatibility complex (MHC) molecule, that lymphocyte receives signals that trigger apoptosis. Thus, the self-reactive cell dies before it can become functionally competent. This process, called **negative selection** (see Chapter 4), is a major mechanism of central tolerance. The process of negative selection affects self-reactive CD4$^+$ T cells and CD8$^+$ T cells, which recognize self peptides displayed by class II MHC and class I MHC molecules, respectively. It is not known why immature lymphocytes die upon receiving strong T cell receptor (TCR) signals in the thymus, whereas mature lymphocytes that get strong TCR signals in the periphery are activated.

Some immature CD4$^+$ T cells that recognize self antigens in the thymus with high affinity do not die but develop into regulatory T cells and enter peripheral tissues (see Fig. 9-2). The functions of regulatory T cells are described later in the chapter. What determines whether a thymic CD4$^+$ T cell that recognizes a self antigen will die or become a regulatory T cell is also not known.

Immature lymphocytes may interact strongly with an antigen if the antigen is present at high concentrations in the thymus and if the lymphocytes express receptors that recognize the antigen with high affinity. Antigens that induce negative selection may include proteins that are abundant throughout the body, such as plasma proteins and common cellular proteins.

Surprisingly, many self proteins that are normally present only in certain peripheral tissues are also expressed in some of the epithelial cells of the thymus. A protein called **AIRE** (autoimmune regulator) is responsible for the thymic expression of these peripheral tissue antigens. Mutations in the *AIRE* gene are the cause of a rare disorder called autoimmune polyendocrine syndrome. In this disorder, several tissue antigens are not expressed in the thymus because of a lack of functional AIRE protein, so immature T cells specific for these antigens are not eliminated and do not develop into regulatory cells, remaining

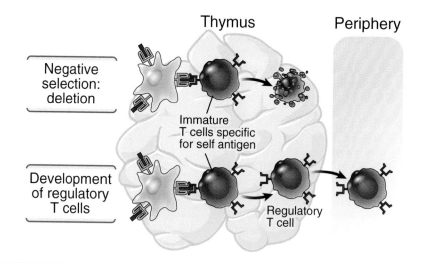

FIGURE 9-2 Central T cell tolerance. Strong recognition of self antigens by immature T cells in the thymus may lead to death of the cells (negative selection, or deletion), or the development of regulatory T cells that enter peripheral tissues.

capable of reacting harmfully against the self antigens. These antigens are expressed normally in the appropriate peripheral tissues (because only thymic expression is under the control of AIRE). Therefore, T cells specific for these antigens emerge from the thymus, encounter the antigens in the peripheral tissues, and attack the tissues and cause disease. It is not clear why endocrine organs are the major targets of this autoimmune attack. Although this rare syndrome illustrates the importance of negative selection in the thymus for maintaining self-tolerance, it is not known if defects in negative selection contribute to common autoimmune diseases.

Negative selection is imperfect, and numerous self-reactive lymphocytes are present in healthy individuals. As discussed next, peripheral mechanisms may prevent the activation of these lymphocytes.

PERIPHERAL T LYMPHOCYTE TOLERANCE

Peripheral tolerance is induced when mature T cells recognize self antigens in peripheral tissues, leading to functional inactivation (anergy) or death, or when the self-reactive lymphocytes are suppressed by regulatory T cells (Fig. 9-3). Each of these mechanisms of peripheral T cell tolerance is described in this section. Peripheral tolerance is clearly important for preventing T cell responses to self antigens that are not present in the thymus, and it also may provide backup mechanisms for preventing autoimmunity in situations where central tolerance is incomplete.

Antigen recognition without adequate costimulation results in T cell anergy or death, or makes T cells sensitive to

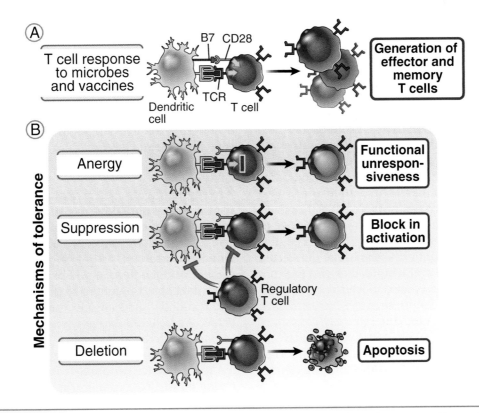

FIGURE 9-3 **Peripheral T cell tolerance. A,** Normal T cell responses require antigen recognition and costimulation. **B,** Three major mechanisms of peripheral T cell tolerance are illustrated: cell-intrinsic anergy, suppression by regulatory T cells, and deletion (apoptotic cell death).

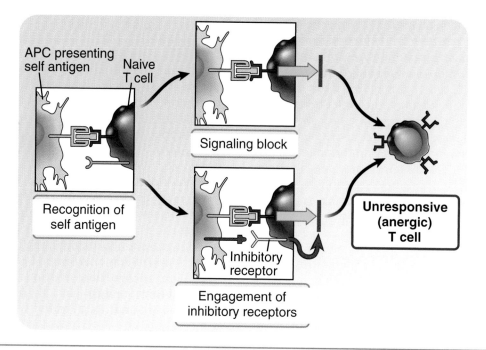

FIGURE 9-4 T cell anergy. If a T cell recognizes antigen without strong costimulation, the T cell receptors may lose their ability to deliver activating signals, or the T cell may engage inhibitory receptors, such as cytotoxic T lymphocyte–associated protein 4 (CTLA-4), that block activation.

suppression by regulatory T cells. As noted in previous chapters, naive T lymphocytes need at least two signals to induce their proliferation and differentiation into effector and memory cells: Signal 1 is always antigen, and signal 2 is provided by costimulators that are expressed on antigen-presenting cells (APCs), typically as part of the innate immune response to microbes (or to damaged host cells) (see Chapter 5, Fig. 5-6). It is believed that dendritic cells in normal uninfected tissues and peripheral lymphoid organs are in a resting (or immature) state, in which they express little or no costimulators, such as B7 proteins (see Chapter 5). These dendritic cells may constantly process and display the self antigens that are present in the tissues. T lymphocytes with receptors for the self antigens are able to recognize the antigens and thus receive signals from their antigen receptors (signal 1), but the T cells do not receive strong costimulation because there is no accompanying innate immune response. The presence or absence of costimulation is a major

factor determining whether T cells are activated or tolerized. Some examples illustrating this concept are discussed below.

Anergy

Anergy in T cells refers to long-lived functional unresponsiveness that is induced when these cells recognize self antigens (Fig. 9-4). Self antigens are normally displayed with low levels of costimulators, as discussed earlier. Antigen recognition without adequate costimulation is thought to be the basis of anergy induction, by mechanisms that are described below. Anergic cells survive but are incapable of responding to the antigen.

The two best-defined mechanisms responsible for the induction of anergy are abnormal signaling by the TCR complex and the delivery of inhibitory signals from receptors other than the TCR complex.

• When T cells recognize antigens without costimulation, the TCR complex may lose its ability to transmit activating signals. In some cases, this is related to the activation of enzymes (ubiquitin ligases) that modify signaling proteins and target them for intracellular destruction by proteases.

- On recognition of self antigens, T cells also may preferentially engage one of the inhibitory receptors of the CD28 family, cytotoxic T lymphocyte–associated antigen 4 (CTLA-4, or CD152) or programmed death protein 1 (PD-1), which were introduced in Chapter 5. Anergic T cells may express higher levels of these inhibitory receptors, which will inhibit responses to subsequent antigen recognition. The functions and mechanisms of action of these receptors are described in more detail below.

Although several experimental animal models support the importance of T cell anergy in the maintenance of self-tolerance, it is still not clear if anergic T cells specific for self antigens are present in most healthy people and if their loss is associated with the development of autoimmunity. Forced expression of high levels of B7 costimulators in a tissue in a mouse, using transgenic technology, results in autoimmune reactions against antigens in that tissue. Thus, artificially providing second signals may break anergy and activate autoreactive T cells.

Regulation of T Cell Responses by Inhibitory Receptors

The concept that immune responses are influenced by a balance between activating and inhibitory receptors is established for all lymphocyte populations, including NK cells (see Chapter 2), B lymphocytes (see Chapter 7), and T cells. In T cells, the best-defined inhibitory receptors are CTLA-4 and PD-1.

- *CTLA-4.* CTLA-4 is expressed transiently on activated CD4$^+$ T cells and constitutively on regulatory T cells (described below). It functions to terminate activation of responding T cells and also mediates the suppressive function of regulatory T cells. CTLA-4 works by blocking and removing B7 molecules from the surface of APCs, thus reducing costimula-

tion and preventing the activation of T cells; CTLA-4 might also deliver inhibitory signals to T cells. It is intriguing that CTLA-4, which is involved in shutting off T cell responses, recognizes the same B7 costimulators that bind to CD28 and initiate T cell activation. One theory to explain how T cells choose CD28 or CTLA-4, with these very different outcomes, is based on the fact that CTLA-4 has a higher affinity for B7 molecules than does CD28. Thus, when B7 levels are low (as would be expected normally when APCs are displaying self antigens), the receptor that is preferentially engaged is the high-affinity CTLA-4, but when B7 levels are high (as in infections), the low-affinity activating receptor CD28 is engaged to a greater extent.

- *PD-1.* PD-1 is expressed on CD4$^+$ and CD8$^+$ T cells after antigen stimulation. It has an immunoreceptor tyrosine-based inhibitory motif (ITIM) typical of receptors that deliver inhibitory signals. PD-1 terminates responses of T cells to self antigens and also to chronic infections, notably virus infections (see Chapter 6, Fig. 6-15).

One of the most impressive therapeutic applications of our understanding of these inhibitory receptors is treatment of cancer patients with antibodies that block these receptors. Such treatment leads to enhanced antitumor immune responses and tumor regression in a significant fraction of the patients (see Chapter 10). This type of therapy has been termed **checkpoint blockade**, because the inhibitory receptors impose checkpoints in immune responses, and the treatment blocks these checkpoints ("removes the brakes" on immune responses). Predictably, patients treated with checkpoint blockade often develop autoimmune reactions, consistent with the idea that the inhibitory receptors are constantly functioning to keep autoreactive T cells in check. In experimental animals, if CTLA-4 or PD-1 molecules are blocked (by treatment with antibodies) or eliminated (by gene knockout), the animals develop autoimmune reactions against their own tissues. Polymorphisms in the *CTLA4* gene have been associated with some autoimmune diseases in humans. Rare patients

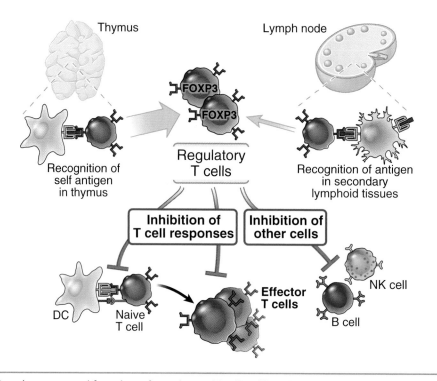

FIGURE 9-5 **Development and function of regulatory T cells.** CD4+ T cells that recognize self antigens may differentiate into regulatory cells in the thymus or peripheral tissues, in a process that is dependent on the transcription factor FoxP3. (The larger arrow from the thymus, compared to the one from peripheral tissues, indicates that most of these cells probably arise in the thymus.) These regulatory cells inhibit the activation of naive T cells and their differentiation into effector T cells by contact-dependent mechanisms or by secreting cytokines that inhibit T cell responses. The generation and maintenance of regulatory T cells also require interleukin-2 (not shown). *DC*, Dendritic cell.

with mutations in one of their two copies of the *CTLA4* gene also develop multiorgan inflammation (and a profound, as yet unexplained, defect in antibody production).

Several other receptors on T cells other than CTLA-4 and PD-1 have been shown to inhibit immune responses and are currently the targets of checkpoint blockade therapy. The role of these receptors in maintaining tolerance to self antigens is not clearly established.

Immune Suppression by Regulatory T Cells

Regulatory T cells develop in the thymus or peripheral tissues on recognition of self antigens and suppress the activation of potentially harmful lymphocytes specific for these self antigens (Fig. 9-5).

The majority of self-reactive regulatory T cells probably develop in the thymus (see Fig. 9-2), but they may also arise in peripheral lymphoid organs. Most regulatory T cells are CD4+ and express high levels of CD25, the α chain of the interleukin-2 (IL-2) receptor. They also express a transcription factor called FoxP3, which is required for the development and function of the cells. Mutations of the gene encoding FoxP3 in humans or in mice cause a systemic, multiorgan autoimmune disease, demonstrating the importance of FoxP3+ regulatory T cells for the maintenance of self-tolerance. The human disease is known by the acronym IPEX, for *immune dysregulation, polyendocrinopathy, enteropathy, X*-linked syndrome. The severe autoimmunity seen in FoxP3-deficient mice and humans is the best evidence for the importance of regulatory T cells in maintaining self-tolerance.

The survival and function of regulatory T cells are dependent on the cytokine IL-2. This role of IL-2 accounts for the severe autoimmune disease that develops in mice in which IL-2 or IL-2 receptor genes are deleted. Recall that we introduced IL-2 in Chapter 5 as a cytokine made by antigen-activated T cells that stimulates proliferation of these cells. Thus, IL-2 is an example of a cytokine that serves two opposite roles: it promotes immune responses by stimulating T cell proliferation, and it inhibits immune responses by maintaining functional regulatory T cells. Numerous clinical trials are testing the ability of IL-2 to promote regulation and control harmful immune reactions, such as graft rejection and inflammation in autoimmune diseases.

The cytokine transforming growth factor β (TGF-β) also plays a role in the generation of regulatory T cells, perhaps by stimulating expression of the FoxP3 transcription factor. Many cell types can produce TGF-β, but the source of TGF-β for inducing regulatory T cells in the thymus or peripheral tissues is not defined.

Regulatory T cells may suppress immune responses by several mechanisms.
- Some regulatory cells produce cytokines (e.g., IL-10, TGF-β) that inhibit the activation of lymphocytes, dendritic cells, and macrophages.
- Regulatory cells express CTLA-4, which, as discussed earlier, may block or remove B7 molecules made by APCs and make these APCs incapable of providing costimulation via CD28 and activating T cells.
- Regulatory T cells, by virtue of the high level of expression of the IL-2 receptor, may bind and consume this essential T cell growth factor, thus reducing its availability for responding T cells.

The great interest in regulatory T cells has in part been driven by the hypothesis that the underlying abnormality in some autoimmune diseases in humans is defective regulatory T cell function or the resistance of pathogenic

T cells to regulation. However, the importance of defects in regulatory T cells in common human autoimmune diseases is not established, perhaps because it has proved difficult to identify regulatory T cells specific for self antigens in humans. There is also growing interest in cellular therapy with regulatory T cells to treat graft-versus-host disease, graft rejection, and autoimmune disorders.

Deletion: Apoptosis of Mature Lymphocytes

Recognition of self antigens may trigger pathways of apoptosis that result in elimination (deletion) of the self-reactive lymphocytes (Fig. 9-6). There are two likely mechanisms of death of mature T lymphocytes induced by self antigens:
- Antigen recognition induces the production of pro-apoptotic proteins in T cells that induce cell death by causing mitochondrial proteins to leak out and activate caspases, cytosolic enzymes that induce apoptosis. In normal immune responses, the activity of these pro-apoptotic proteins is counteracted by anti-apoptotic proteins that are induced by costimulation and by growth factors produced during the responses. However, self antigens, which are recognized without strong costimulation, do not stimulate production of anti-apoptotic proteins, and the relative deficiency of survival signals induces death of the cells that recognize these antigens.
- Recognition of self antigens may lead to the coexpression of death receptors and their ligands. This ligand-receptor interaction generates signals through the death receptor that culminate in the activation of caspases and apoptosis. The best-defined death receptor–ligand pair involved in self-tolerance is a protein called Fas (CD95), which is expressed on many cell types, and Fas ligand (FasL), which is expressed mainly on activated T cells. The Fas pathway may also be involved in death of some B cells in germinal centers, discussed later.

Evidence from genetic studies supports the role of apoptosis in self-tolerance. Eliminating

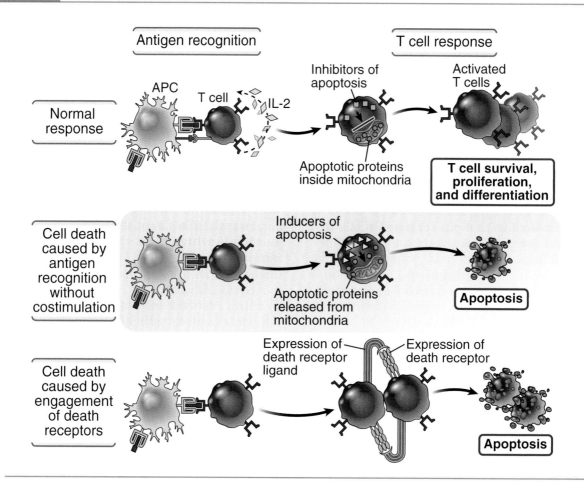

FIGURE 9-6 Mechanisms of apoptosis of T lymphocytes. T cells respond to antigen presented by normal antigen-presenting cells (APCs) by secreting interleukin-2 (IL-2), expressing anti-apoptotic (pro-survival) proteins, and undergoing proliferation and differentiation. The anti-apoptotic proteins prevent the release of mediators of apoptosis from mitochondria. Self antigen recognition by T cells without costimulation may lead to relative deficiency of intracellular anti-apoptotic proteins, and the excess of pro-apoptotic proteins causes cell death by inducing release of mediators of apoptosis from mitochondria (death by the mitochondrial [intrinsic] pathway of apoptosis). Alternatively, self antigen recognition may lead to expression of death receptors and their ligands, such as Fas and Fas ligand (FasL), on lymphocytes, and engagement of the death receptor leads to apoptosis of the cells by the death receptor (extrinsic) pathway.

the mitochondrial pathway of apoptosis in mice results in a failure of deletion of self-reactive T cells in the thymus and also in peripheral tissues. Mice with mutations in the *fas* and *fasl* genes and children with mutations in *FAS* all develop autoimmune diseases with lymphocyte accumulation. Children with mutations in the genes encoding caspase-8 or -10, which are downstream of FAS signaling, also have similar

autoimmune diseases. The human diseases, collectively called the autoimmune lymphoproliferative syndrome, are rare and are the only known examples of defects in apoptosis causing a complex autoimmune phenotype.

From this discussion of the mechanisms of T cell tolerance, it should be clear that self antigens differ from foreign microbial antigens in

Feature of antigen	Tolerogenic self antigens	Immunogenic foreign antigens
	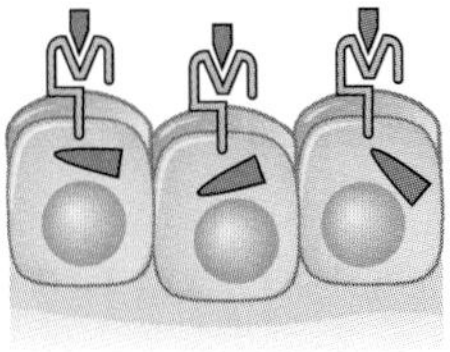 Tissue	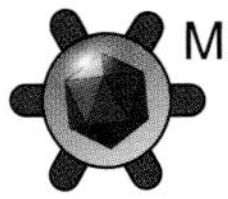 Microbe
Location of antigens	Presence in generative organs (some self antigens) induces negative selection and other mechanisms of central tolerance	Presence in blood and peripheral tissues (most microbial antigens) permits concentration in peripheral lymphoid organs
Costimulation	Deficiency of costimulators may lead to T cell anergy or apoptosis, development of Treg, or sensitivity to suppression by Treg	Expression of costimulators, typically seen with microbes, promotes lymphocyte survival and activation
Duration of antigen exposure	Long-lived persistence (throughout life); prolonged TCR engagement may induce anergy and apoptosis	Short exposure to microbial antigen reflects effective immune response

FIGURE 9-7 Features of protein antigens that influence the choice between T cell tolerance and activation. This figure summarizes some of the characteristics of self and foreign (e.g., microbial) protein antigens that determine why the self antigens induce tolerance and microbial antigens stimulate T cell–mediated immune responses. *TCR*, T cell receptor; *Treg*, T regulatory cells.

several ways, which contribute to the choice between tolerance induced by the former and activation by the latter (Fig. 9-7).

- Self antigens are present in the thymus, where they induce deletion and generate regulatory T cells; by contrast, most microbial antigens tend to be excluded from the thymus, because they are typically captured from their sites of entry and transported into peripheral lymphoid organs (see Chapter 3).
- Self antigens are displayed by resting APCs in the absence of innate immunity and second signals, thus favoring the induction of T cell anergy or death, or suppression by regulatory T cells. By contrast, microbes elicit innate immune reactions, leading to the expression of costimulators and cytokines that promote T cell proliferation and differentiation into effector cells.
- Self antigens are present throughout life and may therefore cause prolonged or repeated TCR

engagement, again promoting anergy, apoptosis, and the development of regulatory T cells.

B LYMPHOCYTE TOLERANCE

Self polysaccharides, lipids, and nucleic acids are T-independent antigens that are not recognized by T cells. These antigens must induce tolerance in B lymphocytes to prevent autoantibody production. Self proteins may not elicit autoantibody responses because of tolerance in helper T cells and in B cells. It is suspected that diseases associated with autoantibody production, such as systemic lupus erythematosus, are caused by defective tolerance in both B lymphocytes and helper T cells.

Central B Cell Tolerance

When immature B lymphocytes interact strongly with self antigens in the bone

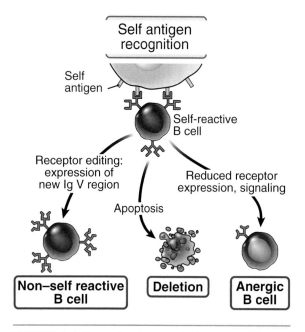

FIGURE 9-8 Central tolerance in immature B lymphocytes. An immature B cell that recognizes self antigen in the bone marrow changes its antigen receptor (receptor editing), dies by apoptosis (negative selection, or deletion), or reduces antigen receptor expression and becomes functionally unresponsive.

marrow, the B cells either change their receptor specificity (receptor editing) or are killed (deletion) (Fig. 9-8).

- *Receptor editing.* Some immature B cells that recognize self antigens in the bone marrow may reexpress RAG genes, resume immunoglobulin (Ig) light-chain gene recombination, and express a new Ig light chain (see Chapter 4). This new light chain associates with the previously expressed Ig heavy chain to produce a new antigen receptor that may no longer be specific for the self antigen. This process of changing receptor specificity, called **receptor editing,** reduces the chance that potentially harmful self-reactive B cells will leave the marrow. It is estimated that 25% to 50% of mature B cells in a normal individual may have undergone receptor editing during their maturation. (There is no evidence that developing T cells can undergo receptor editing.)
- *Deletion.* If editing fails, immature B cells that strongly recognize self antigens receive death signals and die by apoptosis. This process of

deletion is similar to negative selection of immature T lymphocytes. As in the T cell compartment, negative selection of B cells eliminates lymphocytes with high-affinity receptors for abundant, and usually widely expressed, cell membrane or soluble self antigens.
- *Anergy.* Some self antigens, such as soluble proteins, may be recognized in the bone marrow with low avidity. B cells specific for these antigens survive, but antigen receptor expression is reduced, and the cells become functionally unresponsive (anergic).

Peripheral B Cell Tolerance

Mature B lymphocytes that encounter self antigens in peripheral lymphoid tissues become incapable of responding to that antigen (Fig. 9-9). According to one hypothesis, if B cells recognize an antigen and do not receive T cell help (because helper T cells have been eliminated or are tolerant), the B cells become anergic because of a block in signaling from the antigen receptor. Anergic B cells may leave lymphoid follicles and are subsequently excluded from the follicles. These excluded B cells may die because they do not receive necessary survival stimuli. B cells that

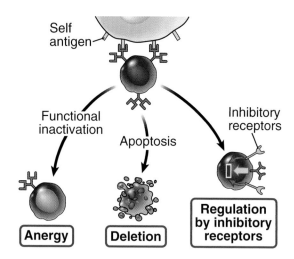

FIGURE 9-9 Peripheral tolerance in B lymphocytes. A mature B cell that recognizes a self antigen without T cell help is functionally inactivated and becomes incapable of responding to that antigen (anergy), or it dies by apoptosis (deletion), or its activation is suppressed by engagement of inhibitory receptors.

recognize self antigens in the periphery may also undergo apoptosis, or inhibitory receptors on the B cells may be engaged, thus preventing activation. As mentioned earlier, regulatory T cells may also contribute to B cell tolerance.

During somatic hypermutation of Ig genes in germinal centers (discussed in Chapter 7), some antigen receptors may be generated that are capable of recognizing self antigens. B cells expressing these autoreactive receptors die either because there are no follicular helper T cells to rescue them or because germinal center B cells express high levels of Fas and are killed by FasL-expressing T cells. The autoimmune disease that results from *FAS* mutations may in part be caused by survival of these self-reactive germinal center B cells.

TOLERANCE TO COMMENSAL MICROBES AND FETAL ANTIGENS

Before concluding our discussion of the mechanisms of immunological tolerance, it is useful to consider two other types of antigens that are not self but are produced by cells or tissues that have to be tolerated by the immune system. These are products of commensal microbes that live in symbiosis with humans and paternally derived antigens in the fetus. Coexistence with these antigens is dependent on many of the same mechanisms that are used to maintain peripheral tolerance to self antigens. Foremost among these mechanisms are regulatory T cells.

Tolerance to Commensal Microbes in the Intestines and Skin

The microbiome of healthy humans consists of about 10^{14} bacteria and viruses (which is 10 times the number of human cells, prompting microbiologists to point out that we are only 10% human and 90% microbial!). These microbes reside in the intestinal and respiratory tracts and on the skin, where they serve many essential functions. For instance, in the gut, the normal bacteria aid in digestion and absorption of foods and prevent overgrowth of potentially harmful organisms. Mature lymphocytes in these tissues are capable of recognizing the organisms but do not react against them, so the microbes are not eliminated, and

harmful inflammation is not triggered. In the gut, several mechanisms account for the inability of the healthy immune system to react against commensal microbes. These mechanisms include an abundance of IL-10–producing regulatory T cells, an unusual property of dendritic cells such that signaling from some Toll-like receptors leads to inhibition rather than activation, and separation of some bacteria from the intestinal immune system by the epithelium. The mechanisms that maintain tolerance to commensal bacteria in the skin are not as well defined.

Tolerance to Fetal Antigens

The evolution of placentation in eutherian mammals allowed the fetus to mature before birth but created the problem that paternal antigens expressed in the fetus, which are foreign to the mother, have to be tolerated by the immune system of the pregnant mother. One mechanism of this tolerance is the generation of peripheral FoxP3+ regulatory T cells specific for these paternal antigens. In fact, during evolution, placentation is strongly correlated with the ability to generate stable peripheral regulatory T cells. It is unclear whether women who suffer recurrent pregnancy losses have a defect in the generation or maintenance of these regulatory T cells. Other mechanisms of fetal tolerance include exclusion of inflammatory cells from the pregnant uterus, poor antigen presentation in the placenta, and an inability to generate harmful Th1 responses in the healthy pregnant uterus.

Now that we have described the principal mechanisms of immunological tolerance, we consider the consequences of the failure of self-tolerance—namely, the development of autoimmunity. The mechanisms of tissue injury in autoimmune diseases and therapeutic strategies for these disorders are described in Chapter 11.

AUTOIMMUNITY

Autoimmunity is defined as an immune response against self (autologous) antigens. It is an important cause of disease, estimated to affect 2% to 5% of the population in developed countries, and the prevalence of several autoimmune diseases

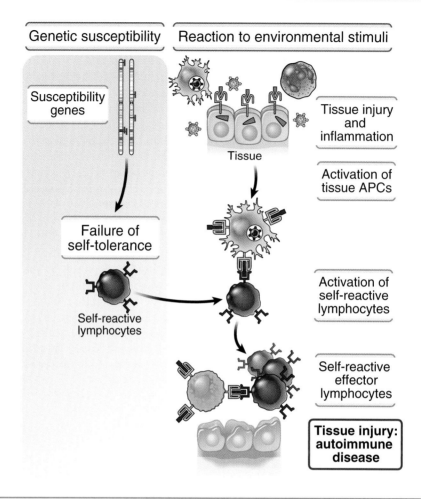

FIGURE 9-10 Postulated mechanisms of autoimmunity. In this proposed model of organ-specific T cell–mediated autoimmunity, various genetic loci may confer susceptibility to autoimmunity, probably by influencing the maintenance of self-tolerance. Environmental triggers, such as infections and other inflammatory stimuli, promote the influx of lymphocytes into tissues and the activation of antigen-presenting cells (APCs) and subsequently of self-reactive T cells, resulting in tissue injury.

is increasing. Different autoimmune diseases may be organ-specific, affecting only one or a few organs, or systemic, with widespread tissue injury and clinical manifestations. Tissue injury in autoimmune diseases may be caused by antibodies against self antigens or by T cells reactive with self antigens (see Chapter 11). A cautionary note is that in many cases, diseases associated with uncontrolled immune responses are called autoimmune without formal evidence that the responses are directed against self antigens.

Pathogenesis

The principal factors in the development of autoimmunity are the inheritance of susceptibility genes and environmental triggers, such as infections (Fig. 9-10). It is postulated that susceptibility genes interfere with pathways of self-tolerance and lead to the persistence of self-reactive T and B lymphocytes. Environmental stimuli may cause cell and tissue injury and inflammation and activate these self-reactive lymphocytes, resulting in the generation

Disease	MHC allele	Relative risk
Ankylosing spondylitis	HLA-B27	90
Rheumatoid arthritis	HLA-DRB1*01/*04/*10	4-12
Type 1 diabetes mellitus	HLA-DRB1*0301/0401	35
Pemphigus vulgaris	HLA-DR4	14

FIGURE 9-11 Association of autoimmune diseases with alleles of the major histocompatibility complex (MHC) locus. Family and linkage studies show a greater likelihood of developing certain autoimmune diseases in persons who inherit particular human leukocyte antigen (HLA) alleles than in persons who lack these alleles (odds ratio or relative risk). Selected examples of HLA-disease associations are listed. For instance, in people who have the HLA-B27 allele, the risk of development of ankylosing spondylitis, an autoimmune diseases of the spine, is 90 to 100 times higher than in B27-negative people; other diseases show various degrees of association with other HLA alleles. Breeding studies in animals have also shown that the incidence of some autoimmune diseases correlates strongly with the inheritance of particular MHC alleles (e.g., type 1 diabetes mellitus with a mouse class II allele called I-A^{g7}).

of effector T cells and autoantibodies that are responsible for the autoimmune disease.

Despite our growing knowledge of the immunological abnormalities that may result in autoimmunity, we still do not know the etiology of common human autoimmune diseases. This lack of understanding results from several factors: autoimmune diseases in humans usually are heterogeneous and multifactorial; the self antigens that are the inducers and targets of the autoimmune reactions often are unknown; and the diseases may manifest clinically long after the autoimmune reactions have been initiated. Recent advances, including the identification of disease-associated genes, better techniques for studying antigen-specific immune responses in humans, and the analysis of animal models that can be extrapolated to clinical situations, hold promise for providing answers to the enigma of autoimmunity.

Genetic Factors

Inherited risk for most autoimmune diseases is attributable to multiple gene loci, of which the largest contribution is made by MHC genes. If an autoimmune disease develops in one of two twins, the same disease is more likely to develop in the other twin than in an unrelated member of the general population.

Furthermore, this increased incidence is greater among monozygotic (identical) twins than among dizygotic twins. These findings prove the importance of genetics in the susceptibly to autoimmunity. Genome-wide association studies have revealed some of the common variations (polymorphisms) of genes that may contribute to different autoimmune diseases. Emerging results suggest that different polymorphisms are more frequent (predisposing) or less frequent (protective) in patients than in healthy controls. Their importance is reinforced by the finding that many of these polymorphisms may affect immune responses, and the same genetic polymorphisms are associated with different autoimmune diseases. However, these polymorphisms are frequently present in healthy individuals, and the individual contribution of each of these genes to the development of autoimmunity is very small. In rare cases, autoimmunity-associated genes are variants (mutations) that are essentially nonexistent in healthy individuals, rather than commonly detected polymorphisms. Such rare variants can have a large impact on the development of autoimmunity.

Many autoimmune diseases in humans and inbred animals are linked to particular MHC alleles (Fig. 9-11). The association between human leukocyte antigen (HLA) alleles and autoimmune diseases in humans was recognized many years ago and was one of the first indications that T cells played an important role in these disorders (because the only known function of MHC molecules is to present peptide antigens to T cells). The incidence of a particular autoimmune disease often is greater among individuals who inherit a particular HLA allele(s) than in the general population. This increased incidence is called the odds ratio or relative risk of an HLA-disease association; the same nomenclature is applicable to the association of any gene with any disease. It is important to point out that although an HLA allele may increase the risk of developing a particular autoimmune disease, the HLA allele is not, by itself, the cause of the disease. In fact, the disease never develops in the vast majority of people who inherit an HLA allele that does confer increased risk of the disease. Despite the clear association of MHC alleles with several autoimmune diseases, how these alleles contribute to the development of the diseases remains unknown. Some hypotheses are that particular MHC alleles may be especially effective at presenting pathogenic self peptides to autoreactive T cells, or they are inefficient at displaying certain self antigens in the thymus, leading to defective negative selection of T cells.

Polymorphisms in non-HLA genes are associated with various autoimmune diseases and may contribute to failure of self-tolerance or abnormal activation of lymphocytes (Fig. 9-12, *A*). Many such disease-associated genetic variants have been described:

- Polymorphisms in the gene encoding the tyrosine phosphatase PTPN22 (protein tyrosine phosphatase N22) may lead to uncontrolled activation of both B and T cells and are associated with numerous autoimmune diseases, including rheumatoid arthritis, systemic lupus erythematosus, and type 1 diabetes mellitus.
- Variants of the innate immune cytoplasmic microbial sensor NOD-2 that cause reduced resistance to intestinal microbes are associated

with Crohn's disease, an inflammatory bowel disease, in some ethnic populations.
- Other polymorphisms associated with multiple autoimmune diseases include genes encoding the IL-2 receptor α chain (CD25), believed to influence the balance of effector and regulatory T cells; the receptor for the cytokine IL-23, which promotes the development of proinflammatory Th17 cells; and CTLA-4, a key inhibitory receptor in T cells discussed earlier.

It is hoped that elucidation of these genetic associations will reveal pathogenic mechanisms or provide new ideas for better prediction and treatment.

Some rare autoimmune disorders are mendelian in origin, caused by mutations in single genes that have high penetrance and lead to autoimmunity in most or all individuals who inherit these mutations. These genes, alluded to earlier, include *AIRE, FOXP3, FAS,* and *CTLA4* see (Fig. 9-12, *B*). Mutations in these genes have been valuable for identifying key molecules and pathways involved in self-tolerance. These mendelian forms of autoimmunity are exceedingly rare, however, and common autoimmune diseases are not caused by mutations in any of these known genes.

Role of Infections and Other Environmental Influences

Infections may activate self-reactive lymphocytes, thereby triggering the development of autoimmune diseases. Clinicians have recognized for many years that the clinical manifestations of autoimmunity sometimes are preceded by infectious prodromes. This association between infections and autoimmune tissue injury has been formally established in animal models.

Infections may contribute to autoimmunity in several ways (Fig. 9-13):
- An infection of a tissue may induce a local innate immune response, which may lead to increased production of costimulators and cytokines by tissue APCs. These activated tissue APCs may be able to stimulate self-reactive

A. Genes that may contribute to genetically complex autoimmune diseases

Gene(s)	Disease association	Mechanism
PTPN22	RA, several others	Abnormal tyrosine phosphatase regulation of T cell selection and activation?
NOD2	Crohn's disease	Defective resistance or abnormal responses to intestinal microbes?
IL23R	IBD, PS, AS	Component of IL-23 receptor; role in generation and maintenance of Th17 cells
CTLA4	T1D, RA	Impaired inhibitory checkpoint and regulatory T cell function
CD25 (IL-2Rα)	MS, type 1 diabetes, others	Abnormalities in effector and/or regulatory T cells?
C2, C4 (Complement proteins)	SLE	Defects in clearance of immune complexes or in B cell tolerance?
FCGRIIB (FCγRIIB)	SLE	Defective feedback inhibition of B cells

B. Single-gene defects that cause autoimmunity (mendelian diseases)

Gene(s)	Disease association	Mechanism
AIRE	Autoimmune polyendocrine syndrome (APS-1)	Reduced expression of peripheral tissue antigens in the thymus, leading to defective elimination of self-reactive T cells
CTLA4	Autosomal dominant immune dysregulation syndrome	Impaired inhibitory checkpoint and regulatory T cell function leading to loss of B and T cell homeostasis
FOXP3	Immune dysregulation, X-linked polyendocrinopathy and enteropathy (IPEX)	Deficiency of regulatory T cells
FAS	Autoimmune lymphoproliferative syndrome (ALPS)	Defective apoptosis of self-reactive T and B cells in the periphery

FIGURE 9-12 Roles of non-MHC genes in autoimmunity. **A,** Select examples of variants (polymorphisms) of genes that confer susceptibility to autoimmune diseases but individually have small or no effects. **B,** Examples of genes whose mutations result in autoimmunity. These are rare examples of autoimmune diseases with mendelian inheritance. The pattern of inheritance varies in the different diseases. APS-1 is autosomal recessive, and in most patients, both alleles of the gene (*AIRE*) have to be abnormal to cause the disease. IPEX is X-linked, so mutation in one allele of the gene (*FOXP3*) is sufficient to cause a defect in boys. ALPS is autosomal dominant with highly variable penetrance, because FAS and FASL are trimeric proteins and mutations in one of the alleles of either gene result in reduced expression of intact trimers. The disease caused by *CTLA4* mutations is also autosomal dominant, perhaps because mutation in one allele reduces the expression of the protein enough to impair its function. *AS,* Ankylosing spondylitis; *IBD,* inflammatory bowel disease; *MS,* multiple sclerosis; *PS,* psoriasis; *RA,* rheumatoid arthritis; *SLE,* systemic lupus erythematosus; *T1D,* type 1 diabetes.

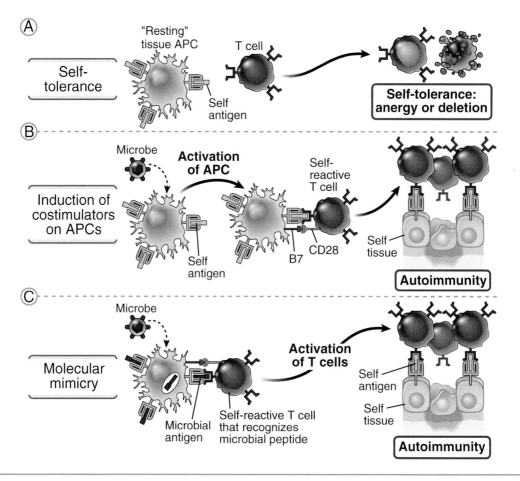

FIGURE 9-13 Mechanisms by which microbes may promote autoimmunity. A, Normally, an encounter of mature T cells with self antigens presented by resting tissue antigen-presenting cells (APCs) results in peripheral tolerance. **B,** Microbes may activate the APCs to express costimulators, and when these APCs present self antigens, the specific T cells are activated, rather than being rendered tolerant. **C,** Some microbial antigens may cross-react with self antigens (mimicry). Therefore, immune responses initiated by the microbes may become directed at self cells and tissues. This figure illustrates concepts as they apply to T cells; molecular mimicry also may apply to self-reactive B lymphocytes.

T cells that encounter self antigens in the tissue. In other words, infection may break T cell tolerance and promote the activation of self-reactive lymphocytes.

- Some infectious microbes may produce peptide antigens that are similar to, and cross-react with, self antigens. Immune responses to these microbial peptides may result in an immune attack against self antigens. Such cross-reactions between microbial and self antigens are termed **molecular mimicry.** Although the contribution of molecular mimicry to autoimmunity has fascinated immunologists, its actual significance in the development of most autoimmune diseases remains unknown. In some rare disorders, antibodies produced against a microbial protein bind to self proteins. In rheumatic fever, antibodies against streptococci cross-react with a myocardial antigen and cause heart disease.

- The innate response to infections may alter the chemical structure of self antigens. For example, some periodontal bacterial infections are associated with rheumatoid arthritis. It is postulated that the acute and chronic inflammatory responses to these bacteria lead to enzymatic conversion of arginines to citrullines in self proteins, and the citrullinated proteins are recognized as nonself and elicit adaptive immune responses.

- Infections also may injure tissues and release antigens that normally are sequestered from the immune system. For example, some sequestered antigens (e.g., in testis and eye) normally are not seen by the immune system and are ignored. Release of these antigens (e.g., by trauma or infection) may initiate an autoimmune reaction against the tissue.

- The abundance and composition of normal commensal microbes in the gut, skin, and other sites (the microbiome) may also influence the health of the immune system and the maintenance of self-tolerance. This possibility has generated a great deal of interest, but normal variations in the microbiome of humans related to environmental exposure and diet make it difficult to define the relationship between particular microbes and the development of autoimmune diseases.

Paradoxically, some infections appear to confer protection from autoimmune diseases. This conclusion is based on epidemiologic data and limited experimental studies. The basis of this protective effect of infections is unknown.

Several other environmental and host factors may contribute to autoimmunity. Many autoimmune diseases are more common in women than in men, but how gender might affect immunological tolerance or lymphocyte activation remains unknown. Exposure to sunlight is a trigger for the development of the autoimmune disease systemic lupus erythematosus (SLE), in which autoantibodies are produced against self nucleic acids and nucleoproteins. It is postulated that these nuclear antigens may be released from cells that die by apoptosis as a consequence of exposure to ultraviolet radiation in sunlight.

■ SUMMARY

- Immunological tolerance is specific unresponsiveness to an antigen induced by exposure of lymphocytes to that antigen. All individuals are tolerant of (unresponsive to) their own (self) antigens. Tolerance against antigens may be induced by administering that antigen in particular ways, and this strategy may be useful for treating immunologic diseases and for preventing the rejection of transplants.

- Central tolerance is induced in immature lymphocytes that encounter antigens in the generative lymphoid organs. Peripheral tolerance results from the recognition of antigens by mature lymphocytes in peripheral tissues.

- Central tolerance of T cells is the result of high-affinity recognition of antigens in the thymus. Some of these self-reactive T cells die (negative selection), thus eliminating the potentially most dangerous T cells, which express high-affinity receptors for self antigens. Other T cells of the CD4 lineage develop into regulatory T cells that suppress self reactivity in the periphery.

- Peripheral tolerance in T cells is induced by multiple mechanisms. Anergy (functional inactivation) results from the recognition of antigens without costimulators (second signals). The mechanisms of anergy include a block in TCR signaling and engagement of inhibitory receptors such as CTLA-4 and PD-1. Self-reactive regulatory T cells suppress potentially pathogenic T cells. Deletion (death by apoptosis) may occur when T cells encounter self antigens.

- In B lymphocytes, central tolerance occurs when immature cells recognize self antigens in the bone marrow. Some of the cells change their receptors (receptor editing), and others die by apoptosis (negative selection, or deletion). Peripheral tolerance is induced when mature B cells recognize self antigens without T cell help, which results in anergy and death of the B cells, or engagement of inhibitory receptors.

■ Autoimmune diseases result from a failure of self-tolerance. Multiple factors contribute to autoimmunity, including the inheritance of susceptibility genes and environmental triggers such as infections.

■ Many genes contribute to the development of autoimmunity. The strongest associations are between HLA genes and various T cell–dependent autoimmune diseases.

■ Infections predispose to autoimmunity by causing inflammation and stimulating the expression of costimulators or because of cross-reactions between microbial and self antigens.

REVIEW QUESTIONS

1. What is immunological tolerance? Why is it important?
2. How is central tolerance induced in T lymphocytes and B lymphocytes?
3. Where do regulatory T cells develop, and how do they protect against autoimmunity?
4. How is functional anergy induced in T cells? How may this mechanism of tolerance fail to give rise to autoimmune disorders?
5. What are the mechanisms that prevent immune responses against commensal microbes and fetuses?
6. What are some of the genes that contribute to autoimmunity? How may MHC genes play a role in the development of autoimmune diseases?
7. What are some possible mechanisms by which infections promote the development of autoimmunity?

Answers to and discussion of the Review Questions are available at https://studentconsult.inkling.com.

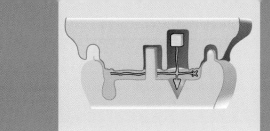

CHAPTER 10

Immune Responses Against Tumors and Transplants

Immunity to Noninfectious Transformed and Foreign Cells

Cancer and organ transplantation are two clinical situations in which the role of the immune system has received a great deal of attention. In cancer, it is widely believed that enhancing immunity against tumors holds much promise for treatment. In organ transplantation, of course, the situation is precisely the reverse: immune responses against the transplants are a barrier to successful transplantation, and learning how to suppress these responses is a major goal of transplant immunologists. Because of the importance of the immune system in host responses to tumors and transplants, tumor immunology and transplantation immunology have become subspecialties in which researchers and clinicians come together to address both fundamental and clinical questions.

Immune responses against tumors and transplants share several characteristics. These are situations in which the immune system is not responding to microbes, as it usually does, but to noninfectious cells that are perceived as foreign. The antigens that mark tumors and transplants as foreign may be expressed in virtually any cell type that is the target of malignant transformation or is grafted from one individual to another. Therefore, the mechanisms for inducing immune responses against tumors must be effective for diverse cell types. Also, a major mechanism by which the immune system kills both tumor cells and the cells of tissue transplants is by cytotoxic T lymphocytes (CTLs). For all these reasons, immunity to tumors and to transplants is discussed together in this chapter. We focus on the following questions:

- What are the antigens in tumors and tissue transplants that are recognized as foreign by the immune system?
- How does the immune system recognize and react to tumors and transplants?
- How can immune responses to tumors and grafts be manipulated to enhance tumor rejection and inhibit graft rejection?

We discuss tumor immunity first and then transplantation, and we point out the principles common to both.

IMMUNE RESPONSES AGAINST TUMORS

For over a century it has been proposed that a physiologic function of the adaptive immune system is to prevent the outgrowth of transformed cells and to destroy these cells before they become harmful tumors. Control and elimination of malignant cells by the immune system is called **immune surveillance.** Several lines of evidence support the idea that immune surveillance against tumors is important for preventing tumor growth (Fig. 10-1). However, the fact that common malignant tumors develop in immunocompetent individuals indicates that tumor immunity is often incapable of preventing tumor growth or is easily overwhelmed by rapidly growing tumors. Furthermore, one of the hallmarks of cancers is their ability to evade immune destruction. This has led to the growing realization that the immune response to tumors is often dominated by tolerance or regulation, not by effective immunity. The field of tumor immunology has focused on defining the types of tumor antigens against which the immune system reacts and the nature of the immune responses, and developing strategies for maximally enhancing antitumor immunity.

Tumor Antigens

Malignant tumors express various types of molecules that may be recognized by the immune system as foreign antigens (Fig. 10-2). If the immune system is able to react against a tumor in the individual, the tumor must express antigens that are seen as nonself by the individual's immune system. Common tumor antigens can be classified into several groups:

- *Products of diverse mutated genes.* Recent sequencing of tumor genomes has revealed that common human tumors harbor a large number of mutations in diverse genes, which play no role in tumorigenesis and are called passenger mutations. The products of many of these altered genes may stimulate an adaptive immune response in the tumor patients. In experimental tumors induced by chemical carcinogens or radiation, the tumor antigens

Evidence	Conclusion
Lymphocytic infiltrates around some tumors and enlargement of draining lymph nodes correlate with better prognosis	Immune responses against tumors inhibit tumor growth
Transplants of a syngeneic tumor are rejected by animals, and more rapidly if the animals have been previously exposed to that tumor; immunity to tumor transplants can be transferred by lymphocytes from a tumor-bearing animal	Tumor rejection shows features of adaptive immunity (specificity, memory) and is mediated by lymphocytes
Immunodeficient individuals have an increased incidence of some types of tumors	The immune system protects against the growth of tumors
Therapeutic blockade of inhibitory receptors such as PD-1 and CTLA-4 leads to tumor remission	Tumors evade immune surveillance in part by engaging inhibitory receptors on T cells

FIGURE 10-1 Evidence supporting the concept that the immune system reacts against tumors. Several lines of clinical and experimental evidence indicate that defense against tumors is mediated by reactions of the adaptive immune system.

are also mutants of normal cellular proteins. Virtually any gene may be mutagenized randomly in different tumors.

- *Products of oncogenes or mutated tumor suppressor genes.* Some tumor antigens are products of mutated or translocated oncogenes or tumor suppressor genes that presumably are involved in the process of malignant transformation, called driver mutations. These types of mutations may encode proteins that are seen as foreign. Novel proteins generated across translocation breakpoints also may serve as tumor antigens.

- *Aberrantly expressed proteins.* In several human tumors, the antigens that elicit immune responses appear to be normal (unmutated) proteins whose expression is dysregulated in the tumors. These structurally normal self antigens would not be expected to elicit immune responses, but their aberrant expression may be enough to make them immunogenic. For example, self proteins that are expressed only in embryonic tissues may not induce tolerance in adults; thus, the same proteins expressed in tumors may be recognized as foreign by the immune system.

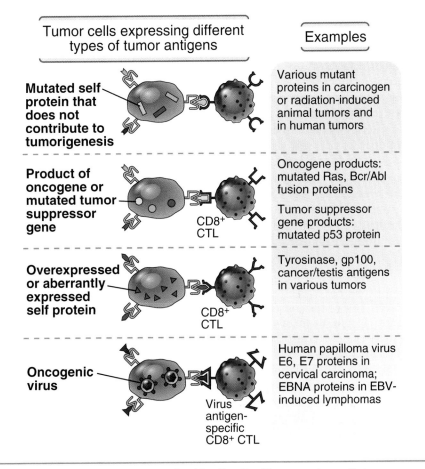

FIGURE 10-2 Types of tumor antigens recognized by T cells. Tumor antigens that are recognized by tumor-specific CD8+ T cells may be mutated forms of various self proteins that do not contribute to malignant behavior of the tumor; products of oncogenes or tumor suppressor genes; self proteins whose expression is increased in tumor cells; and products of oncogenic viruses. Cancer/testis antigens are proteins that are normally expressed in the testis and are also expressed in some tumors. Tumor antigens also may be recognized by CD4+ T cells, but less is known about the role that CD4+ T cells play in tumor immunity. *CTL,* Cytotoxic T lymphocyte; *EBNA,* Epstein-Barr virus nuclear antigen; *EBV,* Epstein-Barr virus; *gp100,* glycoprotein of 100 kD.

- *Viral antigens.* In tumors caused by oncogenic viruses, the tumor antigens may be products of the viruses.

Immune Mechanisms of Tumor Rejection

The principal immune mechanism of tumor eradication is killing of tumor cells by CTLs specific for tumor antigens. A majority of tumor antigens that elicit immune responses in tumor-bearing individuals are endogenously synthesized cytosolic or nuclear proteins that are displayed as class I major histocompatibility complex (MHC)–associated peptides. Therefore, these antigens are recognized by class I MHC–restricted CD8+ CTLs, whose function is to kill cells producing the antigens. The role of CTLs in tumor rejection has been established in animal models: transplants of tumors can be destroyed by transferring tumor-reactive CD8+ T cells into the tumor-bearing animals. Studies of some human tumors indicate that abundant CTL infiltration predicts a more favorable clinical course compared with tumors with sparse CTLs.

CTL responses against tumors are induced by recognition of tumor antigens on host antigen-presenting cells (APCs). The APCs ingest tumor cells or their antigens and present the antigens to T cells (Fig. 10-3). Tumors may arise from virtually any nucleated cell type, and, like all nucleated cells, they express class I MHC molecules, but often they do not express costimulators or class II MHC molecules. We know, however, that the activation of naive CD8+ T cells to proliferate and differentiate into active CTLs requires recognition of antigen (class I MHC–associated peptide) on dendritic cells and also costimulation and/or help from class II MHC–restricted CD4+ T cells (see Chapter 5). How, then, can tumors of different cell types stimulate CTL responses? The likely answer is that tumor cells or their proteins are ingested by the host's dendritic cells, and the antigens of the tumor cells are processed and displayed by class I MHC molecules on the host dendritic cells. This process, called **cross-presentation** or cross-priming, was introduced in Chapter 3 (see Fig. 3-16). Dendritic cells can also present ingested peptides from tumor antigens

on class II MHC molecules. Thus, tumor antigens may be recognized by CD8+ T cells and by CD4+ T cells.

At the same time that dendritic cells are presenting tumor antigens, they may express costimulators that provide signals for the activation of the T cells. It is not known how tumors induce the expression of costimulators on APCs because, as discussed in Chapter 5, the physiologic stimuli for the induction of costimulators are usually microbes, and tumors are generally sterile. One possibility is that tumor cells die if their growth outstrips their blood and nutrient supply, and dying cells release products that stimulate innate responses (damage-associated molecular patterns; see Chapter 2). The activation of APCs to express costimulators is part of these responses.

Once naive CD8+ T cells have differentiated into effector CTLs, they are able to kill tumor cells expressing the relevant antigens without a requirement for costimulation or T cell help. Thus, CTL differentiation may be induced by cross-presentation of tumor antigens by host dendritic cells, but the CTLs are effective against the tumor itself.

Immune mechanisms in addition to CTLs may play a role in tumor rejection. Antitumor CD4+ T cell responses and antibodies have been detected in patients, but whether these responses actually protect individuals against tumor growth has not been established. Experimental studies have shown that activated macrophages and natural killer (NK) cells are capable of killing tumor cells in vitro, but the protective role of these effector mechanisms in tumor-bearing individuals is also largely unknown.

Evasion of Immune Responses by Tumors

Immune responses often fail to check tumor growth because tumors evolve to evade immune recognition or resist immune effector mechanisms. The immune system faces daunting challenges in combating malignant tumors, because immune responses must kill all the tumor cells in order to be effective, and tumors can grow rapidly. Often, the growth of the tumor simply outstrips immune defenses. Immune responses against tumors may be weak because many tumors elicit little inflammation and costimulation and may express few nonself antigens.

Not surprisingly, tumor cells that evade the host immune response are selected to survive and grow. Tumors use several mechanisms to avoid destruction by the immune system (Fig. 10-4):

- Some tumors stop expressing the antigens that are the targets of immune attack. These tumors are called antigen loss variants. If the lost antigen is not involved in maintaining the malignant properties of the tumor, the variant tumor cells continue to grow and spread.
- Other tumors stop expressing class I MHC molecules, so they cannot display antigens

to CD8$^+$ T cells. NK cells recognize molecules expressed on tumor cells, but not on normal cells, and are activated when their target cells lack class I MHC molecules. Therefore, NK cells may provide a mechanism for killing class I MHC–negative tumors.

- Tumors engage pathways that inhibit T cell activation. Some tumors express ligands for T cell inhibitory receptors such as PD-1. Tumors may also induce only low levels of B7 costimulators on APCs, resulting in preferential engagement of the inhibitory receptor CTLA-4 on T

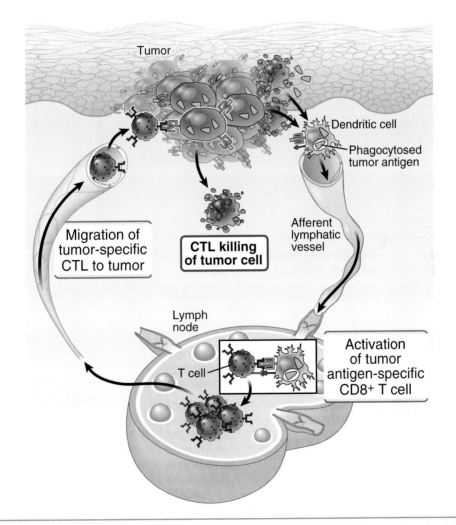

FIGURE 10-3 Immune response against tumors. Tumor antigens are picked up by host dendritic cells, and responses are initiated in peripheral (secondary) lymphoid organs. Tumor-specific CTLs migrate back to the tumor and kill tumor cells. Other mechanisms of tumor immunity are not shown.

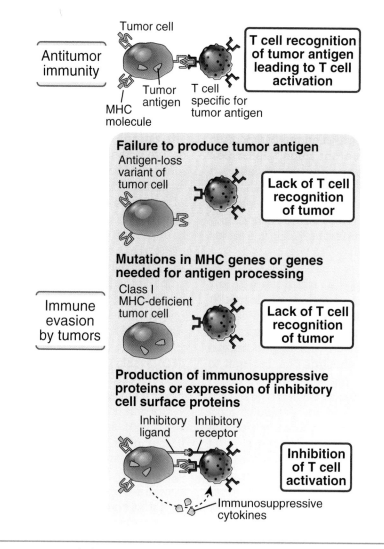

FIGURE 10-4 How tumors evade immune responses. Antitumor immunity develops when T cells recognize tumor antigens and are activated. Tumor cells may evade immune responses by losing expression of antigens or major histocompatibility complex (MHC) molecules or by producing immunosuppressive cytokines or ligands such as PD-L1 for inhibitory receptors on T cells. Tumors may also induce regulatory T cells (not shown).

cells rather than the stimulatory receptor CD28 (see Chapter 9). The net result may be reduced T cell activation upon recognition of tumor antigens. Some tumors may induce regulatory T cells, which also suppress antitumor immune responses.

- Still other tumors may secrete immunosuppressive cytokines, such as transforming growth factor β, or induce regulatory T cells that suppress immune responses.

Cancer Immunotherapy

The main strategies for cancer immunotherapy aim to provide antitumor effectors (antibodies and T cells) to patients, actively immunize patients against their tumors, and stimulate the patients' own antitumor immune responses. At present, most treatment protocols for disseminated cancers, which cannot be cured surgically, rely on chemotherapy and irradiation, both of which

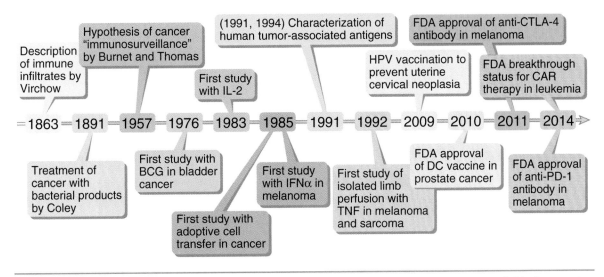

FIGURE 10-5 History of cancer immunotherapy. Some of the important discoveries in the field of cancer immunotherapy are summarized. (Modified from Lesterhuis et al: Cancer immunotherapy—revisited. *Nat Rev Drug Disc* 10:591, 2011.) *BCG,* Bacillus Calmette-Guerin; *CAR,* chimeric antigen receptor; *CTLA-4,* cytotoxic T-lymphocyte-associated protein 4; *DC,* Dendritic cell; *FDA,* Federal Drug Administration; *HPV,* Human papillomavirus; *IFNα,* Intereron-α; *IL-2,* Interleukin -2; *PD-1,* Programmed cell death protein 1; *TNF,* Tumor necrosis factor.

damage normal nontumor tissues and are associated with serious toxicities. Because the immune response is highly specific, it has long been hoped that tumor-specific immunity may be used to selectively eradicate tumors without injuring the patient. Immunotherapy remains a major goal of tumor immunologists, and many approaches have been tried in experimental animals and in humans. The history of cancer immunotherapy illustrates how the initial, often empirical, approaches have been largely supplanted by rational strategies based on our improved understanding of normal immune responses (Fig. 10-5).

Passive Immunotherapy

One strategy for tumor immunotherapy relies on various forms of passive immunization, in which immune effectors are injected into cancer patients (Fig. 10-6, *A*):

- *Antibody therapy.* Monoclonal antibodies against various tumor antigens have been used in many cancers. The antibodies bind to tumor antigens and activate host effector mechanisms, such as phagocytes or the complement system, that destroy the tumor cells. For example, an antibody specific for CD20, which is expressed on B cells, is used to treat B cell tumors, usually in combination with chemotherapy. Because CD20 is not expressed by hematopoietic stem cells, normal B cells are replenished after the antibody treatment is stopped. Other monoclonal antibodies that are used in cancer therapy may work by blocking growth factor signaling (e.g., anti-Her2/Neu for breast cancer and anti–EGF-receptor antibody for various tumors) or by inhibiting angiogenesis (e.g., antibody against the vascular endothelial growth factor for colon cancer and other tumors).

- *Adoptive cellular therapy.* T lymphocytes may be isolated from the blood or tumor infiltrates of a patient, expanded by culture with growth factors, and injected back into the same patient. The T cells presumably contain tumor-specific CTLs, which find the tumor and destroy it. This approach, called adoptive cellular immunotherapy, has been tried as a treatment for several types of metastatic cancers, but results have been variable among different patients and tumors.

- *Chimeric antigen receptors.* In a more recent modification of T cell therapy, a chimeric antigen receptor that recognizes a tumor antigen and coupled to intracellular signaling domains is genetically introduced into a patient's T cells, and the cells are expanded ex vivo and transferred back into the patient. Such therapy has shown remarkable efficacy in some leukemias.

Stimulation of Host Antitumor Immune Responses

The host's immune response against tumors can be promoted by vaccinating with tumor antigens or by blocking inhibitory mechanisms that suppress antitumor immunity.

- *Vaccination.* One way of stimulating active immunity against tumors is to vaccinate patients with their own tumor cells or with antigens from these cells. An important reason for defining tumor antigens is to produce and use

these antigens to vaccinate individuals against their own tumors. Vaccines may be administered as recombinant proteins with adjuvants. In another approach, a tumor patient's dendritic cells are expanded in vitro from blood precursors, the dendritic cells are exposed to tumor cells or a defined tumor antigen, and these tumor-antigen-pulsed dendritic cells are used as vaccines. It is hoped that the dendritic cells bearing tumor antigens will mimic the normal pathway of cross-presentation and will generate CTLs against the tumor cells. Tumor vaccines have achieved only modest success, perhaps because these are therapeutic vaccines that are administered to patients in whom tumors may have established mechanisms that suppress immune responses. Tumors caused by oncogenic viruses can be prevented by vaccinating against these viruses. Two such vaccines

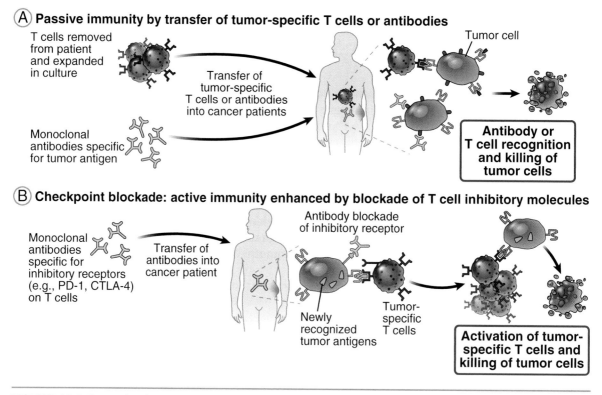

FIGURE 10-6 Strategies for enhancing antitumor immune responses. A, Transfer of antitumor antibodies or T cells, a form of passive immunity. A variation of T cell therapy is to express in patients' T cells an antibody domain that recognizes a tumor antigen; by attaching signaling domains to the antibody, the T cell is activated upon recognition of the tumor. **B,** Blockade of inhibitory pathways to boost endogenous antitumor responses. Not shown are tumor vaccines, sometimes given in the form of autologous dendritic cells incubated with tumor cells or their antigens.

that are proving to be remarkably effective are against hepatitis B virus (the cause of a form of liver cancer) and human papillomavirus (the cause of cervical cancer). These are preventive vaccines given to individuals before they are infected, and thus prevent infection (like all preventive vaccines for infections).

- *Checkpoint blockade.* The realization that tumors activate regulatory mechanisms that suppress immune responses has led to promising recent approaches and a new paradigm in tumor immunotherapy. The principle of this strategy is to boost host immune responses against tumors by blocking normal inhibitory signals for lymphocytes, thus removing the brakes (checkpoints) on the immune response (Fig. 10-6, *B*). An antibody against CTLA-4 was approved for the treatment of melanoma in 2011. Clinical trials of antibodies that block PD-1 or its ligand PD-L1 have shown impressive efficacy in a variety of cancers, and anti–PD-1 for cancer immunotherapy was approved in 2014. The immune response induced by checkpoint blockade is largely specific for peptides produced by mutated genes in the tumors. Predictably, patients treated with these antibodies, especially anti–CTLA-4, develop manifestations of autoimmunity, because the physiologic function of the inhibitory receptors is to maintain tolerance to self antigens (see Chapter 9).

- *Cytokine therapy.* Other ways of boosting antitumor immune responses include treating patients with cytokines that promote lymphocyte activation. The first cytokine to be used in this way was interleukin-2 (IL-2), but its clinical use is limited by serious toxic effects at the high doses that are needed to stimulate antitumor T cell responses. IL-2 also enhances the numbers and functions of regulatory T cells, which may interfere with antitumor immunity. Many other cytokines have been tried for systemic therapy or local administration at sites of tumors, with mostly unimpressive results thus far.

IMMUNE RESPONSES AGAINST TRANSPLANTS

Some of the earliest attempts to replace damaged tissues by transplantation were during World War II, as a way of treating pilots who had received severe skin burns in airplane crashes. It was soon realized that individuals reject tissue grafts from other individuals. Rejection results from inflammatory reactions that damage the transplanted tissues. Studies since the 1940s and 1950s established that graft rejection is mediated by the adaptive immune system, because it shows specificity and memory and it is dependent on lymphocytes (Fig. 10-7). Much of the knowledge

Evidence	Conclusion
Prior exposure to donor MHC molecules leads to accelerated graft rejection	Graft rejection shows memory and specificity, two cardinal features of adaptive immunity
The ability to reject a graft rapidly can be transferred to a naive individual by lymphocytes from a sensitized individual	Graft rejection is mediated by lymphocytes
Depletion or inactivation of T lymphocytes by drugs or antibodies results in reduced graft rejection	Graft rejection requires T lymphocytes

FIGURE 10-7 Evidence indicating that the rejection of tissue transplants is an immune reaction. Clinical and experimental evidence indicates that rejection of grafts is a reaction of the adaptive immune system. *MHC*, Major histocompatibility complex.

about the immunology of transplantation came from experiments with inbred strains of rodents, particularly mice. All members of an inbred strain are genetically identical to one another and different from the members of other strains. These studies showed that grafts among members of one inbred strain are accepted and grafts from one strain to another are rejected, firmly establishing rejection as a process controlled by the animals' genes. Later experiments defined the nature of the genes that control graft rejection and showed that the products of many of these genes are expressed in all tissues.

As mentioned in Chapter 3, the genes that contributed the most to the rejection of grafts exchanged between mice of different inbred strains were called **major histocompatibility complex (MHC)** genes. The language of transplantation immunology evolved from the experimental studies. The individual who provides the graft is called the **donor,** and the individual in whom the graft is placed is the **recipient** or **host.** Animals that are identical to one another (and grafts exchanged among these animals) are said to be **syngeneic;** animals (and grafts) of one species that differ from other animals of the same species are said to be **allogeneic;** and animals (and grafts) of different species are **xenogeneic.** Allogeneic and xenogeneic grafts, also called **allografts** and **xenografts,** are always rejected by a recipient with a normal immune system. The antigens that serve as the targets of rejection are called alloantigens and xenoantigens, and the antibodies and T cells that react against these antigens are alloreactive and xenoreactive, respectively. In the clinical situation, transplants are exchanged between allogeneic individuals, who are members of an outbred species who differ from one another (except for identical twins). Most of the following discussion focuses on immune responses to allografts.

Transplantation Antigens

The antigens of allografts that serve as the principal targets of rejection are proteins encoded in the MHC. Homologous MHC genes and molecules are present in all mammals; the human MHC is called the **human leukocyte antigen** (HLA) complex. It took more than 20 years after the discovery of the MHC to show that the physiologic function of MHC molecules is to display peptide antigens for recognition by T lymphocytes (see Chapter 3). Recall that every person expresses six class I MHC alleles (one allele of HLA-A, -B, and -C from each parent) and usually more than eight class II MHC alleles (one allele of HLA-DQ and -DP and one or two of -DR from each parent, and some combinations of these). MHC genes are highly polymorphic, with over 13,000 HLA alleles among all humans, encoding about 2200 HLA-A proteins, 2900 HLA-B proteins, and 1300 DR B proteins. Because these alleles can be inherited and expressed in virtually any combination, every individual is likely to express some MHC proteins that differ from those of another individual and that therefore appear foreign to another individual's immune system, except in the case of identical twins. Because each HLA locus is inherited as a block, the chance that two siblings will have the same MHC alleles is 1 in 4.

The response to MHC antigens on another individual's cells is one of the strongest immune responses known. T cell receptors (TCRs) for antigens have evolved to recognize MHC molecules, which is essential for surveillance of cells harboring infectious microbes. As a result of positive selection of developing T cells in the thymus, mature T cells that have some affinity for self MHC molecules survive, and many of these will have high affinity for self MHC displaying foreign peptides. Allogeneic MHC molecules containing peptides derived from the allogeneic cells may look like self MHC molecules plus bound foreign peptides (Fig. 10-8). Therefore, recognition of allogeneic MHC molecules in allografts is an example of an immunologic cross-reaction.

There are several reasons why recognition of allogeneic MHC molecules results in strong T cell reactions. Many clones of T cells specific for different foreign peptides bound to the same self MHC molecule may cross-react with any one allogeneic MHC molecule, as long as the allogeneic MHC molecule resembles complexes of self MHC plus foreign peptides. As a result, many self MHC–restricted T cells specific for different peptide antigens may recognize any one allogeneic MHC molecule. Also, the process of negative selection in the thymus eliminates cells that strongly

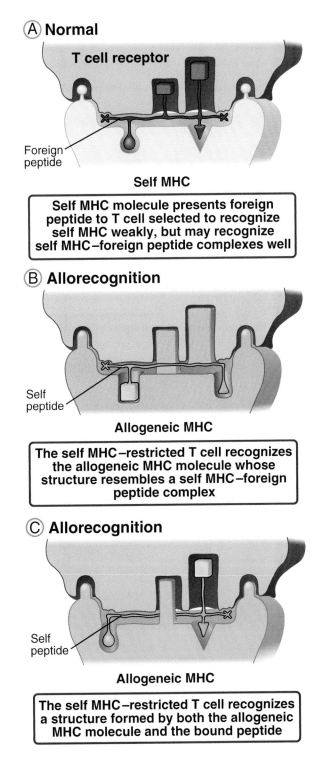

FIGURE 10-8 Recognition of allogeneic major histocompatibility complex (MHC) molecules by T lymphocytes. Recognition of allogeneic MHC molecules may be thought of as a cross-reaction in which a T cell specific for a self MHC molecule–foreign peptide complex **(A)** also recognizes an allogeneic MHC molecule whose structure resembles that of a self MHC molecule–foreign peptide complex **(B and C)**. Peptides derived from the graft or recipient (labeled self peptide) may not contribute to allorecognition **(B)**, or they may form part of the complex that the T cell recognizes **(C)**. The type of T cell recognition depicted in **B** and **C** is direct allorecognition.

recognize self MHC, but there is no mechanism for selectively eliminating T cells whose TCRs have a high affinity for allogeneic MHC molecules, because these are never present in the thymus. Furthermore, a single allogeneic graft cell will express thousands of MHC molecules, every one of which may be recognized as foreign by a graft recipient's T cells. By contrast, in the case of an infected cell, only a small fraction of the self MHC molecules on the cell surface will carry a foreign microbial peptide recognized by the host's T cells. The net result of these features of allorecognition is that as many as 0.1% to 1% of all T cells in a normal individual may react against an allogeneic MHC molecule, much more than the 1 in 10^5 or 10^6 T cells that recognize any microbial antigen.

Although MHC proteins are the major antigens that stimulate graft rejection, other polymorphic proteins also may play a role in rejection.

Non-MHC antigens that induce graft rejection are called minor histocompatibility antigens, and most are normal cellular proteins that differ in sequence between donor and recipient. The rejection reactions that minor histocompatibility antigens elicit usually are not as strong as reactions against foreign MHC proteins. Two clinical situations in which minor antigens are important targets of rejection are blood transfusion and hematopoietic stem cell transplantation, discussed later.

Induction of Immune Responses Against Transplants

In order to elicit antigraft immune responses, alloantigens from the graft are transported by dendritic cells to draining lymph nodes, where they are recognized by alloreactive T cells (Fig. 10-9). The dendritic cells that present alloantigens also

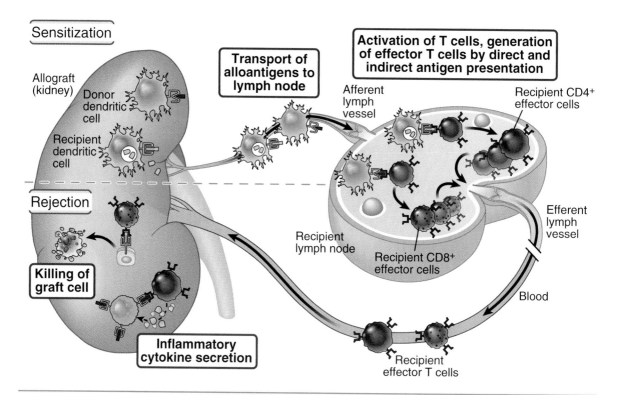

FIGURE 10-9 Immune response against transplants. Graft antigens that are expressed on donor dendritic cells or captured by recipient dendritic cells are transported to peripheral lymphoid organs where alloantigen-specific T cells are activated (the sensitization step). The T cells migrate back into the graft and destroy graft cells (rejection). Antibodies are also produced against graft antigens and can contribute to rejection (not shown). The example shown is that of a kidney graft, but the same general principles apply to all organ grafts.

provide costimulators and can stimulate helper T cells as well as alloreactive CTLs. The effector T cells that are generated circulate back to the transplant and mediate rejection.

T cells may recognize allogeneic MHC molecules in the graft displayed by donor dendritic cells in the graft, or graft alloantigens may be processed and presented by the host's dendritic cells (Fig. 10-10). These two pathways of presentation of graft antigens have different features and names.

- *Direct allorecognition.* Most tissues contain dendritic cells, and when the tissues are transplanted, the dendritic cells are carried in the graft. When T cells in the recipient recognize donor allogeneic MHC molecules on graft dendritic cells, the T cells are activated; this process is called **direct recognition** (or direct presentation) of alloantigens. Direct recognition stimulates the development of alloreactive T cells (e.g., CTLs) that recognize and attack the cells of the graft.

- *Indirect allorecognition.* If graft cells (or alloantigens) are ingested by recipient dendritic cells, donor alloantigens are processed and presented by the self MHC molecules on recipient APCs. This process is called **indirect recognition** (or indirect presentation) and is similar to the cross-presentation of tumor antigens discussed earlier. If alloreactive CTLs are induced by the indirect pathway, these CTLs are specific for donor alloantigens displayed by the recipient's self MHC molecules on the recipient's APCs, so they cannot recognize and kill cells in the graft (which, of course, express donor MHC molecules). When graft alloantigens are recognized by the indirect pathway, the subsequent rejection of the graft likely is mediated mainly by alloreactive CD4+ T cells. These T cells may enter the graft together with host APCs, recognize graft antigens that are picked up and displayed by these APCs, and secrete cytokines that injure the graft by an inflammatory reaction.

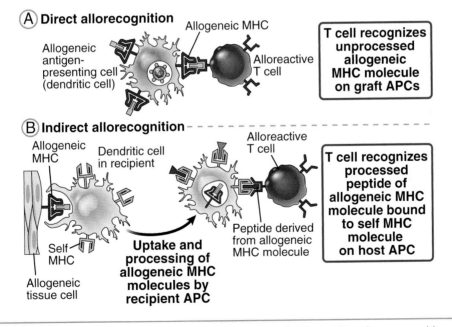

FIGURE 10-10 Direct and indirect recognition of alloantigens. A, Direct alloantigen recognition occurs when T cells bind directly to intact allogeneic major histocompatibility complex (MHC) molecules on antigen-presenting cells (APCs) in a graft, as illustrated in Figure 10-8. **B,** Indirect alloantigen recognition occurs when allogeneic MHC molecules from graft cells are taken up and processed by recipient APCs, and peptide fragments of the allogeneic MHC molecules are presented by recipient (self) MHC molecules. Recipient APCs also may process and present graft proteins other than allogeneic MHC molecules.

We do not know the relative importance of the direct and indirect pathways of allorecognition in the rejection of allografts. The direct pathway may be most important for CTL-mediated acute rejection, and the indirect pathway may play a greater role in chronic rejection, as described later.

T cell responses to allografts require costimulation, but which stimuli in grafts enhance the expression of costimulators on APCs is unclear. As with tumors, graft cells may undergo necrosis, perhaps in the period of ischemia before the transplant is done, and substances released from the injured and dead cells activate APCs by innate immune mechanisms. As we discuss later, blocking costimulation is one therapeutic strategy for promoting graft survival.

The **mixed lymphocyte reaction** (MLR) is an in vitro model of T cell recognition of alloantigens. In this model, T cells from one individual are cultured with leukocytes of another individual, and the responses of the T cells are assayed. The magnitude of this response is proportional to the extent of the MHC differences between these individuals and is a rough predictor of the outcomes of grafts exchanged between these individuals.

Although much of the emphasis on allograft rejection has been on the role of T cells, it is clear that alloantibodies also contribute to rejection. Most of these antibodies are helper T cell–dependent high-affinity antibodies. In order to produce alloantibodies, recipient B cells recognize donor alloantigens and then process and present peptides derived from these antigens to helper T cells (that may have been previously activated by recipient DCs presenting the same donor alloantigen), thus initiating the process of antibody production. This is a good example of indirect presentation of alloantigens, in this case by B lymphocytes.

Immune Mechanisms of Graft Rejection

Graft rejection is classified into hyperacute, acute, and chronic, on the basis of clinical and pathologic features (Fig. 10-11). This historical classification was devised by clinicians based on rejection of kidney allografts, and it has stood the test of time remarkably well.

It also has become apparent that each type of rejection is mediated by a particular type of immune response.

- **Hyperacute rejection** occurs within minutes of transplantation and is characterized by thrombosis of graft vessels and ischemic necrosis of the graft. Hyperacute rejection is mediated by circulating antibodies that are specific for antigens on graft endothelial cells and that are present before transplantation. These preformed antibodies may be natural IgM antibodies specific for blood group antigens, or they may be antibodies specific for allogeneic MHC molecules that are induced by exposure to allogeneic cells due to previous blood transfusions, pregnancy, or organ transplantation. Almost immediately after transplantation, the antibodies bind to antigens on the graft vascular endothelium and activate the complement and clotting systems, leading to injury to the endothelium and thrombus formation. Hyperacute rejection is not a common problem in clinical transplantation, because every donor and recipient are matched for blood type and potential recipients are tested for antibodies against the cells of the prospective donor. (The test for antibodies is called a cross-match.) However, hyperacute rejection is the major barrier to xenotransplantation, as discussed later.

- **Acute rejection** occurs within days or weeks after transplantation and is the principal cause of early graft failure. Acute rejection is mediated by T cells and antibodies specific for alloantigens in the graft. The T cells may be CD8+ CTLs that directly destroy graft cells or CD4+ cells that secrete cytokines and induce inflammation, which destroys the graft. T cells may also react against cells in graft vessels, leading to vascular damage. Antibodies contribute especially to the vascular component of acute rejection. Antibody-mediated injury to graft vessels is caused mainly by complement activation by the classical pathway. Current immunosuppressive therapy is designed mainly to prevent and reduce acute rejection by blocking the activation of alloreactive T cells.

- **Chronic rejection** is an indolent form of graft damage that occurs over months or years, leading to progressive loss of graft function. Chronic rejection may be manifested as fibrosis of the graft and by gradual narrowing of graft blood vessels, called graft arteriosclerosis. In both lesions, the culprits are believed to be T cells that react against graft alloantigens and secrete cytokines, which stimulate the proliferation and activities of fibroblasts and vascular smooth muscle cells in the graft. Alloantibodies also contribute to chronic rejection. Although treatments to prevent or curtail acute rejection have steadily improved, leading to better 1-year survival of transplants, chronic rejection is refractory to most of these therapies and is becoming the principal cause of graft failure.

Prevention and Treatment of Graft Rejection

The mainstay of preventing and treating the rejection of organ transplants is immunosuppression, designed mainly to inhibit T cell activation and effector functions (Fig. 10-12). The development of immunosuppressive drugs launched the modern era of organ transplantation, because these drugs made it feasible to transplant organs from donors that were not HLA-matched with recipients, especially in situations when such matching was impractical, such as transplantation of heart, lung, and liver.

One of the most useful classes of immunosuppressive drugs in clinical transplantation has been the calcineurin inhibitors cyclosporine and tacrolimus (FK506), which function by blocking the phosphatase calcineurin. This enzyme is required to activate the transcription factor NFAT (nuclear factor of activated T cells), and blocking its activity inhibits the transcription of cytokine genes in the T cells. Cyclosporine was the first clinically useful immunosuppressive drug that inhibited the major mediators of graft rejection, T cells. Another widely used drug is rapamycin, which inhibits a kinase called mTOR required for T cell activation. Many other immunosuppressive agents are now used as adjuncts to or instead of calcineurin and mTOR inhibitors (see Fig. 10-12).

All of these immunosuppressive drugs carry the problem of nonspecific immunosuppression (i.e., the drugs inhibit responses to more than the graft). Therefore, patients receiving these drugs as part of their post-transplantation treatment regimen become susceptible to infections, particularly infections by intracellular microbes, and demonstrate an increased incidence of cancer, especially tumors caused by oncogenic viruses.

The matching of donor and recipient HLA alleles by tissue typing had an important role in minimizing graft rejection before cyclosporine became available for clinical use. Although MHC matching is critical for the success of transplantation of some types of tissues (e.g., hematopoietic stem cell transplants) and improves survival of other types of organ grafts (e.g., renal allografts), modern immunosuppression is so effective that HLA matching is not considered necessary for many types of organ transplants (e.g., heart and liver), mainly because the number of donors is limited and the recipients often are too sick to wait for well-matched organs to become available.

The long-term goal of transplant immunologists is to induce immunological tolerance specifically for the graft alloantigens. If this is achieved, it will allow graft acceptance without shutting off other immune responses in the host. Experimental and clinical attempts to induce graft-specific tolerance are ongoing.

A major problem in transplantation is the shortage of suitable donor organs. **Xenotransplantation** has been considered a possible solution for this problem. Experimental studies show that hyperacute rejection is a frequent cause of xenotransplant loss. The reasons for the high incidence of hyperacute rejection of xenografts are that individuals often contain antibodies that react with cells from other species and the xenograft cells lack regulatory proteins that can inhibit human complement activation. These antibodies, similar to antibodies against blood group antigens, are called natural antibodies because their production does not require prior exposure to the xenoantigens. It is thought that these antibodies are produced against bacteria that

(A) Hyperacute rejection

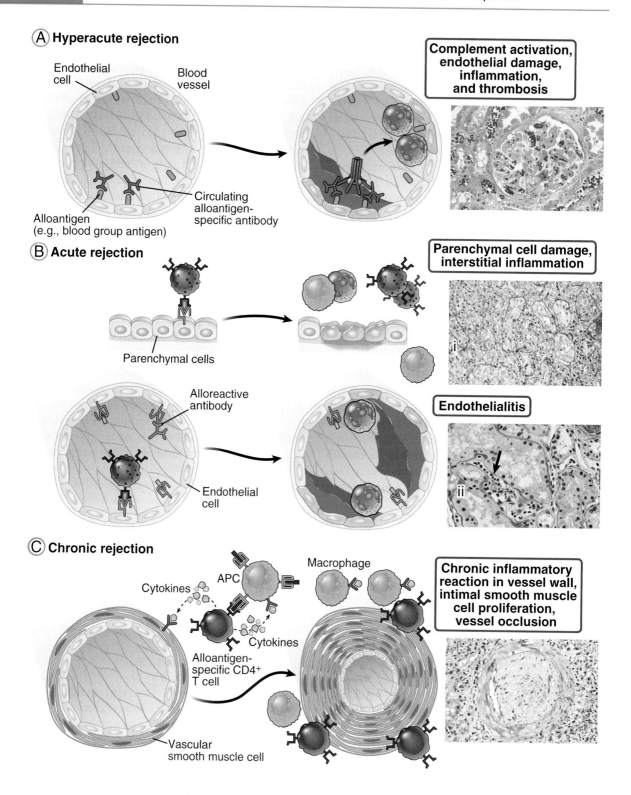

Endothelial cell

Blood vessel

Circulating alloantigen-specific antibody

Alloantigen (e.g., blood group antigen)

Complement activation, endothelial damage, inflammation, and thrombosis

(B) Acute rejection

Parenchymal cells

Alloreactive antibody

Endothelial cell

Parenchymal cell damage, interstitial inflammation

i

Endothelialitis

ii

(C) Chronic rejection

Cytokines

APC

Macrophage

Alloantigen-specific CD4+ T cell

Cytokines

Vascular smooth muscle cell

Chronic inflammatory reaction in vessel wall, intimal smooth muscle cell proliferation, vessel occlusion

FIGURE 10-11 Mechanisms and histopathology of graft rejection. A representative histologic appearance of each type of rejection is shown on the right. **A,** In hyperacute rejection, preformed antibodies react with alloantigens on the vascular endothelium of the graft, activate complement, and trigger rapid intravascular thrombosis and necrosis of the vessel wall. **B,** In acute rejection, CD8+ T lymphocytes reactive with alloantigens on graft endothelial cells and parenchymal cells or antibodies reactive with endothelial cells cause damage to these cell types. Inflammation of the endothelium is called endothelialitis. The histology shows acute cellular rejection in i and humoral (antibody-mediated) rejection in ii. **C,** In chronic rejection with graft arteriosclerosis, T cells reactive with graft alloantigens may produce cytokines that induce inflammation and proliferation of intimal smooth muscle cells, leading to luminal occlusion.

normally inhabit the gut and that the antibodies cross-react with cells of other species. Xenografts also are subject to acute rejection, much like allografts but often even more severe than rejection of allografts. Because of the problem of rejection, and difficulty in procuring organs from animals that are evolutionarily close to humans, clinical xenotransplantaion remains a distant goal.

Transplantation of Blood Cells and Hematopoietic Stem Cells

Transplantation of blood cells, called **transfusion,** is the oldest form of transplantation in clinical medicine. The major barrier to transfusion is the presence of foreign **blood group antigens,** the prototypes of which are the ABO antigens (Fig. 10-13). These antigens are expressed on red blood cells, endothelial cells, and many other cell types. ABO antigens are carbohydrates on membrane glycoproteins or glycosphingolipids; they contain a core glycan that may have an additional terminal sugar. Blood group antigens A and B have different terminal sugars (*N*-acetylgalactosamine and galactose, respectively); AB individuals express both terminal sugars on different glycolipid molecules; and individuals with blood group O express the core glycan but neither of the terminal sugars.

Individuals expressing one blood group antigen are tolerant of that antigen but have antibodies against the other; O group individuals make both anti-A and anti-B antibodies. These antibodies are produced against antigens that are expressed by intestinal microbes and that

cross-react with the ABO blood group antigens. The preformed antibodies react against transfused blood cells expressing the target antigens, and the result may be a severe **transfusion reaction.** This problem is avoided by matching blood donors and recipients, a standard practice in medicine. Because the blood group antigens are sugars, they do not elicit T cell responses.

Blood group antigens other than the ABO antigens also are involved in transfusion reactions, and these usually are less severe. One important example is the Rh antigen, which is a red cell membrane protein that can be the target of maternal antibodies that may attack a developing fetus when the fetus expresses paternal Rh and the mother lacks the protein.

Hematopoietic stem cell transplantation is being used increasingly to correct hematopoietic defects, to restore bone marrow cells damaged by irradiation and chemotherapy for cancer, and to treat leukemias. Either bone marrow cells or, more often, hematopoietic stem cells mobilized in a donor's blood are injected into the circulation of a recipient, and the cells home to the marrow. The transplantation of hematopoietic stem cells poses many special problems. Before transplantation, some of the bone marrow of the recipient has to be destroyed to create space to receive the transplanted stem cells, and this depletion of the recipient's marrow inevitably causes deficiency of blood cells, including immune cells, resulting in potentially serious immune deficiencies. The immune system reacts strongly against allogeneic hematopoietic stem cells, so successful transplantation requires careful HLA matching of donor and recipient. HLA

Drug	Mechanism of action
Cyclosporine and tacrolimus	Blocks T cell cytokine production by inhibiting the phosphatase calcineurin and thus blocking activation of the NFAT transcription factor
Mycophenolate mofetil	Blocks lymphocyte proliferation by inhibiting guanine nucleotide synthesis in lymphocytes
Rapamycin	Blocks lymphocyte proliferation by inhibiting mTOR and IL-2 signaling
Corticosteroids	Reduce inflammation by effects on multiple cell types
Antithymocyte globulin	Binds to and depletes T cells by promoting phagocytosis or complement-mediated lysis (used to treat acute rejection)
Anti–IL-2 receptor (CD25) antibody	Inhibits T cell proliferation by blocking IL-2 binding; may also opsonize and help eliminate activated IL-2R–expressing T cells
CTLA4-Ig (belatacept)	Inhibits T cell activation by blocking B7 costimulator binding to T cell CD28
Anti-CD52 (alemtuzumab)	Depletes lymphocytes by complement-mediated lysis

FIGURE 10-12 Treatments for graft rejection. Agents used to treat rejection of organ grafts and their mechanisms of action. Like cyclosporine, tacrolimus (FK506) is a calcineurin inhibitor, but it is not as widely used. *CTLA4-Ig*, Cytotoxic T lymphocyte–associated protein 4–immunoglobulin (fusion protein); *IL*, interleukin; *NFAT*, nuclear factor of activated T cells.

matching also prevents rejection of transplanted stem cells by natural killer cells, which are inhibited by recognition of self MHC molecules (see Chapter 2). If mature allogeneic T cells are transplanted with the stem cells, these mature T cells can attack the recipient's tissues, resulting in a clinical reaction called **graft-versus-host disease.** Because HLA matching is always done for these transplants, this reaction is likely directed against minor histocompatibility antigens. The same reaction is exploited to kill leukemia cells, and hematopoietic stem cell transplantation is now commonly used to treat leukemias resistant to chemotherapy. NK cells in the marrow inoculum may also contribute to the destruction of leukemia cells.

Even if the graft is successful, recipients often are severely immunodeficient while their immune systems are being reconstituted. Despite these problems, hematopoietic stem cell transplantation is a successful therapy for a wide variety of diseases affecting the hematopoietic and lymphoid systems.

▮ SUMMARY

- ▪ A physiologic function of the immune system is to eradicate tumors and prevent the growth of tumors.
- ▪ Tumor antigens may be products of oncogenes or tumor suppressor genes, mutated cellular proteins that do not contribute to the malignant phenotype, overexpressed or aberrantly expressed structurally normal molecules, or products of oncogenic viruses.
- ▪ Tumor rejection is mediated mainly by CTLs recognizing peptides derived from tumor antigens. The induction of CTL responses against tumor antigens often involves ingestion of tumor cells or their antigens by dendritic cells and presentation of the antigens to T cells.
- ▪ Tumors may evade immune responses by losing expression of their antigens, shutting off expression of MHC molecules or molecules involved in antigen processing, expressing ligands for T cell inhibitory receptors, and inducing regulatory T cells or secreting cytokines that suppress immune responses.

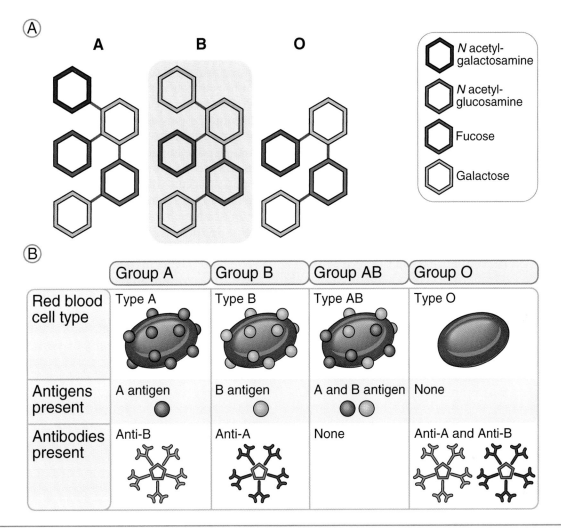

FIGURE 10-13 ABO blood group antigens. **A,** Chemical structure of ABO antigens. **B,** Figure shows the antigens and antibodies present in people with the major ABO blood groups.

- Immunotherapy for cancer aims to enhance antitumor immunity by passively providing immune effectors to patients or by actively boosting the host's own effectors. Approaches for active boosting include vaccination with tumor antigens or with tumor antigen-pulsed dendritic cells, and treatment of cancer patients with antibodies that block T cell inhibitory receptors.
- Transplants of foreign tissues are rejected by the immune system, and the major antigen targets of rejection are MHC molecules.

- The antigens of allografts that are recognized by T cells are allogeneic MHC molecules that resemble peptide-loaded self MHC molecules that the T cells are selected to recognize. Graft antigens either are directly presented to recipient T cells or are picked up and presented by host APCs.
- Grafts may be rejected by different mechanisms. Hyperacute rejection is mediated by preformed antibodies to blood group antigens or HLA molecules, which cause endothelial injury and thrombosis of blood vessels in the

graft. Acute rejection is mediated by T cells, which injure graft cells and endothelium, and by antibodies that bind to the endothelium. Chronic rejection is caused by T cells that produce cytokines that stimulate growth of vascular smooth muscle cells and tissue fibroblasts.

■ Treatment for graft rejection is designed to suppress T cell responses and inflammation. The mainstay of treatment has been immunosuppressive drugs, including corticosteroids and cyclosporine; many other agents are in clinical use now.

■ Hematopoietic stem cell transplants elicit strong rejection reactions, carry the risk of graft-versus-host disease, and often lead to temporary immunodeficiency in recipients.

REVIEW QUESTIONS

1. What are the main types of tumor antigens that the immune system reacts against?
2. What is the evidence that tumor rejection is an immunologic phenomenon?
3. How do naive CD8$^+$ T cells recognize tumor antigens, and how are these cells activated to differentiate into effector CTLs?
4. What are some of the mechanisms by which tumors may evade the immune response?
5. What are some strategies for enhancing host immune responses to tumor antigens?
6. Why do normal T cells, which recognize foreign peptide antigens bound to self MHC molecules, react strongly against the allogeneic MHC molecules of a graft?
7. What are the principal mechanisms of rejection of allografts?
8. How is the likelihood of graft rejection reduced in clinical transplantation?
9. What are some of the problems associated with the transplantation of hematopoietic stem cells?

Answers to and discussion of the Review Questions are available at https://studentconsult. inkling.com.

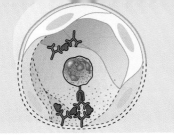

CHAPTER 11

Hypersensitivity

Disorders Caused by Immune Responses

The concept that the immune system is required for defending the host against infections has been emphasized throughout this book. However, immune responses are themselves capable of causing tissue injury and disease. Injurious, or pathologic, immune reactions are called **hypersensitivity reactions.** An immune response to an antigen may result in sensitivity to challenge with that antigen, and therefore hypersensitivity is a reflection of excessive or aberrant immune responses. Hypersensitivity reactions may occur in two situations. First, responses to foreign antigens (microbes and noninfectious environmental antigens) may cause tissue injury, especially if the reactions are repetitious or poorly controlled. Second, the immune responses may be directed against self (autologous) antigens, as a result of the failure of self-tolerance (see Chapter 9). Responses against self antigens are termed **autoimmunity,** and disorders caused by such responses are called **autoimmune diseases.**

This chapter describes the important features of hypersensitivity reactions and the resulting diseases, focusing on their pathogenesis. Their clinicopathologic features are described only briefly and can be found in other medical textbooks. The following questions are addressed:
- What are the mechanisms of different types of hypersensitivity reactions?
- What are the major clinical and pathologic features of diseases caused by these reactions, and what principles underlie treatment of such diseases?

TYPES OF HYPERSENSITIVITY REACTIONS

Hypersensitivity reactions are classified on the basis of the principal immunologic mechanism that is responsible for tissue injury and disease (Fig. 11-1). We prefer the more informative descriptive designations rather

231

Type of hypersensitivity	Pathologic immune mechanisms	Mechanisms of tissue injury and disease
Immediate hypersensitivity (Type I)	Th2 cells, IgE antibody, mast cells, eosinophils 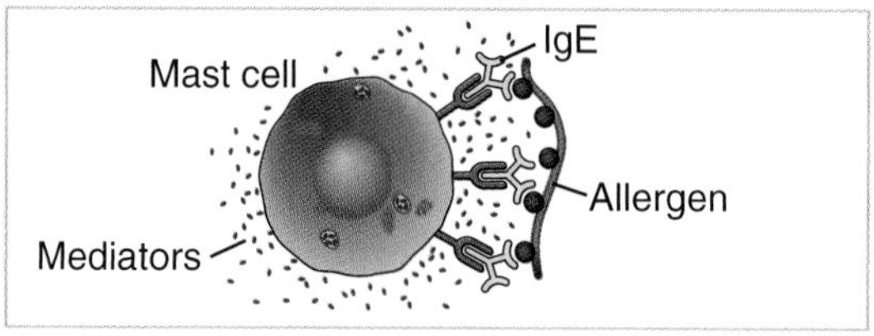	Mast cell-derived mediators (vasoactive amines, lipid mediators, cytokines) Cytokine-mediated inflammation (eosinophils, neutrophils, lymphocytes)
Antibody-mediated (Type II)	IgM, IgG antibodies against cell surface or extracellular matrix antigens 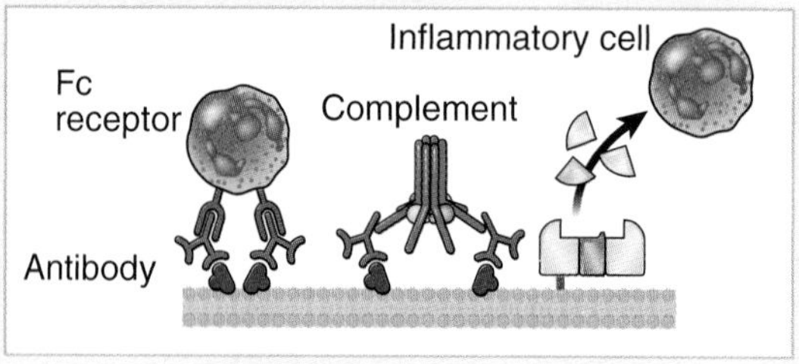	Complement- and Fc receptor-mediated recruitment and activation of leukocytes (neutrophils, macrophages) Opsonization and phagocytosis of cells Abnormalities in cellular function (e.g., hormone or neurotransmitter receptor signaling)
Immune complex-mediated (Type III)	Immune complexes of circulating antigens and IgM or IgG antibodies deposited in vascular basement membrane 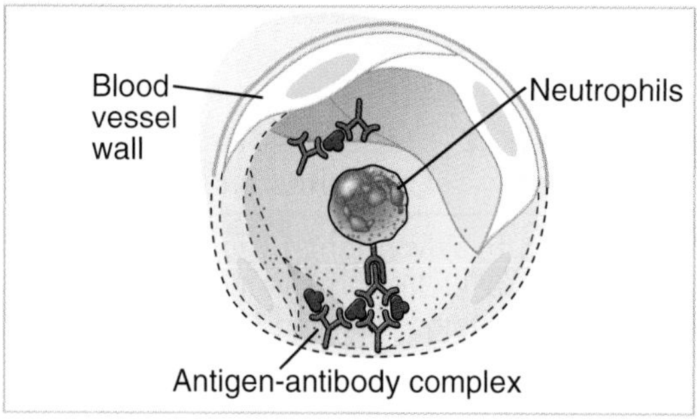	Complement- and Fc receptor-mediated recruitment and activation of leukocytes, and tissue damage secondary to impaired blood flow
T cell-mediated (Type IV)	1. CD4+ T cells (cytokine-mediated inflammation) 2. CD8+ CTLs (T cell-mediated cytolysis) 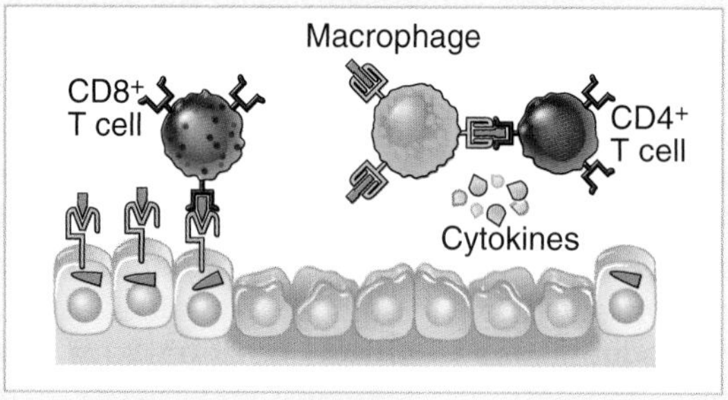	1. Macrophage activation, cytokine-mediated inflammation 2. Direct target cell lysis, cytokine-mediated inflammation

FIGURE 11-1 Types of hypersensitivity reactions. In the four major types of hypersensitivity reactions, different immune effector mechanisms cause tissue injury and disease. *CTLs*, Cytotoxic T lymphocytes; *Ig*, immunoglobulin.

than numeric terms, so these descriptors are used throughout this chapter.

- Immediate hypersensitivity, or type I hypersensitivity, is a type of pathologic reaction that is caused by the release of mediators from mast cells. This reaction most often depends on the production of immunoglobulin E (IgE) antibody against environmental antigens and the binding of IgE to mast cells in various tissues.
- Antibodies other than IgE that are directed against cell or tissue antigens can damage these cells or tissues or can impair their function. These diseases are said to be antibody mediated and represent type II hypersensitivity.
- Antibodies against soluble antigens may form complexes with the antigens, and the immune complexes may deposit in blood vessels in various tissues, causing inflammation and tissue injury. Such diseases are called immune complex diseases and represent type III hypersensitivity.
- Some diseases result from the reactions of T lymphocytes, often against self antigens in tissues. These T cell–mediated diseases represent type IV hypersensitivity.

This classification scheme is useful because it distinguishes the mechanisms of immune-mediated tissue injury. In many human immunologic diseases, however, the damage may result from a combination of antibody-mediated and T cell–mediated reactions, so it is often difficult to classify these diseases neatly into one type of hypersensitivity.

IMMEDIATE HYPERSENSITIVITY

Immediate hypersensitivity is an IgE antibody– and mast cell–mediated reaction to certain antigens that causes rapid vascular leakage and mucosal secretions, often followed by inflammation. Disorders in which IgE-mediated immediate hypersensitivity is prominent are also called **allergy**, or **atopy**, and individuals with a propensity to develop these reactions are said to be atopic. Immediate hypersensitivity may affect various tissues and may be of varying severity in different individuals. Common types of allergies include hay fever, food allergies, bronchial

asthma, and anaphylaxis. Allergies are the most frequent disorders of the immune system, estimated to affect 10% to 20% of people, and the incidence of allergic diseases has been increasing in industrialized societies.

The sequence of events in the development of immediate hypersensitivity reactions begins with the activation of Th2 and IL-4–secreting follicular helper T (Tfh) cells, which stimulate the production of IgE antibodies in response to an antigen, binding of the IgE to specific Fc receptors of mast cells, then on subsequent exposure to the antigen, cross-linking of the bound IgE by the antigen, and release of mast cell mediators (Fig. 11-2). Some mast cell mediators cause a rapid increase in vascular permeability and smooth muscle contraction, resulting in many of the symptoms of these reactions (Fig. 11-3). This vascular and smooth muscle reaction may occur within minutes of reintroduction of antigen into a previously sensitized individual, hence the name *immediate* hypersensitivity. Other mast cell mediators are cytokines that recruit neutrophils and eosinophils to the site of the reaction over several hours. This inflammatory component is called the **late-phase reaction**, and it is mainly responsible for the tissue injury that results from repeated bouts of immediate hypersensitivity.

With this background, we proceed to a discussion of the steps in immediate hypersensitivity reactions.

Activation of Th2 Cells and Production of IgE Antibody

In individuals who are prone to allergies, exposure to some antigens results in the activation of Th2 and Tfh cells and the production of IgE antibody (see Fig. 11-2). Most individuals do not mount strong Th2 responses to environmental antigens. For unknown reasons, when some individuals encounter certain antigens, such as proteins in pollen, certain foods, insect venoms, or animal dander, or if they are treated with certain drugs such as penicillin, there is a strong Th2 response. Immediate hypersensitivity develops as a consequence of

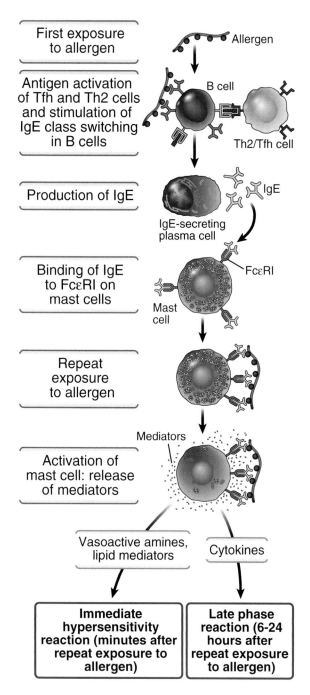

First exposure to allergen

Antigen activation of Tfh and Th2 cells and stimulation of IgE class switching in B cells

Allergen

B cell

Th2/Tfh cell

Production of IgE

IgE

IgE-secreting plasma cell

Binding of IgE to FcεRI on mast cells

FcεRI

Mast cell

Repeat exposure to allergen

Mediators

Activation of mast cell: release of mediators

Vasoactive amines, lipid mediators

Cytokines

Immediate hypersensitivity reaction (minutes after repeat exposure to allergen)

Late phase reaction (6-24 hours after repeat exposure to allergen)

FIGURE 11-2 The sequence of events in immediate hypersensitivity. Immediate hypersensitivity reactions are initiated by the introduction of an allergen, which stimulates Th2 and IL-4/IL-13–producing Tfh cells and immunoglobulin E (IgE) production. IgE binds to Fc receptors (FcεRI) on mast cells, and subsequent exposure to the allergen activates the mast cells to secrete the mediators that are responsible for the pathologic reactions of immediate hypersensitivity.

the activation of Th2 cells in response to protein antigens or chemicals that bind to proteins. Antigens that elicit immediate hypersensitivity (allergic) reactions often are called allergens. Any atopic individual may be allergic to one or more of these antigens. It is not understood why only a small subset of common environmental antigens elicit Th2-mediated reactions and IgE production, or what characteristics of these antigens are responsible for their behavior as allergens.

Two of the cytokines secreted by Th2 cells or by Tfh cells activated by the same antigen are IL-4 and IL-13. These cytokines stimulate B lymphocytes to switch to IgE-producing plasma cells. Therefore, atopic individuals produce large amounts of IgE antibody in response to antigens that do not elicit IgE responses in other people. The propensity toward development of IL-4–producing T cells, IgE production, and immediate hypersensitivity has a strong genetic basis; a major known risk for developing allergies is a family history of atopic disease. Many different genes appear to play contributory roles, but the mechanisms by which these genes influence the development of allergies are poorly understood.

Activation of Mast Cells and Secretion of Mediators

IgE antibody produced in response to an allergen binds to high-affinity Fc receptors, specific for the ε heavy chain, that are expressed on mast cells (see Fig. 11-2). Thus, in an atopic individual, mast cells are coated with IgE antibody specific for the antigen(s) to which the individual is allergic. This process of coating

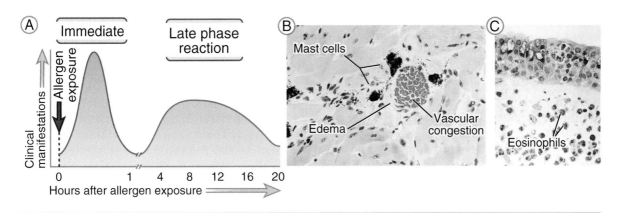

FIGURE 11-3 Immediate hypersensitivity. **A,** Kinetics of the immediate and late-phase reactions. The immediate vascular and smooth muscle reaction to allergen develops within minutes after challenge (allergen exposure in a previously sensitized individual), and the late-phase reaction develops 2 to 24 hours later. **B,** Morphology of the immediate reaction is characterized by vasodilation, congestion, and edema. **C,** The late-phase reaction is characterized by an inflammatory infiltrate rich in eosinophils, neutrophils, and T cells. (Micrographs courtesy Dr. Daniel Friend, Department of Pathology, Brigham and Women's Hospital, Boston.)

mast cells with IgE is called sensitization, because coating with IgE specific for an antigen makes the mast cells sensitive to activation by subsequent encounter with that antigen. In normal individuals, by contrast, mast cells may carry IgE molecules of many different specificities, because many antigens may elicit small IgE responses, and the amount of IgE specific for any one antigen is not enough to cause immediate hypersensitivity reactions upon exposure to that antigen.

Mast cells are present in all connective tissues, especially under epithelia, and they are usually located adjacent to blood vessels. Which of the body's mast cells are activated by cross-linking of allergen-specific IgE often depends on the route of entry of the allergen. For example, inhaled allergens activate mast cells in the submucosal tissues of the bronchus, whereas ingested allergens activate mast cells in the wall of the intestine.

The high-affinity receptor for IgE, called FcεRI, consists of three polypeptide chains, one of which binds the Fc portion of the ε heavy chain very strongly, with a K_d of approximately 10^{-11} M. (The concentration of IgE in the plasma is approximately 10^{-9} M, which explains why even in normal individuals, mast cells are always coated with IgE bound to FcεRI.) The other two chains of the receptor are signaling proteins. The same FcεRI is

also present on basophils, which are circulating cells with many of the features of mast cells, but the role of basophils in immediate hypersensitivity is not as well established as the role of mast cells.

When mast cells sensitized by IgE are exposed to the allergen, the cells are activated to secrete their mediators (Fig. 11-4). Mast cell activation results from binding of the allergen to two or more IgE antibodies on the cell. When this happens, the FcεRI molecules that are carrying the IgE are cross-linked, triggering biochemical signals from the signal-transducing chains of FcεRI. The signals lead to three types of responses in the mast cell: rapid release of granule contents (degranulation), synthesis and secretion of lipid mediators, and synthesis and secretion of cytokines.

The most important mediators produced by mast cells are vasoactive amines and proteases stored in and released from granules, newly generated and secreted products of arachidonic acid metabolism, and cytokines (see Fig. 11-4). These mediators have different actions. The major amine, histamine, causes the dilation of small blood vessels, increases vascular permeability, and stimulates the transient contraction of smooth muscles. Proteases may cause damage to local tissues. Arachidonic acid metabolites include prostaglandins, which

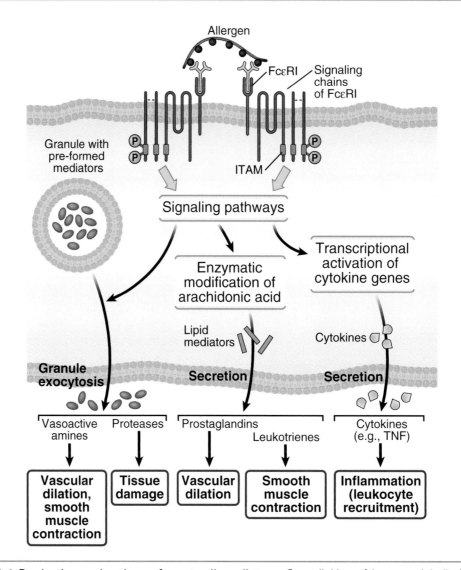

FIGURE 11-4 Production and actions of mast cell mediators. Cross-linking of immunoglobulin E (IgE) on a mast cell by an allergen stimulates phosphorylation of immunoreceptor tyrosine-based activation motifs (ITAMs) in the signaling chains of the IgE Fc receptor (FcεRI), which then initiates multiple signaling pathways. These signaling pathways stimulate the release of mast cell granule contents (amines, proteases), the synthesis of arachidonic acid metabolites (prostaglandins, leukotrienes), and the synthesis of various cytokines. *TNF*, Tumor necrosis factor.

cause vascular dilation, and leukotrienes, which stimulate prolonged smooth muscle contraction. Cytokines induce local inflammation (the late-phase reaction, described next). Thus, mast cell mediators are responsible for acute vascular and smooth muscle reactions and inflammation, the hallmarks of immediate hypersensitivity.

Cytokines produced by mast cells stimulate the recruitment of leukocytes, which cause the late-phase reaction. The principal leukocytes involved in this reaction are eosinophils, neutrophils, and Th2 cells. Mast cell–derived tumor necrosis factor (TNF) and IL-4 promote neutrophil- and eosinophil-rich

Clinical syndrome	Clinical and pathological manifestations
Allergic rhinitis, sinusitis (hay fever)	Increased mucus secretion; inflammation of upper airways, sinuses
Food allergies	Increased peristalsis due to contraction of intestinal muscles
Bronchial asthma	Airway obstruction caused by bronchial smooth muscle hyperactivity; inflammation and tissue injury caused by late-phase reaction
Anaphylaxis (may be caused by drugs, bee sting, food)	Fall in blood pressure (shock) caused by vascular dilation; airway obstruction due to bronchoconstriction and laryngeal edema

FIGURE 11-5 Clinical manifestations of immediate hypersensitivity reactions. Immediate hypersensitivity may be manifested in many other ways, as in development of skin lesions (e.g., urticaria, eczema).

inflammation. Chemokines produced by mast cells and by epithelial cells in the tissues also contribute to leukocyte recruitment. Eosinophils and neutrophils liberate proteases, which cause tissue damage, and Th2 cells may exacerbate the reaction by producing more cytokines. Eosinophils are prominent components of many allergic reactions and are an important cause of tissue injury in these reactions. These cells are activated by the cytokine IL-5, which is produced by Th2 cells, innate lymphoid cells, and mast cells.

Clinical Syndromes and Therapy

Immediate hypersensitivity reactions have diverse clinical and pathologic features, all of which are attributable to mediators produced by mast cells in different amounts and in different tissues (Fig. 11-5).

- Some mild manifestations, such as allergic rhinitis and sinusitis, which are common in **hay fever**, are reactions to inhaled allergens, such as a protein of ragweed pollen. Mast cells in the nasal mucosa produce histamine, and Th2 cells produce IL-13, and these two mediators cause increased production of mucus. Late-phase reactions may lead to more prolonged inflammation.
- In **food allergies**, ingested allergens trigger mast cell degranulation, and the released histamine causes increased peristalsis, resulting in vomiting and diarrhea.
- **Bronchial asthma** is most often a form of respiratory allergy in which inhaled allergens (often undefined) stimulate bronchial mast cells to release mediators, including leukotrienes, which cause repeated bouts of bronchial constriction and airway obstruction. In chronic asthma, large numbers of eosinophils accumulate in the bronchial mucosa, excessive secretion of mucus occurs in the airways, and the bronchial smooth muscle becomes hypertrophied and hyperreactive to various stimuli. Some cases of asthma are not associated with IgE production, although all are caused by mast cell activation. In some patients, asthma may be triggered by cold or exercise; how either of these causes mast cell activation is unknown.
- The most severe form of immediate hypersensitivity is **anaphylaxis,** a systemic reaction characterized by edema in many tissues, including the larynx, accompanied by a fall in blood pressure and bronchoconstriction. Some of the most frequent inducers of anaphylaxis include bee stings, injected or ingested penicillin-family antibiotics, and ingested nuts or shellfish. The reaction is caused by widespread mast cell degranulation in response to the systemic distribution of the antigen, and it is life threatening because of the sudden fall in blood pressure and airway obstruction.

The therapy for immediate hypersensitivity diseases is aimed at inhibiting mast cell degranulation, antagonizing the effects of mast cell mediators, and reducing inflammation (Fig. 11-6). Common drugs include antihistamines for hay fever, agents that relax bronchial

Syndrome	Therapy	Mechanism of action
Anaphylaxis	Epinephrine	Causes vascular smooth muscle cell contraction, increases cardiac output (to counter shock), and inhibits bronchial smooth muscle cell contraction
Bronchial asthma	Corticosteroids	Reduce inflammation
	Leukotriene antagonists	Relax bronchial smooth muscle and reduce inflammation
	Phosphodiesterase inhibitors	Relax bronchial smooth muscles
Various allergic diseases	Desensitization (repeated administration of low doses of allergens)	Unknown; may inhibit IgE production and increase production of other Ig isotypes; may induce T cell tolerance
	Anti-IgE antibody	Neutralizes and eliminates IgE
	Antihistamines	Block actions of histamine on vessels and smooth muscles
	Cromolyn	Inhibits mast cell degranulation

FIGURE 11-6 **Treatment of immediate hypersensitivity reactions.** The figure summarizes the principal mechanisms of action of the various drugs used to treat allergic disorders. *Ig*, Immunoglobulin.

smooth muscles in asthma, and epinephrine in anaphylaxis. In diseases with inflammation as an important pathologic component, such as asthma, corticosteroids are used to inhibit inflammation. Many patients benefit from repeated administration of small doses of allergens, called desensitization or allergen-specific immunotherapy. This treatment may work by changing the T cell response away from Th2 dominance or the antibody response away from IgE, by inducing tolerance in allergen-specific T cells, or by stimulating regulatory T cells (Tregs).

Before concluding the discussion of immediate hypersensitivity, it is important to address the question of why evolution has preserved an IgE antibody– and mast cell–mediated immune response whose major effects are pathologic. There is no definitive answer to this puzzle, but immediate hypersensitivity reactions likely evolved to protect against pathogens or toxins. It is known that IgE antibody and eosinophils are important mechanisms of defense against helminthic infections, and mast cells play a role in innate immunity against some bacteria and in destroying venomous toxins.

DISEASES CAUSED BY ANTIBODIES AND ANTIGEN-ANTIBODY COMPLEXES

Antibodies other than IgE may cause disease by binding to their target antigens in cells and tissues or by forming immune complexes

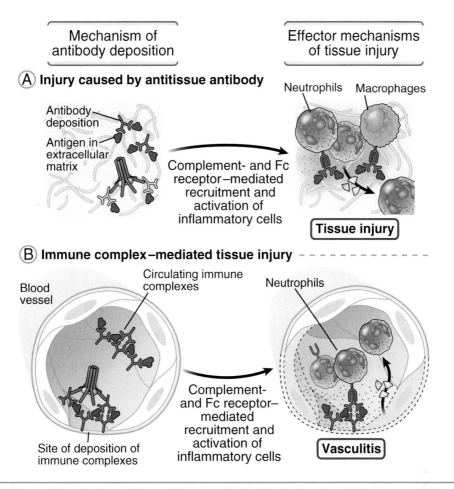

FIGURE 11-7 Types of antibody-mediated diseases. Antibodies (other than IgE) may cause tissue injury and disease by: **A,** binding directly to their target antigens on the surface of cells and in the extracellular matrix (type II hypersensitivity) or **B,** by forming immune complexes that deposit mainly in blood vessels (type III hypersensitivity).

that deposit in blood vessels (Fig. 11-7). Antibody-mediated hypersensitivity reactions have long been recognized as the basis of many chronic immunologic diseases in humans. Antibodies against cells or extracellular matrix components may deposit in any tissue that expresses the relevant target antigen. Diseases caused by such antibodies usually are specific for a particular tissue. Immune complexes often deposit in blood vessels, including vessels through which plasma is filtered at high pressure (e.g., in renal glomeruli and joint synovium). Therefore, immune complex diseases tend to be systemic and often manifest as widespread vasculitis, arthritis, and nephritis.

Etiology of Antibody-Mediated Diseases

The antibodies that cause disease most often are autoantibodies against self antigens and less commonly are specific for foreign (e.g., microbial) antigens. The production of autoantibodies results from a failure of self-tolerance. In Chapter 9 we discussed the mechanisms by which self-tolerance may fail, but why this happens in any human autoimmune disease is still not understood. Autoantibodies may bind to self antigens in tissues or may form immune complexes with circulating self antigens.

Two of the best-described diseases caused by antibodies produced against microbial antigens are rare, late sequelae of streptococcal infections. After such infections, some individuals produce antistreptococcal antibodies that cross-react with an antigen in heart tissues. Deposition of these antibodies in the heart triggers an inflammatory disease called rheumatic fever, which can lead to acute heart failure or slow scarring of valves and late-onset heart failure. Other individuals make antistreptococcal antibodies that deposit in kidney glomeruli, causing an inflammatory process called poststreptococcal glomerulonephritis that can lead to renal failure. Some immune complex diseases are caused by complexes of antimicrobial antibodies and microbial antigens. This may occur in patients with chronic infections with certain viruses (e.g., the hepatitis virus) or parasites (e.g., malaria).

Mechanisms of Tissue Injury and Disease

Antibodies specific for cell and tissue antigens may deposit in tissues and cause injury by inducing local inflammation, they may induce phagocytosis and destruction of cells, or they interfere with normal cellular functions (Fig. 11-8).

- *Inflammation.* Antibodies against tissue antigens and immune complexes deposited in vessels induce inflammation by attracting and activating leukocytes. IgG antibodies of the IgG1 and IgG3 subclasses bind to neutrophil and macrophage Fc receptors and activate these leukocytes, resulting in inflammation (see Chapter 8). The same antibodies, as well as IgM, activate the complement system by the classical pathway, resulting in the production of complement byproducts that recruit leukocytes and induce inflammation. When leukocytes are activated at sites of antibody deposition, these cells release reactive oxygen species and lysosomal enzymes that damage the adjacent tissues.
- *Opsonization and phagocytosis.* If antibodies bind to cells, such as erythrocytes and platelets, the cells are opsonized and may be ingested and destroyed by host phagocytes.
- *Abnormal cellular responses.* Some antibodies may cause disease without directly inducing tissue injury. For example, antibodies against hormone receptors may inhibit receptor function; in some cases of myasthenia gravis, antibodies against the acetylcholine receptor inhibit neuromuscular transmission, causing paralysis. Other antibodies may directly activate receptors, mimicking their physiologic ligands. In a form of hyperthyroidism called Graves disease, antibodies against the receptor for thyroid-stimulating hormone stimulate thyroid cells even in the absence of the hormone.

Clinical Syndromes and Therapy

Many chronic hypersensitivity disorders in humans are caused by, or are associated with, antibodies against cells and tissues (Fig. 11-9) and immune complexes (Fig. 11-10). The first immune complex disease studied was serum sickness, seen in subjects who repeatedly received animal serum for the treatment of infections. This illness could be re-created in experimental animals. **Serum sickness** is induced by systemic administration of a protein antigen, which elicits an antibody response and leads to the formation of circulating immune complexes. Systemic lupus erythematosus is another example of a well-studied systemic immune complex disease.

A localized immune complex reaction called the **Arthus reaction** was first studied in experimental animals. It is induced by subcutaneous administration of a protein antigen to a previously immunized animal; it results in the formation of immune complexes at the site of antigen injection and a local vasculitis. In a small percentage of vaccine recipients who have previously been vaccinated or already have antibodies against the vaccine antigen, a painful swelling that develops at the injection site represents a clinically relevant Arthus reaction.

Therapy for antibody-mediated diseases is intended mainly to limit inflammation and its injurious consequences, with drugs such as corticosteroids. In severe cases, plasmapheresis is used to reduce levels of circulating antibodies or immune complexes. Some of these diseases respond well to treatment with intravenous IgG (IVIG) pooled from healthy donors. How IVIG works is not known; it may induce the expression of and bind to the inhibitory Fc receptor on myeloid cells and B cells (see Chapter 7, Fig. 7-15), or it may reduce the half-life of pathogenic antibodies by competing for binding to the neonatal Fc receptor in endothelial

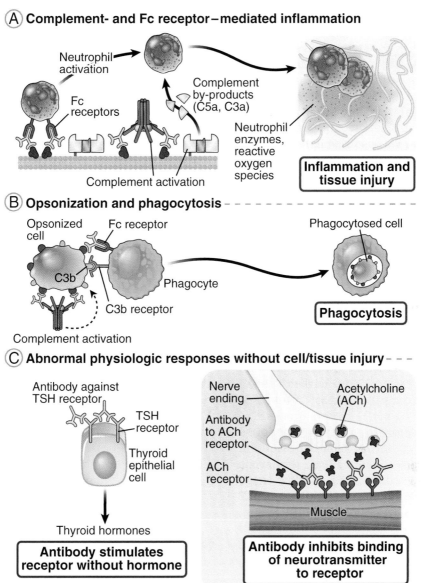

FIGURE 11-8 Effector mechanisms of antibody-mediated diseases. Antibodies cause disease by **A,** inducing inflammation at the site of deposition; **B,** opsonizing cells for phagocytosis; and **C,** interfering with normal cellular functions, such as hormone receptor signaling. All three mechanisms are seen with antibodies that bind directly to their target antigens, but immune complexes cause disease mainly by inducing inflammation (**A**). *TSH,* Thyroid-stimulating hormone.

and other cells (see Chapter 8, Fig. 8-2). Treatment of patients with an antibody specific for CD20, a surface protein of mature B cells, results in depletion of the B cells and may be useful for treating some antibody-mediated disorders.

Other approaches being tried for inhibiting the production of autoantibodies include treating patients with antibodies that block CD40 or its ligand and thus inhibit helper T cell–dependent B cell activation and antibodies to block cytokines that promote

Antibody-mediated disease	Target antigen	Mechanisms of disease	Clinicopathologic manifestations
Autoimmune hemolytic anemia	Erythrocyte membrane proteins (Rh blood group antigens, I antigen)	Opsonization and phagocytosis of erythrocytes	Hemolysis, anemia
Autoimmune (idiopathic) thrombocytopenic purpura	Platelet membrane proteins (gpIIb/IIIa integrin)	Opsonization and phagocytosis of platelets	Bleeding
Goodpasture syndrome	Noncollagenous protein in basement membranes of kidney glomeruli and lung alveoli	Complement and Fc receptor–mediated inflammation	Nephritis, lung hemorrhage
Graves disease (hyperthyroidism)	Thyroid stimulating hormone (TSH) receptor	Antibody-mediated stimulation of TSH receptors	Hyperthyroidism
Myasthenia gravis	Acetylcholine receptor	Antibody inhibits acetycholine binding, down-modulates receptors	Muscle weakness, paralysis
Pemphigus vulgaris	Proteins in intercellular junctions of epidermal cells (desmoglein)	Antibody-mediated activation of proteases, disruption of intercellular adhesions	Skin vesicles (bullae)
Pernicious anemia	Intrinsic factor of gastric parietal cells	Neutralization of intrinsic factor, decreased absorption of vitamin B_{12}	Abnormal erythropoiesis, anemia
Rheumatic fever	Streptococcal cell wall antigen; antibody cross-reacts with myocardial antigen	Inflammation, macrophage activation	Myocarditis, arthritis

FIGURE 11-9 Human antibody-mediated diseases (type II hypersensitivity). The figure lists examples of human diseases caused by antibodies. In most of these diseases, the role of antibodies is inferred from the detection of antibodies in the blood or the lesions, and in some cases by similarities with experimental models in which the involvement of antibodies can be formally established by transfer studies.

the survival of B cells and plasma cells. There is also interest in inducing tolerance in cases in which the autoantigens are known.

DISEASES CAUSED BY T LYMPHOCYTES

The role of T lymphocytes in human immunologic diseases has been increasingly recognized with improved methods for identifying and isolating these cells from lesions and through animal models of human disease in which a pathogenic role of T cells is established by experiments. In fact, much of the recent interest in the pathogenesis and treatment of human autoimmune diseases has focused on disorders in which tissue injury is caused mainly by T lymphocytes.

Immune complex disease	Antibody specificity	Clinicopathologic manifestations
Systemic lupus erythematosus	DNA, nucleoproteins, others	Nephritis, arthritis, vasculitis
Polyarteritis nodosa	In some cases, microbial antigens (e.g., hepatitis B virus surface antigen); most cases unknown	Vasculitis
Poststreptococcal glomerulonephritis	Streptococcal cell wall antigen(s)	Nephritis
Serum sickness (clinical and experimental)	Various protein antigens	Systemic vasculitis, nephritis, arthritis
Arthus reaction (experimental)	Various protein antigens	Cutaneous vasculitis

FIGURE 11-10 Immune complex diseases (type III hypersensitivity). Examples of human diseases caused by the deposition of immune complexes, as well as two experimental models. In the diseases, immune complexes are detected in the blood or in the tissues that are the sites of injury. In all the disorders, injury is caused by complement-mediated and Fc receptor–mediated inflammation.

Etiology of T Cell–Mediated Diseases

The major causes of T cell–mediated hypersensitivity reactions are autoimmunity and exaggerated or persistent responses to environmental antigens. The autoimmune reactions usually are directed against cellular antigens with restricted tissue distribution. Therefore, T cell–mediated autoimmune diseases tend to be limited to a few organs and usually are not systemic. Examples of T cell–mediated hypersensitivity reactions against environmental antigens include contact sensitivity to chemicals (e.g., various therapeutic drugs and substances found in plants such as poison ivy). Tissue injury also may accompany T cell responses to microbes. For example, in tuberculosis, a T cell–mediated immune response develops against protein antigens of *Mycobacterium tuberculosis,* and the response becomes chronic because the infection is difficult to eradicate. The resultant granulomatous inflammation causes injury to normal tissues at the site of infection.

Excessive polyclonal T cell activation by certain microbial toxins produced by some bacteria and viruses can lead to production of large amounts of inflammatory cytokines, causing a syndrome similar to septic shock. These toxins are called **superantigens** because they stimulate large numbers of T cells. Superantigens bind to invariant parts of T cell receptors on many different clones of T cells, regardless of antigen specificity, thereby activating these cells.

Mechanisms of Tissue Injury

In different T cell–mediated diseases, tissue injury is caused by inflammation induced by cytokines that are produced mainly by CD4+ T cells or by killing of host cells by CD8+ CTLs (Fig. 11-11). These mechanisms of tissue injury are the same as the mechanisms used by T cells to eliminate cell-associated microbes.

CD4+ T cells may react against cell or tissue antigens and secrete cytokines that induce local inflammation and activate macrophages. Different diseases may be associated with activation of Th1 and Th17 cells. Th1 cells are the source of

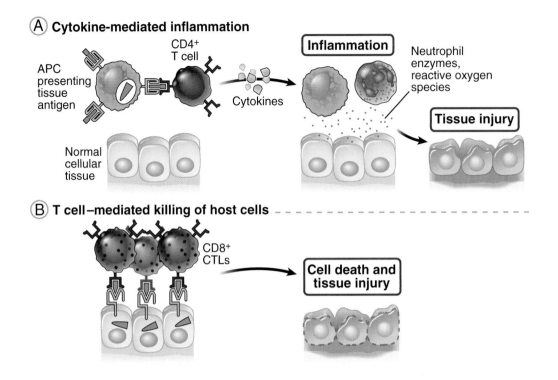

FIGURE 11-11 Mechanisms of T cell–mediated tissue injury (type IV hypersensitivity). T cells may cause tissue injury and disease by two mechanisms. **A,** Inflammation may be triggered by cytokines produced mainly by CD4+ T cells in which tissue injury is caused by activated macrophages and inflammatory cells; *APC,* Antigen-presenting cell. **B,** Direct killing of target cells is mediated by CD8+ cytotoxic T lymphocytes (CTLs).

interferon-γ (IFN-γ), the principal macrophage-activating cytokine, and Th17 cells are responsible for the recruitment of leukocytes, including neutrophils. The actual tissue injury in these diseases is caused mainly by the macrophages and neutrophils.

The typical reaction mediated by T cell cytokines is **delayed-type hypersensitivity** (DTH), so called because it occurs 24 to 48 hours after an individual previously exposed to a protein antigen is challenged with the antigen (i.e., the reaction is delayed). The delay occurs because it takes several hours for circulating effector T lymphocytes to home to the site of antigen challenge, respond to the antigen at this site, and secrete cytokines that induce a detectable reaction. DTH reactions are manifested by infiltrates of T cells and blood monocytes in the tissues, edema and fibrin deposition caused by increased vascular permeability in response to cytokines produced by CD4+ T cells, and tissue damage induced by leukocyte products, mainly from macrophages that are activated by the T cells (Fig. 11-12). DTH reactions often are used to determine if people have been previously exposed to and have responded to an antigen. For example, a DTH reaction to a mycobacterial antigen, PPD (purified protein derivative), is an indicator of a T cell response to the mycobacteria. This is the basis for the PPD skin test, used to detect past or active mycobacterial infection.

CD8+ T cells specific for antigens on host cells may directly kill these cells. CD8+ T cells also produce cytokines that induce inflammation, but they are usually not the major sources of cytokines in immune reactions. In many T cell–mediated autoimmune diseases, both CD4+ T cells and CD8+ T cells specific for self antigens are present, and both contribute to tissue injury.

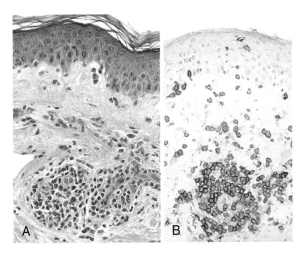

FIGURE 11-12 Delayed-type hypersensitivity reaction in the skin. **A,** Perivascular accumulation (cuffing) of mononuclear inflammatory cells (lymphocytes and macrophages), with associated dermal edema and fibrin deposition. **B,** Immunoperoxidase staining reveals a predominantly perivascular cellular infiltrate that marks positively with anti-CD4 antibodies. (**B,** Courtesy Dr. Louis Picker, Department of Pathology, Oregon Health Sciences University, Portland.)

Clinical Syndromes and Therapy

Many organ-specific autoimmune diseases in humans are believed to be caused by T cells, based on the identification of these cells in lesions and similarities with animal models in which the diseases are known to be T cell mediated (Fig. 11-13). These disorders typically are chronic and progressive, in part because T cell reactions tend to be prolonged and often self-perpetuating, and because the inciting antigens, such as tissue antigens or proteins expressed by resident microbes, are often never cleared. Also, tissue injury causes release and alteration of self proteins, which may result in reactions against these newly encountered proteins. This phenomenon has been called epitope spreading to indicate that the initial immune response against one or a few self antigen epitopes may expand to include responses against many more self antigens. Chronic inflammatory diseases that are initiated by immune reactions are sometimes called immune-mediated inflammatory diseases.

The therapy for T cell–mediated hypersensitivity disorders is designed to reduce inflammation and to inhibit T cell responses. The mainstay of treatment of such diseases has been the potent antiinflammatory steroids, but these drugs have significant side effects. The development of more targeted therapies based on understanding of the fundamental mechanisms of these diseases has been one of the most impressive accomplishments of immunology. Antagonists of TNF have proved to be beneficial in patients with rheumatoid arthritis and inflammatory bowel disease by reducing inflammation. Newer agents developed to inhibit T cell responses include drugs that block costimulators such as B7, and antagonists against cytokines or their receptors such as IL-1, IL-6, and IL-17. B cell depletion with anti-CD20 has also been effective in rheumatoid arthritis and multiple sclerosis; it is not clear if this is because antibodies contribute to the diseases or because B cells function as antigen-presenting cells to promote T cell activation. There also is great hope for inducing tolerance in pathogenic T cells, but no successful clinical trials have been reported.

▌ SUMMARY

- Immune responses that cause tissue injury are called hypersensitivity reactions, and the diseases caused by these reactions are called hypersensitivity diseases or immune-mediated inflammatory diseases.
- Hypersensitivity reactions may arise from uncontrolled or abnormal responses to foreign antigens or autoimmune responses against self antigens.
- Hypersensitivity reactions are classified according to the mechanism of tissue injury.
- Immediate hypersensitivity (type I, commonly called allergy) is caused by the activation of Th2 cells and IL-4-producing Tfh cells and production of IgE antibody against environmental antigens or drugs (allergens), sensitization of mast cells by the IgE, and degranulation of these mast cells on subsequent encounter with the allergen.

Disease	Specificity of pathogenic T cells	Clinicopathologic manifestations
Multiple sclerosis	Myelin proteins	Demyelination in the central nervous system, sensory and motor dysfunction
Rheumatoid arthritis	Unknown antigens in joint	Inflammation of synovium and erosion of cartilage and bone in joints
Type 1 (insulin-dependent) diabetes mellitus	Pancreatic islet antigens	Impaired glucose metabolism, vascular disease
Crohn's disease	Unknown, ? role of intestinal microbes	Inflammation of the bowel wall; abdominal pain, diarrhea, hemorrhage
Contact sensitivity (e.g., poison ivy reaction)	Modified skin proteins	DTH reaction in skin, rash
Chronic infections (e.g., tuberculosis)	Microbial proteins	Chronic (e.g., granulomatous) inflammation
Viral hepatitis (HBV, HCV)	Virally encoded proteins	CTL-mediated hepatocyte death, liver dysfunction; fibrosis
Superantigen-mediated diseases (toxic shock syndrome)	Polyclonal (microbial superantigens activate many T cells of different specificities)	Fever, shock related to systemic inflammatory cytokine release

FIGURE 11-13 T cell–mediated diseases. Diseases in which T cells play a dominant role in causing tissue injury; antibodies and immune complexes may also contribute. Note that multiple sclerosis, rheumatoid arthritis, and type 1 diabetes are autoimmune disorders. Crohn's disease, an inflammatory bowel disease, is likely caused by reactions against microbes in the intestine and may have a component of autoimmunity. The other diseases are caused by reactions against foreign (microbial or environmental) antigens. In most of these diseases, the role of T cells is inferred from the detection and isolation of T cells reactive with various antigens from the blood or lesions, and from the similarity with experimental models in which the involvement of T cells has been established by a variety of approache diseases. The specificity of pathogenic T cells has been defined in animal models and in some of the human diseases. Viral hepatitis and toxic shock syndrome are disorders in which T cells play an important pathogenic role, but these are not considered examples of hypersensitivity. CTL, Cytotoxic T lymphocyte; DTH, delayed-type hypersensitivity; HBV, hepatitis B virus; HCV, hepatitis C virus.

- Clinicopathologic manifestations of immediate hypersensitivity result from the actions of mediators secreted by the mast cells: amines dilate vessels and contract smooth muscles, arachidonic acid metabolites also contract muscles, and cytokines induce inflammation, the hallmark of the late-phase reaction. Treatment of allergies is designed to inhibit the production of mediators, antagonize their actions, and counteract their effects on end organs.

- Antibodies against cell and tissue antigens may cause tissue injury and disease (type II hypersensitivity). IgM and IgG antibodies promote the phagocytosis of cells to which they bind, induce inflammation by complement-mediated and Fc receptor–mediated leukocyte recruitment, and may interfere with the functions of cells by binding to essential molecules and receptors.

- In immune complex diseases (type III hypersensitivity), antibodies may bind to circulating antigens to form immune complexes, which deposit in vessels, leading to inflammation in the vessel wall (vasculitis), which secondarily causes tissue injury due to impaired blood flow.

- T cell–mediated diseases (type IV hypersensitivity) result from inflammation caused by cytokines produced by CD4+ Th1 and Th17 cells, or killing of host cells by CD8+ CTLs.

▌REVIEW QUESTIONS

1. What are the major types of hypersensitivity reactions?

2. What types of antigens may induce immune responses that cause hypersensitivity reactions?

3. What is the sequence of events in a typical immediate hypersensitivity reaction? What is the late-phase reaction, and how is it caused?

4. What are some examples of immediate hypersensitivity disorders, what is their pathogenesis, and how are they treated?

5. How do antibodies cause tissue injury and disease?

6. What are some examples of diseases caused by antibodies specific for cell surface or tissue matrix antigens?

7. How do immune complexes cause disease, and how are the clinical manifestations different from most diseases caused by antibodies specific for cell surface or tissue matrix proteins?

8. What are some examples of diseases caused by T cells, what is their pathogenesis, and what are their principal clinical and pathologic manifestations?

Answers to and discussion of the Review Questions are available at https://studentconsult.inkling.com.

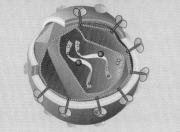

CHAPTER 12

Congenital and Acquired Immunodeficiencies

Diseases Caused by Defective Immunity

Defects in the development and functions of the immune system result in increased susceptibility to newly acquired infections; reactivation of latent infections such as cytomegalovirus, Epstein-Barr virus, and tuberculosis, in which the normal immune response keeps the infection in check but does not eradicate it; and increased incidence of certain cancers. These consequences of defective immunity are predictable because, as emphasized throughout this book, the normal function of the immune system is to defend individuals against infections and some cancers. Disorders caused by defective immunity are called **immunodeficiency diseases.** Some of these diseases may result from genetic abnormalities in one or more components of the immune system; these are called **congenital** (or **primary**) **immunodeficiencies.** Other defects in the immune system may result from infections, nutritional abnormalities, or medical treatments that cause loss or inadequate function of various components of the immune system; these are called **acquired** (or **secondary**) **immunodeficiencies.**

In this chapter we describe the causes and pathogenesis of congenital and acquired immunodeficiencies. Among the acquired diseases, we emphasize acquired immunodeficiency syndrome (AIDS), which results from infection by human immunodeficiency virus (HIV) and is one of the most devastating health problems worldwide. We address the following questions:

- What are the mechanisms by which immunity is compromised in the most common congenital immunodeficiency diseases?
- How does HIV cause the clinical and pathologic abnormalities of AIDS?
- What approaches are being used to treat immunodeficiency diseases?

Information about the clinical features of these disorders can be found in textbooks of pediatrics and medicine.

CONGENITAL (PRIMARY) IMMUNODEFICIENCIES

Congenital immunodeficiencies are caused by genetic defects that lead to blocks in the maturation or functions of different components of the immune system. It is estimated that as many as 1 in 500 individuals in the United States and Europe suffer from congenital immune deficiencies of varying severity. These immunodeficiencies share several features, the most common being infectious complications (Fig. 12-1). Congenital immunodeficiency diseases may, however, differ considerably in clinical and pathologic manifestations. Some of these disorders result in greatly increased susceptibility to infections that may manifest early after birth and may be fatal unless the immunologic defects are corrected. Other congenital immunodeficiencies lead to mild infections and may first be detected in adult life.

The following discussion summarizes the pathogenesis of select immunodeficiencies, several of which are mentioned in earlier chapters to illustrate the physiologic importance of various components of the immune system. Congenital deficiencies in molecules involved in self-tolerance are manifested as autoimmune diseases, as discussed in Chapter 9.

Defects in Lymphocyte Maturation

Many congenital immunodeficiencies are the result of genetic abnormalities that cause blocks in the maturation of B lymphocytes, T lymphocytes, or both (Figs. 12-2 and 12-3).

Severe Combined Immunodeficiency

Disorders manifesting as defects in both the B cell and T cell arms of the adaptive immune system are classified as **severe combined immunodeficiency (SCID).** Several different genetic abnormalities may cause SCID.

- *X-SCID caused by γc mutations.* About half of the cases of SCID are X-linked, affecting only male children. More than 99% of cases of **X-linked SCID** are caused by mutations in the common γ (γc) chain signaling subunit of the

Type of immunodeficiency	Histopathology and laboratory abnormalities	Common infectious consequences
B cell deficiencies	Absent or reduced follicles and germinal centers in lymphoid organs Reduced serum Ig levels	Pyogenic bacterial infections, enteric bacterial and viral infections
T cell deficiencies	May be reduced T cell zones in lymphoid organs Reduced DTH reactions to common antigens Defective T cell proliferative responses to mitogens in vitro	Viral and other intracellular microbial infections (e.g., *Pneumocystis jiroveci*, other fungi, nontuberculous mycobacteria) Virus-associated malignancies (e.g., EBV-associated lymphomas)
Innate immune deficiencies	Variable, depending on which component of innate immunity is defective	Variable; pyogenic bacterial and viral infections

FIGURE 12-1 Features of immunodeficiency diseases. The figure summarizes the important diagnostic features and clinical manifestations of immunodeficiencies affecting different components of the immune system. Within each group, different diseases, and even different patients with the same disease, may show considerable variation. Reduced numbers of circulating B or T cells are often detected in some of these diseases. *DTH,* Delayed-type hypersensitivity; *EBV,* Epstein-Barr virus; *Ig,* immunoglobulin.

receptors for several cytokines, including interleukin-2 (IL-2), IL-4, IL-7, IL-9, IL-15, and IL-21. (Because the γc chain was first identified as one of the three chains of the IL-2 receptor, it is also called the IL-2Rγ chain.) When the γc chain is not functional, immature lymphocytes, especially pro-T cells, cannot proliferate in response to IL-7, which is the major growth factor for these cells. Defective responses to IL-7 result in reduced survival and maturation of lymphocyte precursors. In humans, the defect affects mainly T cell maturation (whereas in mice, B cells are also reduced). The consequence of this developmental block is a profound decrease in the numbers of mature T cells, deficient cell-mediated immunity, and defective humoral immunity because of absent T cell help (even though B cells may mature almost normally). Natural killer (NK) cells also are deficient, because the γc chain is part of the receptor for IL-15, the major cytokine involved in NK cell proliferation and maturation.

- *ADA and PNP deficiencies.* Mutations in autosomal genes that encode proteins involved in nucleic acid metabolism cause many cases of SCID. About half the cases of autosomal recessive SCID are caused by mutations in an enzyme called **adenosine deaminase (ADA)**, which is involved in the breakdown of adenosine. Deficiency of ADA leads to the accumulation of toxic purine metabolites in cells that are actively synthesizing DNA—namely, proliferating cells. Lymphocytes are particularly susceptible to injury by purine metabolites because these cells undergo tremendous proliferation during their maturation. ADA deficiency results in a block in T cell maturation more than in B cell maturation; defective humoral immunity is largely a consequence of the lack of T cell helper function. A similar phenotype is seen in individuals who have a deficiency in **purine nucleotide phosphorylase (PNP).**
- *Other mutations.* Another important autosomal recessive form of SCID is caused by mutation of the gene encoding a kinase called

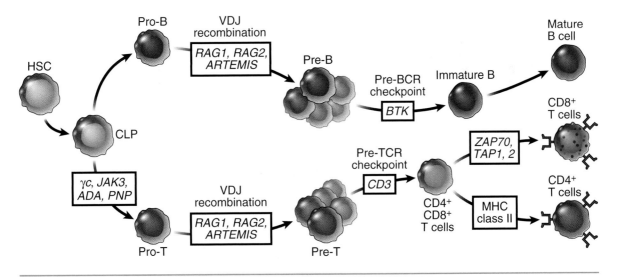

FIGURE 12-2 Congenital immunodeficiencies caused by genetic defects in lymphocyte maturation. Lymphocyte maturation pathways are described in Chapter 4. JAK3 (Janus kinase 3) is a kinase involved in signaling by many cytokine receptors; ARTEMIS is a protein involved in antigen receptor gene recombination; BTK (Bruton tyrosine kinase) is a kinase that delivers signals from the pre–B cell receptor (BCR) and BCR; ZAP70 is a kinase involved in TCR signaling; and TAP proteins transport peptides for presentation by class I MHC molecules. *ADA*, Adenosine deaminase; *CLP*, common lymphoid progenitor; *HSC*, hematopoietic stem cell; *PNP*, purine nucleoside phosphorylase; *RAG*, recombination-activating gene.

JAK3 that is involved in signaling by the γc cytokine receptor chain. Such mutations result in the same abnormalities as those in X-linked SCID caused by γc mutations, described previously. Rare cases of autosomal recessive SCID are caused by mutations in the *RAG1* or *RAG2* gene, which encode the VDJ recombinase that is required for immunoglobulin (Ig) and T cell receptor gene recombination and lymphocyte maturation (see Chapter 4).

With increasing application of newborn screening to identify congenital immunodeficiencies, other causes of SCID are being discovered.

Severe combined immunodeficiency (SCID)

Disease	Functional deficiencies	Mechanism of defect
X-linked SCID	Markedly decreased T cells; normal or increased B cells; reduced serum Ig	Cytokine receptor common γ chain gene mutations, defective T cell maturation due to lack of IL-7 signals
Autosomal recessive SCID due to ADA, PNP deficiency	Progressive decrease in T and B cells (mostly T)	ADA or PNP deficiency leads to accumulation of toxic metabolites in lymphocytes
Autosomal recessive SCID due to other causes	Decreased T and B cells; reduced serum Ig	Defective maturation of T and B cells; may be mutations in *RAG* genes and other genes involved in VDJ recombination or IL-7R signaling

B cell immunodeficiencies

Disease	Functional deficiencies	Mechanism of defect
X-linked agammaglobulinemia	Decrease in all serum Ig isotypes; reduced B cell numbers	Block in maturation beyond pre–B cells, because of mutation in Bruton tyrosine kinase (BTK)
Ig heavy chain deficiencies	Deficiency of IgG subclasses; sometimes associated with absent IgA or IgE	Chromosomal deletion involving Ig heavy-chain locus at 14q32

Disorders of T cell maturation

Disease	Functional deficiencies	Mechanism of defect
DiGeorge syndrome	Decreased T cells; normal B cells; normal or decreased serum Ig	Anomalous development of 3rd and 4th branchial pouches, leading to thymic hypoplasia

FIGURE 12-3 Features of congenital immunodeficiencies caused by defects in lymphocyte maturation. The figure summarizes the principal features of the most common congenital immunodeficiencies in which the genetic blocks are known. *ADA,* Adenosine deaminase; *Ig,* immunoglobulin; *IL-7R,* interleukin-7 receptor; *PNP,* purine nucleoside phosphorylase; *RAG,* recombination-activating gene.

Defects in Maturation of B or T Lymphocytes

Some congenital immunodeficiencies are caused by defects affecting either B or T cells.

- *X-Linked Agammaglobulinemia.* The most common clinical syndrome caused by a block in B cell maturation is **X-linked agammaglobulinemia** (first described as Bruton's agammaglobulinemia). In this disorder, pre-B cells in the bone marrow fail to expand, resulting in a marked decrease or absence of mature B lymphocytes and serum immunoglobulins. The disease is caused by mutations in the gene encoding a kinase called Bruton tyrosine kinase (BTK), resulting in defective production or function of the enzyme. The enzyme is activated by the pre-B cell receptor expressed in pre-B cells, and it delivers signals that promote the survival, proliferation, and maturation of these cells. The *BTK* gene is located on the X chromosome. Therefore, women who carry a mutant *BTK* allele on one of their X chromosomes are carriers of the disease, but male offspring who inherit the abnormal X chromosome are affected. In about a fourth of patients with X-linked agammaglobulinemia, autoimmune diseases, notably arthritis, develop as well. A link between an immunodeficiency and autoimmunity seems paradoxical. One possible explanation for this association is that BTK contributes to B cell receptor signaling and is required for central B cell tolerance, so defective BTK may result in the accumulation of autoreactive B cells.

- *DiGeorge Syndrome.* Selective defects in T cell maturation are quite rare. Of these, **DiGeorge syndrome** is the most frequent. It results from incomplete development of the thymus (and parathyroid glands). Patients with DiGeorge syndrome fail to develop mature T cells. The condition tends to improve with age, probably because the small amount of thymic tissue that does develop is able to support some T cell maturation.

Defects in Lymphocyte Activation and Function

Better understanding of the molecules involved in lymphocyte activation and function has led to the recognition of mutations and other abnormalities in these molecules that result in immunodeficiency disorders (Fig. 12-4). This section describes some of the diseases in which lymphocytes mature normally but the activation and effector functions of the cells are defective.

Defects in B Cell Responses

Defective antibody production may result from abnormalities in B cells or in helper T cells.

- *Hyper-IgM Syndrome.* The **X-linked hyper-IgM syndrome** is characterized by defective B cell heavy-chain isotype (class) switching, so IgM is the major serum antibody, and by deficient cell-mediated immunity against intracellular microbes. The disease is caused by mutations in the X chromosome gene encoding CD40 ligand (CD40L), the helper T cell protein that binds to CD40 on B cells, dendritic cells, and macrophages and thus mediates T cell–dependent activation of these cells (see Chapters 6 and 7). Failure to express functional CD40L leads to defective T cell–dependent B cell responses, such as isotype switching and affinity maturation, in humoral immunity, and to defective T cell–dependent macrophage activation in cell-mediated immunity. Boys with this disease are especially susceptible to infection by *Pneumocystis jiroveci*, a fungus that survives within phagocytes in the absence of T cell help. A rare autosomal recessive form of hyper-IgM syndrome is seen in subjects with mutations affecting the enzyme activation-induced deaminase (AID), which is involved in isotype switching and somatic hypermutation (see Chapter 7).

- Genetic deficiencies in the production of selected Ig isotypes are quite common. IgA deficiency is believed to affect as many as 1 in 700 people but causes no clinical problems in most patients. The defect causing these deficiencies is not known in a majority of cases; rarely, the deficiencies may be caused by mutations of Ig heavy-chain constant (C) region genes.

- **Common variable immunodeficiency** (CVID) is a heterogeneous group of disorders that represent a common form of primary immunodeficiency. These disorders are characterized by poor antibody responses to infections

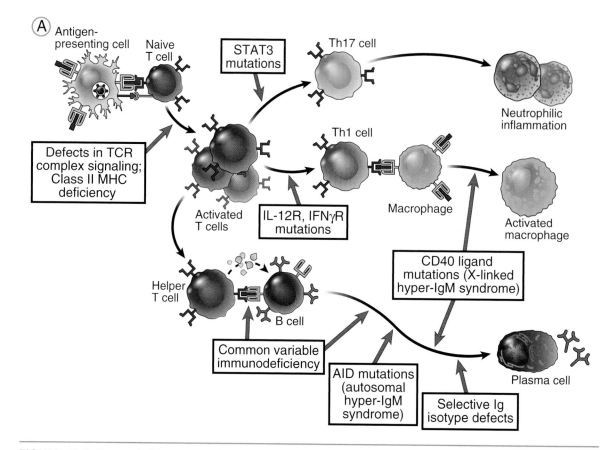

FIGURE 12-4 Congenital immunodeficiencies associated with defects in lymphocyte activation and effector functions. Congenital immunodeficiencies may be caused by genetic defects in the expression of molecules required for antigen presentation to T cells, T or B lymphocyte antigen receptor signaling, helper T cell activation of B cells and macrophages, and differentiation of antibody-producing B cells. **A,** Examples showing the sites at which immune responses may be blocked. *AID,* Activation-induced deaminase; *IL-12R,* IL-12 receptor; *IFNγR,* IFN-γ receptor.

and reduced serum levels of IgG, IgA, and often IgM. The underlying causes of CVID include defects in various genes involved in B cell maturation and activation. Some patients have mutations in genes encoding receptors for B cell growth factors or costimulators that play a role in T cell–B cell interactions. Patients have recurrent infections, autoimmune disease, and lymphomas.

Defective Activation of T Lymphocytes

A variety of inherited abnormalities may interfere with T cell activation.

- The **bare lymphocyte syndrome** is a disease caused by a failure to express class II major

histocompatibility complex (MHC) molecules, as a result of mutations in the transcription factors that normally induce class II MHC expression. Recall that class II MHC molecules display peptide antigens for recognition by CD4+ T cells and this recognition is critical for maturation and activation of the T cells. The disease is manifested by a profound decrease in CD4+ T cells because of defective maturation of these cells in the thymus and poor activation of the cells in peripheral lymphoid organs.

- Rare cases of selective T cell deficiency are caused by mutations affecting various signaling pathways or cytokines and receptors involved in differentiation of naive T cells into

Disease	Functional Deficiencies	Mechanisms of Defect
X-linked hyper-IgM syndrome	Defects in helper T cell–dependent B cell and macrophage activation	Mutations in CD40 ligand
Common variable immunodeficiency	Reduced or no production of selective isotypes or subtypes of immunoglobulins; susceptibility to bacterial infections or no clinical problems	Mutations in receptors for B cell growth factors, costimulators
Defective class II MHC expression: the bare lymphocyte syndrome	Lack of class II MHC expression and impaired CD4+ T cell activation; defective cell-mediated immunity and T cell–dependent humoral immunity	Mutations in genes encoding transcription factors required for class II MHC gene expression
Defects in T cell receptor complex expression or signaling	Decreased T cells or abnormal ratios of CD4+ and CD8+ subsets; decreased cell-mediated immunity	Rare cases due to mutations or deletions in genes encoding CD3 proteins, ZAP-70
Defects in Th1 differentiation	Decreased T cell–mediated macrophage activation; susceptibility to infection	Rare cases due to mutations encoding the receptors for IL-12 or interferon-γ
Defects in Th17 differentiation	Decreased T cell–mediated inflammatory responses; mucocutaneous candidiasis, bacterial skin abscesses	Rare cases due to mutations in genes encoding STAT3, IL-17, IL-17R
X-linked lymphoproliferative syndrome	Uncontrolled EBV-induced B cell proliferation and CTL activation; defective NK cell and CTL function and antibody responses	Mutations in gene encoding SAP (an adaptor protein involved in signaling in lymphocytes)

FIGURE 12-4, cont'd B, This table summarizes the features of select congenital immunodeficiency disorders. Note that abnormalities in class II MHC expression and TCR complex signaling can cause defective T cell maturation (see Fig. 12-2), as well as defective activation of the cells that do mature, as shown here. *CTL,* Cytotoxic T lymphocyte; *EBV,* Epstein-Barr virus; *NK,* natural killer; *SAP,* SLAM-associated protein; *ZAP-70,* ζ chain–associated protein of 70 kD.

effector cells. Depending on the mutation and the extent of the defect, affected patients show severe T cell deficiency or deficiency in particular arms of T cell–mediated immunity, such as in Th1 responses (associated with nontuberculous mycobacterial infections) and Th17 responses (associated with fungal and bacterial infections). These defects have revealed the importance of various pathways of T cell activation, but these are rare disorders.

Defects in Innate Immunity

Abnormalities in two components of innate immunity, phagocytes and the complement system, are important causes of immunodeficiency (Fig. 12-5).

• **Chronic granulomatous disease** is caused by mutations in genes encoding subunits of the enzyme phagocyte oxidase, which catalyzes the production of microbicidal reactive oxygen species in lysosomes (see Chapter 2).

Disease	Functional Deficiencies	Mechanisms of Defect
Chronic granulomatous disease	Defective production of reactive oxygen intermediates by phagocytes	Mutations in genes encoding components of the phagocyte oxidase enzyme, most often cytochrome b558
Leukocyte adhesion deficiency-1	Absent or deficient expression of β2 integrins causing defective leukocyte adhesion-dependent functions	Mutations in gene encoding the β chain (CD18) of β2 integrins
Leukocyte adhesion deficiency-2	Absent or deficient expression of leukocyte ligands for endothelial E- and P-selectins, causing failure of leukocyte migration into tissues	Mutations in gene encoding a protein required for synthesis of the sialyl-Lewis X component of E- and P-selectin ligands
Complement C3 deficiency	Defect in complement cascade activation	Mutations in the C3 gene
Complement C2, C4 deficiency	Deficient activation of classical pathway of complement leading to failure to clear immune complexes and development of lupus-like disease	Mutations in C2 or C4 gene
Chediak-Higashi syndrome	Defective lysosomal function in neutrophils, macrophages, and dendritic cells, and defective granule function in natural killer cells	Mutation in a gene encoding a lysosomal trafficking regulatory protein
Herpes simplex virus 1 (HSV-1) encephalitis	Defective antiviral immunity in the central nervous system	Mutations in TLR3 gene
Recurrent pyogenic bacterial infections	Defective innate immune responses to pyogenic bacteria	Mutations in MyD88 gene

FIGURE 12-5 Congenital immunodeficiencies caused by defects in innate immunity. The figure lists immunodeficiency diseases caused by defects in various components of the innate immune system.

As a result, neutrophils and macrophages are unable to kill the microbes they phagocytose. The immune system tries to compensate for this defective microbial killing by calling in more macrophages and by activating T cells, which stimulate recruitment and activation of phagocytes. Therefore, collections of phagocytes accumulate around foci of infections by intracellular microbes, but the microbes cannot be destroyed effectively. These collections resemble granulomas, giving rise to the name of this disease. The most common form of chronic granulomatous disease is X-linked, caused by mutations in a subunit of the phagocyte oxidase enzyme that is encoded by a gene on the X chromosome.

- **Leukocyte adhesion deficiency** is caused by mutations in genes encoding integrins, molecules required for the expression of ligands for selectins, or signaling molecules activated by chemokine receptors required to activate integrins. Integrins and selectin ligands are involved in the adhesion of leukocytes to other cells. As a result of these mutations, blood leukocytes do not bind firmly to vascular endothelium and are not recruited normally to sites of infection.

- Deficiencies of almost every complement protein, and many complement regulatory proteins, have been described (see Chapter 8). C3 deficiency results in severe infections and may be fatal. Deficiencies of C2 and C4, two components of the classical pathway of complement activation, may result in increased bacterial or viral infection or increased incidence of systemic lupus erythematosus, presumably because of defective clearance of immune complexes. Deficiencies of complement regulatory proteins lead to various syndromes associated with excessive complement activation.
- The **Chédiak-Higashi syndrome** is an immunodeficiency disease in which the lysosomal granules of leukocytes do not function normally. The immune defect is thought to affect phagocytes and NK cells and manifests as increased susceptibility to bacterial infection.
- Rare patients have been described with mutations affecting Toll-like receptors (TLRs) or signaling pathways downstream of TLRs, including molecules required for activation of the nuclear factor κB (NF-κB) transcription factor. Somewhat surprisingly, several of these mutations make patients susceptible to only a limited set of infections. For example, mutations affecting MyD88, an adaptor protein downstream of many TLRs, are associated with severe bacterial (most often pneumococcal) pneumonias, and mutations affecting TLR3 are associated with recurrent herpesvirus encephalitis but apparently not other viral infections. These quite restricted clinical phenotypes suggest considerable redundancy in host defense mechanisms, so defects in one pathway can be compensated by other pathways, and patients are not susceptible to a wide variety of infections.

Lymphocyte Abnormalities Associated with Other Diseases

Some systemic diseases that involve multiple organ systems, and whose major manifestations are not immunologic, may have a component of immunodeficiency.

- **Wiskott-Aldrich syndrome** is characterized by eczema, reduced blood platelets, and immunodeficiency. This X-linked disease is caused by a mutation in a gene that encodes a protein that binds to various adaptor molecules and cytoskeletal components in hematopoietic cells. Because of the absence of this protein, platelets and leukocytes do not develop normally, are small, and fail to migrate normally.
- **Ataxia-telangiectasia** is characterized by gait abnormalities (ataxia), vascular malformations (telangiectasia), and immunodeficiency. The disease is caused by mutations in a gene whose product is involved in DNA repair. Defects in this protein lead to abnormal DNA repair (e.g., during recombination of antigen receptor gene segments), resulting in defective lymphocyte maturation.

Therapy of Congenital Immunodeficiencies

Treatment of primary immunodeficiencies varies with the disease. SCID is fatal in early life unless the patient's immune system is reconstituted. The most widely used treatment is hematopoietic stem cell transplantation, with careful matching of donor and recipient to avoid potentially serious graft-versus-host disease. For selective B cell defects, patients may be given intravenous injections of pooled immunoglobulin (IVIG) from healthy donors to provide passive immunity. IVIG replacement therapy has provided enormous benefit in patients with X-linked agammaglobulinemia. Although the ideal treatment for all congenital immunodeficiencies is to replace the defective gene, this remains a distant goal for most diseases. Successful gene therapy has been reported in patients with X-linked SCID; a normal γc gene was introduced into their bone marrow stem cells, which were then transplanted back into the patients. In some of these patients, however, T cell leukemia has subsequently developed, apparently because the introduced γc gene was inserted near an oncogene and activated it. In all patients with these diseases, infections are treated with antibiotics as needed.

ACQUIRED (SECONDARY) IMMUNODEFICIENCIES

Deficiencies of the immune system often develop because of abnormalities that are not genetic but are acquired during life (Fig. 12-6). The most serious of these abnormalities worldwide is HIV infection, as described later. The most frequent causes of secondary immunodeficiencies in developed countries are cancers involving the bone marrow and various therapies. Cancer treatment with chemotherapeutic drugs and irradiation may damage proliferating cells, including precursors of leukocytes in the bone marrow and mature lymphocytes, resulting in immunodeficiency. Immunosuppressive drugs used to prevent graft rejection and drugs for inflammatory diseases, including some of the newer therapies (e.g., TNF antagonists, costimulation blockade), are designed to blunt immune responses. Therefore, immunodeficiency is a complication of such therapies. Protein-calorie malnutrition results in deficiencies of virtually all components of the immune system and is a common cause of immunodeficiency in developing countries.

ACQUIRED IMMUNODEFICIENCY SYNDROME

Although acquired immunodeficiency syndrome (AIDS) was first recognized as a distinct entity in the 1980s, it has become one of the most devastating afflictions in history. AIDS is caused by infection with HIV. Of the estimated 35 million HIV-infected people worldwide, about 70% are in Africa and 20% in Asia. More than 25 million deaths are attributable to HIV/AIDS, with 1 to 2 million deaths annually. Effective antiretroviral drugs have been developed, but the infection continues to spread in parts of the world where these therapies are not widely available, and in some African countries, more than 30% of the population has HIV infection. This section describes the important features of HIV, how it infects humans, and the disease it causes, ending with a brief discussion of the current status of therapy and vaccine development.

Cause	Mechanism
Human immunodeficiency virus infection	Depletion of CD4+ helper T cells
Irradiation and chemotherapy treatments for cancer	Decreased bone marrow precursors for all leukocytes
Immunosuppression for graft rejection and inflammatory diseases	Depletion or functional impairment of lymphocytes
Involvement of bone marrow by cancers (metastases, leukemias)	Reduced site of leukocyte development
Protein-calorie malnutrition	Metabolic derangements inhibit lymphocyte maturation and function
Removal of spleen	Decreased phagocytosis of microbes

FIGURE 12-6 Acquired (secondary) immunodeficiency. The figure lists the most common causes of acquired immunodeficiency diseases and how they lead to defects in immune responses.

Human Immunodeficiency Virus

Human immunodeficiency virus (HIV) is a retrovirus that infects cells of the immune system, mainly CD4+ T lymphocytes, and causes progressive destruction of these cells. An infectious HIV particle consists of two RNA strands within a protein core, surrounded by a lipid envelope derived from infected host cells but containing viral proteins (Fig. 12-7). The viral RNA encodes structural proteins, various enzymes, and proteins that regulate transcription of viral genes and the viral life cycle.

The life cycle of HIV consists of the following sequential steps: infection of cells, production of a DNA copy of viral RNA and its integration into the host genome, expression of viral genes, and production of viral particles (Fig. 12-8). HIV infects cells by virtue of its major envelope glycoprotein, called gp120 (for 120-kD glycoprotein), which binds to CD4 and to particular chemokine receptors on human cells (mainly CXCR4 and CCR5). The major cell types that may be infected by HIV are CD4+ T lymphocytes, macrophages, and dendritic cells. After binding to cellular receptors, the viral membrane fuses with the host cell membrane, and the virus enters the cell's cytoplasm. Here the virus is uncoated by viral protease, and its RNA is released. A DNA copy of the viral RNA is synthesized by the viral reverse transcriptase enzyme (a process characteristic of all retroviruses), and the DNA integrates into the host cell's DNA by the action of the integrase enzyme. The integrated viral DNA is called a provirus. If the infected T cell, macrophage, or dendritic cell is activated by some extrinsic stimulus, such as another infectious microbe, the cell responds by turning on the transcription of many of its own genes and often by producing cytokines. A negative consequence of this normal protective response is that the cytokines, and the process of cellular activation itself, also may activate the provirus, leading to production of viral RNAs and then proteins. The virus is then able to form a core structure, which migrates to the cell membrane, acquires a lipid envelope from the host, and is shed as an infectious viral particle, ready to infect another cell. The integrated HIV provirus may remain latent within infected cells for months or years, hidden from the patient's immune system (and even from antiviral therapies, discussed later).

Most cases of AIDS are caused by HIV-1 (i.e., HIV type 1). A related virus, HIV-2, causes some cases of the disease.

Pathogenesis of AIDS

AIDS develops over many years as latent HIV becomes activated and destroys cells of the immune system. Virus production leads to death of infected cells, as well as to death of uninfected lymphocytes, subsequent immune deficiencies, and clinical AIDS (Fig. 12-9). HIV infection is acquired by sexual intercourse, sharing contaminated needles used by intravenous drug users, transplacental transfer, or transfusion of infected blood or blood products. After infection there may be a brief, acute viremia, when the virus is detected in the blood, and the host may respond as in any mild viral infection. The virus infects CD4+ T cells, dendritic cells, and macrophages at sites of entry through epithelia; in lymphoid organs such as lymph nodes; and in the circulation. In mucosal tissues at the sites of entry, there may be considerable destruction of infected T cells. Because a large fraction of the body's lymphocytes, and especially memory T cells, reside in these tissues, the result of the local destruction may be a significant functional deficit that is not reflected in the presence of infected cells in the blood or the depletion of circulating T cells. Dendritic cells may capture the virus as it enters through mucosal epithelia and transport it to peripheral lymphoid organs, where it infects T cells. Rare individuals with *CCR5* mutations that do not permit HIV entry into CD4+ T cells can remain disease free for years after HIV infection. The integrated provirus may be activated in infected cells, as described previously, leading to production of viral particles and spread of the infection. During the course of HIV infection, the major source of infectious viral particles is activated CD4+ T cells; dendritic cells and macrophages are reservoirs of infection.

FIGURE 12-7 Structure and genes of the human immunodeficiency virus (HIV). A, An HIV-1 virion is shown next to a T cell surface. HIV-1 consists of two identical strands of RNA (the viral genome) and associated enzymes, including reverse transcriptase, integrase, and protease, packaged in a cone-shaped core composed of the p24 capsid protein with a surrounding p17 protein matrix, all surrounded by a phospholipid membrane envelope derived from the host cell. Virally encoded envelope proteins (gp41 and gp120) bind to CD4 and chemokine receptors on the host cell surface. **B,** The HIV-1 genome consists of genes whose positions are indicated here as different-colored blocks. Some genes contain sequences that overlap with sequences of other genes, as shown by overlapping blocks, but are read differently by host cell RNA polymerase. Similarly shaded blocks separated by lines (*tat, rev*) indicate genes whose coding sequences are separated in the genome and require RNA splicing to produce functional messenger RNA. The major functions of the proteins encoded by different viral genes are listed. *MHC,* Major histocompatibility complex. (**A,** Adapted from front cover, The new face of AIDS. *Science* 272:1841-2102, 1996. © Terese Winslow. **B,** Adapted from Greene WC: *AIDS and the immune system.* © 1993 by Scientific American, Inc. All rights reserved.)

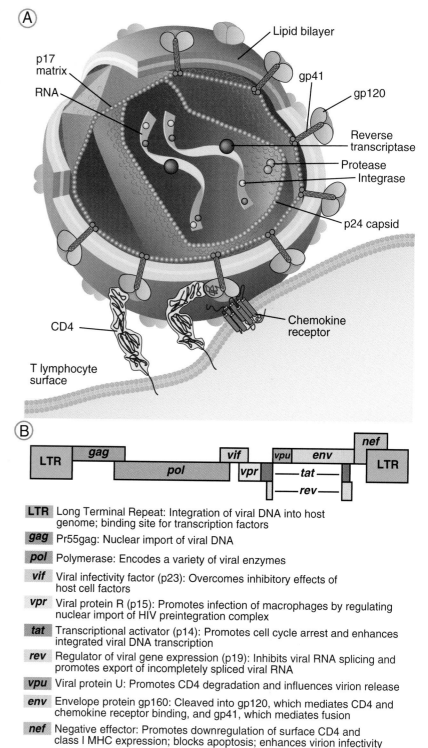

(A)

Lipid bilayer
p17 matrix
RNA
gp41
gp120
Reverse transcriptase
Protease
Integrase
p24 capsid
CD4
Chemokine receptor
T lymphocyte surface

(B)

| LTR | gag | pol | vif | vpr | vpu | env | tat | rev | nef | LTR |

LTR Long Terminal Repeat: Integration of viral DNA into host genome; binding site for transcription factors

gag Pr55gag: Nuclear import of viral DNA

pol Polymerase: Encodes a variety of viral enzymes

vif Viral infectivity factor (p23): Overcomes inhibitory effects of host cell factors

vpr Viral protein R (p15): Promotes infection of macrophages by regulating nuclear import of HIV preintegration complex

tat Transcriptional activator (p14): Promotes cell cycle arrest and enhances integrated viral DNA transcription

rev Regulator of viral gene expression (p19): Inhibits viral RNA splicing and promotes export of incompletely spliced viral RNA

vpu Viral protein U: Promotes CD4 degradation and influences virion release

env Envelope protein gp160: Cleaved into gp120, which mediates CD4 and chemokine receptor binding, and gp41, which mediates fusion

nef Negative effector: Promotes downregulation of surface CD4 and class I MHC expression; blocks apoptosis; enhances virion infectivity

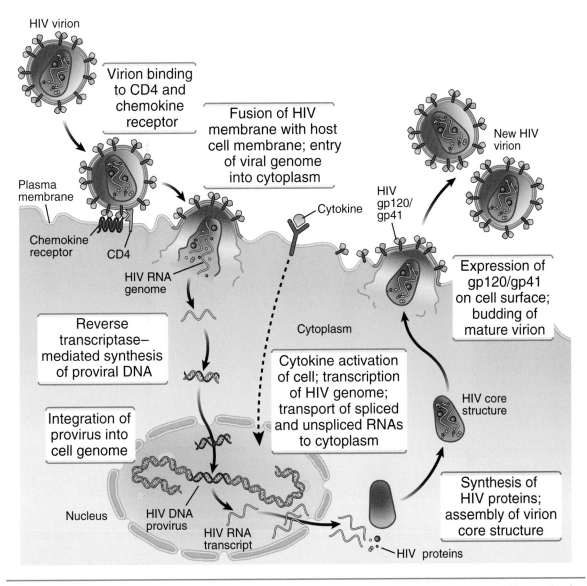

FIGURE 12-8 Life cycle of human immunodeficiency virus (HIV-1). The sequential steps in HIV reproduction are shown, from initial infection of a host cell to release of new virus particles (virions).

The depletion of CD4⁺ T cells after HIV infection is caused by a cytopathic effect of the virus, resulting from production of viral particles in infected cells, as well as death of uninfected cells. Active viral gene expression and protein production may interfere with the synthetic machinery of the T cells. Therefore, infected T cells in which the virus is replicating are killed during this process. The number of

T cells lost during the progression to AIDS is greater than the number of infected cells. The mechanism of this T cell loss remains poorly defined. One possibility is that T cells are chronically activated, perhaps by infections that are common in these patients, and the chronic stimulation culminates in apoptosis.

Other infected cells, such as dendritic cells and macrophages, may also die, resulting in destruction

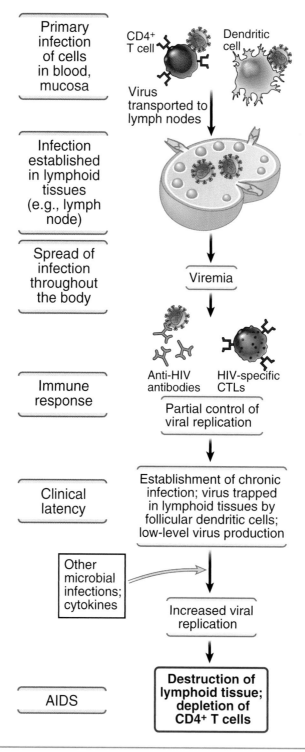

Primary
infection
of cells
in blood,
mucosa

CD4+
T cell

Dendritic
cell

Virus
transported to
lymph nodes

Infection
established
in lymphoid
tissues
(e.g., lymph
node)

Spread of
infection
throughout
the body

Viremia

Immune
response

Anti-HIV
antibodies

HIV-specific
CTLs

Partial control of
viral replication

Clinical
latency

Establishment of chronic
infection; virus trapped
in lymphoid tissues by
follicular dendritic cells;
low-level virus production

Other
microbial
infections;
cytokines

Increased viral
replication

AIDS

Destruction of
lymphoid tissue;
depletion of
CD4+ T cells

FIGURE 12-9 Pathogenesis of disease caused by human immunodeficiency virus (HIV). The development of HIV disease is associated with the spread of HIV from the initial site of infection to lymphoid tissues throughout the body. The immune response of the host temporarily controls acute infection but does not prevent establishment of chronic infection of cells in lymphoid tissues. Cytokines produced in response to HIV and other microbes serve to enhance HIV production and progression to acquired immunodeficiency syndrome (AIDS). *CTLs,* Cytotoxic T lymphocytes.

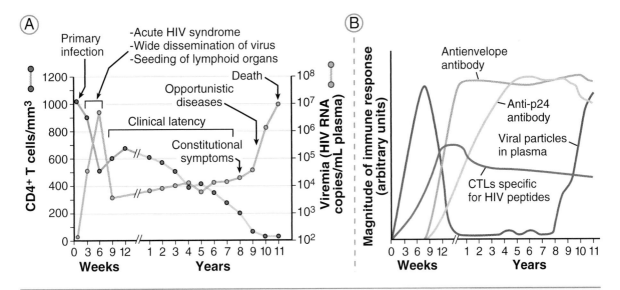

FIGURE 12-10 Clinical course of HIV disease. **A,** Blood-borne virus (plasma viremia) is detected early after infection and may be accompanied by systemic symptoms typical of acute HIV syndrome. The virus spreads to lymphoid organs, but plasma viremia falls to very low levels (detectable only by sensitive reverse transcriptase–polymerase chain reaction assays) and stays this way for many years. CD4+ T cell counts steadily decline during this clinical latency period because of active viral replication and T cell destruction in lymphoid tissues. As the level of CD4+ T cells falls, there is increasing risk of infection and other clinical components of acquired immunodeficiency syndrome (AIDS). **B,** Magnitude and kinetics of immune responses, shown in arbitrary relative units. *CTLs,* Cytotoxic T lymphocytes. (Reproduced with permission from Pantaleo G, Graziosi C, Fauci A: The immunopathogenesis of human immunodeficiency virus infection. *N Engl J Med* 328:327-335, 1993.)

of the architecture of lymphoid organs. Many studies have suggested that immune deficiency results not only from depletion of T cells but, in addition, from various functional abnormalities in T lymphocytes and other immune cells (dendritic cells and macrophages). The significance of these functional defects has not been established, however, and loss of T cells (followed by a fall in the blood CD4+ T cell count) remains the most reliable indicator of disease progression.

Clinical Features of HIV Infection and AIDS

The clinical course of HIV infection is characterized by several phases, culminating in immune deficiency (Fig. 12-10, *A*).

- *Acute HIV syndrome.* Early after HIV infection, patients may experience a mild acute illness with fever and malaise, correlating with the initial viremia. This illness subsides within a few days, and the disease enters a period of clinical latency.

- *Latency.* During latency, there may be few clinical problems but usually there is a progressive loss of CD4+ T cells in lymphoid tissues and destruction of the architecture of these tissues. Eventually, the blood CD4+ T cell count begins to decline, and when the count falls below 200 cells per mm³ (normal level about 1500 cells/mm³), patients become susceptible to infections and are diagnosed as having AIDS.

- *Clinical AIDS.* **The clinicopathologic manifestations of full-blown AIDS are primarily the result of increased susceptibility to infections and some cancers, as a consequence of immune deficiency.** Patients not given antiretroviral drugs often are infected by intracellular microbes, such as viruses, the fungal pathogen *Pneumocystis jiroveci,* and nontuberculous mycobacteria, all of which normally are combated by T cell–mediated immunity. Many of these microbes are present in the environment, but they do not infect healthy persons with intact immune systems. Because these infections are seen in immunodeficient persons, in whom the microbes have an opportunity to establish infection, these types of infections are said to be opportunistic. Many of the opportunistic infections are caused by viruses, such as cytomegalovirus. Patients with AIDS show defective cytotoxic T lymphocyte (CTL) responses to viruses, even though HIV does not infect CD8$^+$ T cells. The CTL responses are defective probably because CD4$^+$ helper T cells (the main targets of HIV) are required for full CD8$^+$ CTL responses against many viral antigens (see Chapters 5 and 6). AIDS patients are at increased risk for infections by extracellular bacteria, probably because of impaired helper T cell–dependent antibody responses to bacterial antigens. Patients also become susceptible to cancers caused by oncogenic viruses. The two most common types of cancers are B cell lymphomas, caused by the Epstein-Barr virus, and a tumor of small blood vessels called Kaposi's sarcoma, caused by a herpesvirus. Patients with advanced AIDS often have a wasting syndrome with significant loss of body mass, caused by altered metabolism and reduced caloric intake. The dementia that develops in some patients with AIDS is likely caused by infection of macrophages (microglial cells) in the brain.

The clinical course of HIV/AIDS has been dramatically changed by effective antiretroviral drug therapy. With appropriate treatment, patients exhibit much slower progression of the disease, fewer opportunistic infections, and greatly reduced incidence of cancers and dementia.

The immune response to HIV is ineffective in controlling spread of the virus and its pathologic effects. Infected patients produce antibodies and CTLs against viral antigens, and the responses help to limit the early, acute HIV syndrome (see Fig. 12-10, *B*). But these immune responses usually do not prevent progression of the disease. Antibodies against envelope glycoproteins, such as gp120, may be ineffective because the virus rapidly mutates the region of gp120 that is the target of most antibodies. CTLs often are ineffective in killing infected cells because the virus inhibits the expression of class I MHC molecules by the infected cells. Immune responses to HIV may paradoxically promote spread of the infection. Antibody-coated viral particles may bind to Fc receptors on macrophages and follicular dendritic cells in lymphoid organs, thus increasing virus entry into these cells and creating additional reservoirs of infection. If CTLs are able to kill infected cells, the dead cells may be cleared by macrophages, which can migrate to other tissues and spread the infection. By infecting and thus interfering with the function of immune cells, the virus is able to prevent its own eradication.

A small fraction of patients control HIV infection without therapy; these individuals are often referred to as elite controllers or long-term nonprogressors. There has been great interest in defining the genes that may protect these individuals, because elucidation of these genes may suggest therapeutic approaches. The presence of certain HLA alleles, such as HLA-B57 and HLA-B27, seems to be protective, perhaps because these HLA molecules are particularly efficient at presenting HIV peptides to CD8$^+$ T cells.

Therapy and Vaccination Strategies

The current treatment for AIDS is aimed at controlling replication of HIV and the infectious complications of the disease. Combinations of drugs that block the activity of the viral reverse transcriptase, protease, and integrase enzymes are now being administered early in the course of the infection. This therapeutic approach is called highly active antiretroviral therapy (HAART) or combination antiretroviral therapy (ART). It has changed the clinical course of HIV infection, such that opportunistic infections (e.g. by *Pneumocystis*) and some tumors (e.g. Kaposi's sarcoma, EBV-induced lymphoma), which were devastating complications in the past, are now rarely seen. In fact, treated patients are living quite long life spans and are dying of cardiovascular and other diseases that also afflict individuals who age without HIV (although they may be accelerated as a consequence of HIV infection, for unknown reasons). Even these highly effective drugs do not completely eradicate HIV infection. The virus is capable of mutating its genes, which may render it resistant to the drugs used, and reservoirs of latent virus are not eradicated by these drugs. Additional drugs that inhibit fusion of the virus with host cells have been developed.

The development of effective vaccines will likely be necessary for control of HIV infection worldwide. A successful vaccine probably needs to induce high titers of neutralizing antibodies and a strong T cell response, as well as mucosal immunity. It has proved difficult to achieve all these goals with current vaccination strategies. An additional challenge is the ability to protect against all subtypes of HIV. Early efforts focused on gp120 as an immunogen but were largely unsuccessful because of the high rate of mutations in gp120. More recent attempts have involved combinations of DNA immunization and recombinant poxviruses encoding several different HIV proteins. So far, vaccine trials for HIV have proved disappointing.

SUMMARY

- Immunodeficiency diseases are caused by defects in various components of the immune system that result in increased susceptibility to infections and some cancers. Congenital (primary) immunodeficiency diseases are caused by genetic abnormalities. Acquired (secondary) immunodeficiencies are the result of infections, cancers, malnutrition, or treatments for other conditions that adversely affect the cells of the immune system.

- Severe combined immunodeficiency results from blocks in lymphocyte maturation. It may be caused by mutations in the cytokine receptor γc chain that reduce the IL-7–driven proliferation of immature lymphocytes, by mutations in enzymes involved in purine metabolism, or by other defects in lymphocyte maturation.

- Selective B cell maturation defects are seen in X-linked agammaglobulinemia, caused by abnormalities in an enzyme involved in B cell maturation (BTK), and selective T cell maturation defects are seen in the DiGeorge syndrome, in which the thymus does not develop normally.

- Some immunodeficiency diseases are caused by defects in lymphocyte activation. The X-linked hyper-IgM syndrome is caused by mutations in the gene encoding CD40 ligand, resulting in defective helper T cell–dependent B cell responses (e.g., Ig heavy chain class switching) and T cell–dependent macrophage activation. The bare lymphocyte syndrome is caused by reduced expression of class II MHC proteins, resulting in impaired maturation and activation of CD4+ T cells.

- Acquired immunodeficiency syndrome is caused by the retrovirus HIV, which infects CD4+ T cells, macrophages, and dendritic cells by using an envelope protein (gp120) to bind to CD4 and chemokine receptors. The viral RNA is reverse transcribed, and the resulting DNA integrates into the host genome, where it may be activated to produce infectious virus. Infected cells die during this process of virus replication, and death of cells of the immune system is the principal mechanism by which the virus causes immune deficiency.

- The clinical course of HIV infection typically consists of acute viremia, clinical latency with progressive destruction of CD4+ T cells and dissolution of lymphoid tissues, and ultimately AIDS, with severe immunodeficiency resulting in opportunistic infections, some cancers, weight loss, and occasionally dementia. Treatment of HIV infection is designed to interfere with the life cycle of the virus. Vaccine development is ongoing.

REVIEW QUESTIONS

1. What are the most common clinicopathologic manifestations of immunodeficiency diseases?
2. What are some of the proteins affected by mutations that may block the maturation of T and B lymphocytes in human immunodeficiency diseases?

3. What are some of the mutations that may block activation or effector functions of both mature CD4$^+$ T cells and B cells, and what are the clinicopathologic consequences of these mutations?

4. How does HIV infect cells and replicate inside infected cells?

5. What are the principal clinical manifestations of advanced HIV infection, and what is the pathogenesis of these manifestations?

Answers to and discussion of the Review Questions are available at https://studentconsult. inkling.com.

SELECTED READINGS

The references listed below are a guide for students interested in learning about particular areas of immunology in depth. The reference list is not intended to be comprehensive or complete in terms of topics and authors.

Chapter 1
General Introduction and Foundations of Immunology

Burnet FM: A modification of Jerne's theory of antibody production using the concept of clonal selection, *Australian Journal of Science* 20:67–69, 1957.

Jerne NK: The natural-selection theory of antibody formation, *Proceedings of the National Academy of Sciences of the United States of America* 41:849–857, 1955.

Silverstein AM: *Paul Ehrlich's Receptor Immunology: The Magnificent Obsession*, Academic Press, New York, 2001.

Lymphocytes: Life History and Functions

Roederer M, Quaye L, Mangino M, et al.: The genetic architecture of the human immune system: a bioresource for autoimmunity and disease pathogenesis, *Cell* 161:387–403, 2015.

Surh CD, Sprent J: Homeostasis of naive and memory T cells, *Immunity* 29:848–862, 2008.

Cells and Tissues of the Immune System

Boehm T: Thymus development and function, *Current Opinion in Immunology* 20:178–184, 2008.

Bronte V, Pittet MJ: The spleen in local and systemic regulation of immunity, *Immunity* 39:806–818, 2013.

Drayton DL, Liao S, Mounzer RW, Ruddle NH: Lymphoid organ development: from ontogeny to neogenesis, *Nature Immunology* 7:344–353, 2006.

Lymphocyte Migration

Masopust D, Schenkel JM: The integration of T cell migration, differentiation and function, *Nature Reviews Immunology* 13:309–320, 2013.

Chapter 2
Pattern Recognition Receptors and Their Ligands

Blasius AL, Beutler B: Intracellular Toll-like receptors, *Immunity* 32:305–315, 2010.

Brubaker SW, Bonham KS, Zanoni I, Kagan JC: Innate immune pattern recognition: a cell biological perspective, *Annual Review of Immunology* 33:257–290, 2015.

Chen G, Shaw MH, Kim YG, Nuñez G: Nod-like receptors: role in innate immunity and inflammatory disease, *Annual Review of Pathology* 4:365–398, 2009.

Franchi L, Munoz-Planilla R, Nunez G: Sensing and reacting to microbes through the inflammasomes, *Nature Immunology* 13:325–332, 2012.

Netea MG, van de Veerdonk FL, van der Meer JW, Dinarello CA, Joosten LA: Inflammasome-dependent regulation of IL1-family cytokines, *Annual Review of Immunology* 33:49–77, 2015.

Takeuchi O, Akira S: Pattern recognition receptors and inflammation, *Cell* 140:805–820, 2010.

Vanaja SK, Rathinam VA, Fitzgerald KA. Mechanisms of inflammasome activation: recent advances and novel insights, *Trends in Cell Biology* 25:308–315, 2015.

Yin Q, Fu T-M, Li J, Wu H: Structural biology of innate immunity, *Annual Review of Immunology* 33:393–416, 2015.

Cells of the Innate Immune System

Amulic B, Cazalet C, Hayes GL, et al.: Neutrophil function: from mechanisms to disease, *Annual Review of Immunology* 30:459–489, 2012.

Dale DC, Boxer L, Liles WC: The phagocytes: neutrophils and monocytes, *Blood* 112:935–945, 2008.

Eberl G, Colonna M, Di Santo JP, McKenzie ANJ: Innate lymphoid cells: a new paradigm in immunology, *Science* 348:aaa6566, 2015.

Flannagan RS, Jaumouille V, Grinstein S: The cell biology of phagocytosis, *Annual Review of Pathology: Mechanisms of Disease* 7:61–98, 2012.

Lanier LL: NK cell recognition, *Annual Review of Immunology* 23:225–274, 2005.

Mócsai A: Diverse novel functions of neutrophils in immunity, inflammation, and beyond, *Journal of Experimental Medicine* 10:1283–1299, 2013.

Selsted ME, Ouellette AJ: Mammalian defensins in the anti-microbial immune response, *Nature Immunology* 6:551–557, 2005.

Varol C, Mildner A, Jung S: Macrophages: development and tissue specialization, *Annual Review of Immunology* 33:643–675, 2015.

Vivier E, Tomasello E, Baratin M, et al.: Functions of natural killer cells, *Nature Immunology* 9:503–510, 2008.

Acute Inflammation

Ley K, Laudanna C, Cybulsky MI, et al.: Getting to the site of inflammation: the leukocyte adhesion cascade updated, *Nature Reviews Immunology* 7:678–689, 2007.

Rock KL, Latz E, Ontiveros F, et al.: The sterile inflammatory response, *Annual Review of Immunology* 28:321–342, 2010.

Sokol CL, Luster AD: The chemokine system in innate immunity, *Cold Spring Harbor Perspectives in Biology* 7:1–18, 2015.

Zlotnik A, Yoshie O: The chemokine superfamily revisited, *Immunity* 36:705–716, 2012.

Antiviral Innate Immunity

Klotman ME, Chang TL: Defensins in innate antiviral immunity, *Nature Reviews Immunology* 6:447–456, 2006.

Pichlmair A, Reis e Sousa C: Innate recognition of viruses, *Immunity* 27:370–383, 2007.

Other Functions of Innate Immunity

Iwasaki A, Medzhitov R: Control of adaptive immunity by the innate immune system, *Nature Immunology* 16:343–353, 2015.

Diseases of Innate Immunity

Angus DC, van der Poll T: Severe sepsis and septic shock, *New England Journal of Medicine* 369:840–851, 2013.

de Jesus AA, Canna SW, Liu Y, Goldbach-Mansky R: Molecular mechanisms in genetically defined autoinflammatory diseases: disorders of amplified danger signaling, *Annual Review of Immunology* 33:823–874, 2015.

Chapter 3
Dendritic Cells in Antigen Capture and Presentation

Bousso P: T-cell activation by dendritic cells in the lymph node: lessons from the movies, *Nature Reviews Immunology* 8:675–684, 2008.

Collin M, McGovern N, Haniffa M: Human dendritic cell subsets, *Immunology* 140:22–30, 2013.

Durand M, Segura E: The known unknowns of the human dendritic cell network, *Frontiers in Immunology* 6:1–7, 2015.

Heath WR, Carbone FR: Dendritic cell subsets in primary and secondary T cell responses at body surfaces, *Nature Immunology* 10:1237–1244, 2009.

Merad M, Sathe P, Helft J, et al.: The dendritic cell lineage: ontogeny and function of dendritic cells and their subsets in the steady state and inflamed setting, *Annual Review of Immunology* 31:563–604, 2013.

Mildner A, Jung S: Development and function of dendritic cell subsets, *Immunity* 40:642–645, 2014.

Shortman K, Sathe P, Vremec D, et al.: Plasmacytoid dendritic cell development, *Advances in Immunology* 120:105–126, 2013.

Structure of MHC Genes, MHC Molecules, and Peptide-MHC Complexes

Bjorkman PJ, Saper MA, Samraoui B, et al.: Structure of the human class I histocompatibility antigen HLA-A2, *Nature* 329:506–512, 1987.

Horton R, Wilming L, Rand V, et al.: Gene map of the extended human MHC, *Nature Reviews Genetics* 5:889–899, 2004.

Protein Antigen Processing and MHC-Associated Presentation of Peptide Antigens

Basler M, Kirk CJ, Groettrup M: The immunoproteasome in antigen processing and other immunological functions, *Current Opinion in Immunology* 25:74–80, 2013.

Blum JS, Wearsch PA, Cresswell P: Pathways of antigen processing, *Annual Review of Immunology* 31:443–473, 2013.

Purcell AW, Elliott T: Molecular machinations of the MHC-I peptide loading complex, *Current Opinion in Immunology* 20:75–81, 2008.

Roche PA, Furuta K: The ins and outs of MHC class II-mediated antigen processing and presentation, *Nature Reviews Immunology* 15:203–216, 2015.

Trombetta ES, Mellman I: Cell biology of antigen processing in vitro and in vivo, *Annual Review of Immunology* 23:975–1028, 2005.

van de Weijer ML, Luteijn RD, Wiertz EJ: Viral immune evasion: lessons in MHC class I antigen presentation, *Seminars in Immunology* 27:125–137, 2015.

Cross-Presentation

Schuette V, Burgdorf S: The ins-and-outs of endosomal antigens for cross-presentation, *Current Opinion in Immunology* 26:63–68, 2014.

Segura E, Amigorena S: Cross-presentation by human dendritic cell subsets, *Immunology Letters* 158:73–78, 2014.

Non-Classical Antigen Presentation

Adams EJ, Luoma AM: The adaptable major histocompatibility complex (MHC) fold: structure and function of nonclassical and MHC class I-like molecules, *Annual Review of Immunology* 31:529–561, 2013.

Cohen NR, Garg S, Brenner MB: Antigen presentation by CD1: lipids, T cells, and NKT cells in microbial immunity, *Advances in Immunology* 102:1–94, 2009.

Chapter 4
Structure and Function of Antibodies

Corti D, Lanzavecchia A: Broadly neutralizing antiviral antibodies, *Annual Review of Immunology* 31:705–742, 2013.

Fagarasan S: Evolution, development, mechanism and function of IgA in the gut, *Current Opinion in Immunology* 20:170–177, 2008.

Law M, Hengartner L: Antibodies against viruses: passive and active immunization, *Current Opinion in Immunology* 20:486–492, 2008.

Structure and Function of the T Cell Receptor for Antigen

Davis SJ, Ikemizu S, Evans EJ, et al.: The nature of molecular recognition by T cells, *Nature Immunology* 4:217–224, 2003.

Klein L, Hinterberger M, Wirnsberger G, et al.: Antigen presentation in the thymus for positive selection and central tolerance induction, *Nature Reviews Immunology* 9:833–844, 2009.

Kuhns MS, Davis MM, Garcia KC: Deconstructing the form and function of the TCR/CD3 complex, *Immunity* 24:133–139, 2006.

Rossjohn J, Gras S, Miles JJ, et al.: T cell antigen receptor recognition of antigen-presenting molecules, *Annual Review of Immunology* 33:169–200, 2015.

Rudolph MG, Stanfield RL, Wilson IA: How TCRs bind MHCs, peptides, and coreceptors, *Annual Review of Immunology* 24:419–466, 2006.

B and T Lymphocyte Development

Boehm T: Thymus development and function, *Current Opinion in Immunology* 20:178–184, 2008.

Jung D, Giallourakis C, Mostoslavsky R, et al.: Mechanism and control of V(D)J recombination at the immunoglobulin heavy chain locus, *Annual Review of Immunology* 24:541–570, 2006.

Klein L, Kyewski B, Allen PM, et al.: Positive and negative selection of the T cell repertoire: what thymocytes see (and don't see), *Nature Reviews Immunology* 14:377–391, 2014.

Lo WL, Allen PM: Self-peptides in TCR repertoire selection and peripheral T cell function, *Current Topics in Microbiology and Immunology* 373:49–67, 2014.

Matthews AG, Oettinger MA: RAG: a recombinase diversified, *Nature Immunology* 10:817–821, 2009.

Reth M, Nielsen P: Signaling circuits in early B-cell development, *Advances in Immunology* 122:129–175, 2014.

Schatz DG, Ji Y: Recombination centers and the orchestration of V(D)J recombination, *Nature Reviews Immunology* 11:251–263, 2011.

Stritesky GL, Jameson SC, Hogquist K: Selection of self-reactive T cells in the thymus, *Annual Review of Immunology* 30:95–114, 2012.

Taniuchi I, Ellmeier W: Transcriptional and epigenetic regulation of CD4/CD8 lineage choice, *Advances in Immunology* 110:71–110, 2011.

Chapter 5
T Cell Antigen Recognition and Costimulation

Chen L, Flies DB: Molecular mechanisms of T cell costimulation and co-inhibition, *Nature Reviews Immunology* 13:227–242, 2013.

Fooksman DR, Vardhana S, Vasiliver-Shamis G, et al.: Functional anatomy of T cell activation and synapse formation, *Annual Review of Immunology* 28:79–105, 2010.

Greenwald RJ, Freeman GJ, Sharpe AH: The B7 family revisited, *Annual Review of Immunology* 23:515–548, 2005.

Huppa JB, Davis MM: The interdisciplinary science of T-cell recognition, *Advances in Immunology* 119:1–50, 2013.

Malissen B, Bongrand P: Early T cell activation: integrating biochemical, structural, and biophysical cues, *Annual Review of Immunology* 33:539–561, 2015.

Biochemical Signals in T Cell Activation

Chakraborty A, Weiss A: Insights into the initiation of TCR signaling, *Nature Immunology* 15:798–807, 2014.

Gallo EM, Cante-Barrett K, Crabtree GR: Lymphocyte calcium signaling from membrane to nucleus, *Nature Immunology* 7:25–32, 2006.

Malissen B, Gregoire C, Malissen M, et al.: Integrative biology of T cell activation, *Nature Immunology* 15:790–797, 2014.

Functional Responses to T Cell Activation

Boyman O, Sprent J: The role of interleukin-2 during homeostasis and activation of the immune system, *Nature Reviews Immunology* 12:180–190, 2012.

Zhu J, Yamane H, Paul WE: Differentiation of effector CD4 T cell populations, *Annual Review of Immunology* 28:445–489, 2010.

Memory T Cells

Farber DL, Yudanin NA, Restifo NP: Human memory T cells: generation, compartmentalization and homeostasis, *Nature Reviews Immunology* 14:24–35, 2014.

Mueller SN, Gebhardt T, Carbone FR, et al.: Memory T cell subsets, migration patterns, and tissue residence, *Annual Review of Immunology* 31:137–161, 2013.

Pepper M, Jenkins MK: Origin of CD4+ effector and central memory T cells, *Nature Immunology* 12:467–471, 2011.

Sallusto F, Lanzavecchia A: Heterogeneity of CD4+ memory T cells: functional modules for tailored immunity, *European Journal of Immunology* 39:2076–2082, 2009.

Sprent J, Surh CD: Normal T cell homeostasis: the conversion of naive cells into memory-phenotype cells, *Nature Immunology* 12:478–484, 2011.

T Cell Migration

Bajénoff M, Egen JG, Qi H, et al.: Highways, byways and breadcrumbs: directing lymphocyte traffic in the lymph node, *Trends in Immunology* 28:346–352, 2007.

Bromley SK, Mempel TR, Luster AD: Orchestrating the orchestrators: chemokines in control of T cell traffic, *Nature Immunology* 9:970–980, 2008.

Masopust D, Schenkel JM: The integration of T cell migration, differentiation and function, *Nature Reviews Immunology* 13:309–320, 2013.

Chapter 6
CD4+ Helper T Cell Subsets

Annunziato F, Romagnani S: Heterogeneity of human effector CD4+ T cells, *Arthritis Research and Therapy* 11:257–264, 2009.

Gordon S, Martinez FO: Alternative activation of macrophages: mechanisms and functions, *Immunity* 32:593–604, 2010.

Kanno Y, Golnaz V, Hirahara K, et al.: Transcriptional and epigenetic control of T helper cell specification: molecular mechanisms underlying commitment and plasticity, *Annual Review of Immunology* 30:707–731, 2012.

Korn T, Bettelli E, Oukka M, et al.: IL-17 and TH17 cells, *Annual Review of Immunology* 27:485–517, 2009.

Littman DR, Rudensky AY: Th17 and regulatory T cells in mediating and restraining inflammation, *Cell* 140:845–858, 2010.

Murphy KM, Stockinger B: Effector T cell plasticity: flexibility in the face of changing circumstances, *Nature Immunology* 11:674–680, 2010.

O'Shea JJ, Paul WE: Mechanisms underlying lineage commitment and plasticity of helper CD4+ T cells, *Science* 327:1098–1102, 2010.

Pulendran B, Artis D: New paradigms in type 2 immunity, *Science* 337:431–435, 2012.

Reiner SL: Development in motion: helper T cells at work, *Cell* 129:33–36, 2007.

Van Dyken SJ, Locksley RM: Interleukin-4- and interleukin-13-mediated alternatively activated macrophages: roles in homeostasis and disease, *Annual Review of Immunology* 31:317–343, 2013.

Zhu J, Yamane H, Paul WE: Differentiation of effector CD4 T cell populations, *Annual Review of Immunology* 28:445–489, 2010.

CD8+ Cytotoxic T Lymphocytes

Kaech SM, Cui W: Transcriptional control of effector and memory CD8+ T cell differentiation, *Nature Reviews Immunology* 12:749–761, 2012.

Williams MA, Bevan MJ: Effector and memory CTL differentiation, *Annual Review of Immunology* 25:171–192, 2007.

Zhang N, Bevan MJ: CD8(+) T cells: foot soldiers of the immune system, *Immunity* 35:161–168, 2011.

Chapter 7
Helper T Cell–Dependent Antibody Responses

Crotty S: T follicular helper cell differentiation, function, and roles in disease, *Immunity* 41:529–542, 2014.

De Silva NS, Klein U: Dynamics of B cells in germinal centres, *Nature Reviews Immunology* 15:137–148, 2015.

Gonzalez SF, Degn SE, Pitcher LA, et al.: Trafficking of B cell antigen in lymph nodes, *Annual Review of Immunology* 29:215–233, 2011.

Goodnow CC, Vinuesa CG, Randall KL, et al.: Control systems and decision making for antibody production, *Nature Immunology* 11:681–688, 2010.

Heesters BA, Myers RC, Carroll MC: Follicular dendritic cells: dynamic antigen libraries, *Nature Reviews Immunology* 14:495–504, 2014.

McHeyzer-Williams M, Okitsu S, Wang N, et al.: Molecular programming of B cell memory, *Nature Reviews Immunology* 12:24–34, 2012.

Nutt SL, Hodgkin PD, Tarlinton DM, et al.: The generation of antibody-secreting plasma cells, *Nature Reviews Immunology* 15:160–171, 2015.

Peled JU, Kuang FL, Iglesias-Ussel MD, et al.: The biochemistry of somatic hypermutation, *Annual Review of Immunology* 26:481–511, 2008.

Shlomchik MJ, Weisel F: Germinal center selection and the development of memory B and plasma cells, *Immunology Reviews* 247:52–63, 2012.

Stavnezer J, Schrader CE: IgH chain class switch recombination: mechanism and regulation, *Journal of Immunology* 193:5370–5378, 2014.

Takemori T, Kaji T, Takahashi Y, et al.: Generation of memory B cells inside and outside germinal centers, *European Journal of Immunology* 44:1258–1264, 2014.

Ueno H, Banchereau J, Vinuesa CG: Pathophysiology of T follicular helper cells in humans and mice, *Nature Immunology* 16:142–152, 2015.

Victora GD, Nussenzweig MC: Germinal centers, *Annual Review of Immunology* 30:429–457, 2012.

T-Independent B Cell Responses

Cerutti A, Cols M, Puga I: Marginal zone B cells: virtues of innate-like antibody-producing lymphocytes, *Nature Reviews Immunology* 13:118–132, 2013.

Chapter 8
Antibody Effector Functions and Fc Receptors

Nimmerjahn F, Ravetch JV: FcγRs in health and disease, *Current Topics in Microbiology and Immunology* 350:105–125, 2011.

Schwab I, Nimmerjahn F: Intravenous immunoglobulin therapy: how does IgG modulate the immune system? *Nature Reviews Immunology* 13:176–189, 2013.

Vidarsson 1, Dekkers G, Rispens T: IgG subclasses and allotypes: from structure to effector functions, *Frontiers in Immunology* 5:520, 2014.

Ward ES: Acquiring maternal immunoglobulin: different receptors, similar functions, *Immunity* 20:507–508, 2004.

Complement

Carroll MV, Sim RB: Complement in health and disease, *Advances in Drug Delivery Reviews* 63:965–975, 2011.

Holers VM: Complement and its receptors: new insights into human disease, *Annual Review of Immunology* 32:433–459, 2015.

Liszewski M, Atkinson JP: Complement regulators in human disease: lessons from modern genetics, *Journal of Internal Medicine* 277:294–305, 2015.

Ricklin D, Lambris JD: Complement in immune and inflammatory disorders, *Journal of Immunology* 190:3831–3847, 2013.

Chapter 9
Immunological Tolerance: General Mechanisms

Baxter AG, Hodgkin PD: Activation rules: the two-signal theories of immune activation, *Nature Reviews Immunology* 2:439–446, 2002.

Goodnow CC, Sprent J, Fazekas de St Groth B, et al.: Cellular and genetic mechanisms of self tolerance and autoimmunity, *Nature* 435:590–597, 2005.

Mueller DL: Mechanisms maintaining peripheral tolerance, *Nature Immunology* 11:21–27, 2010.

Redmond WL, Sherman LA: Peripheral tolerance of CD8 T lymphocytes, *Immunity* 22:275–284, 2005.

Schwartz RH: Historical overview of immunological tolerance, *Cold Spring Harbor Perspectives in Biology* 4:a006908, 2012.

Shlomchik MJ: Sites and stages of autoreactive B cell activation and regulation, *Immunity* 28:18–28, 2008.

Central Tolerance

Hogquist KA, Baldwin TA, Jameson SC: Central tolerance: learning self-control in the thymus, *Nature Reviews Immunology* 5:772–782, 2005.

Kyewski B, Klein L: A central role for central tolerance, *Annual Review of Immunology* 24:571–606, 2006.

Laan M, Peterson P: The many faces of Aire in central tolerance, *Frontiers in Immunology* 4:1–6, 2013.

Mathis D, Benoist C: Aire. *Annual Review of Immunology* 27:287–312, 2009.

Nemazee D: Receptor editing in lymphocyte development and central tolerance, *Nature Reviews Immunology* 6:728–740, 2006.

Von Boehmer H, Melchers F: Checkpoints in lymphocyte development and autoimmune disease, *Nature Immunology* 11:14–20, 2010.

Anergy; Inhibitory Receptors

Okazaki T, Chikuma S, Iwai Y, et al.: A rheostat for immune responses: the unique properties of PD-1 and their advantages for clinical applications, *Nature Immunology* 14:1212–1218, 2013.

Walker LS, Sansom DM: The emerging role of CTLA-4 as a cell-extrinsic regulator of T cell responses, *Nature Reviews Immunology* 11:852–863, 2011.

Wells AD: New insights into the molecular basis of T cell anergy: anergy factors, avoidance sensors, and epigenetic imprinting, *Journal of Immunology* 182:7331–7341, 2009.

Apoptosis

Arakaki R, Yamada A, Kudo Y, et al.: Mechanism of activation-induced cell death of T cells and regulation of FasL expression, *Critical Reviews of Immunology* 34:301–314, 2014.

Bidere N, Su HC, Lenardo MJ: Genetic disorders of programmed cell death in the immune system, *Annual Review of Immunology* 24:321–352, 2006.

Griffith TS, Ferguson TA: Cell death in the maintenance and abrogation of tolerance: the five Ws of dying cells, *Immunity* 35:456–466, 2011.

Regulatory T Cells

Bilate AM, Lafaille JJ: Induced CD4+Foxp3+ regulatory T cells in immune tolerance, *Annual Review of Immunology* 30:733–758, 2012.

Burzyn D, Benoist C, Mathis D: Regulatory T cells in non-lymphoid tissues, *Nature Immunology* 14:1007–1013, 2013.

Josefowicz SZ, Lu L-F, Rudensky Y: Regulatory T cells: mechanisms of differentiation and function, *Annual Review of Immunology* 30:531–564, 2012.

Ohkura N, Kitagawa Y, Sakaguchi S: Development and maintenance of regulatory T cells, *Immunity* 38:414–423, 2013.

Mechanisms of Autoimmunity: Genetics and Environment

Bluestone JA, Bour-Jordan H, Cheng M, Anderson M: T cells in the control of organ-specific autoimmunity, *Journal of Clinical Investigation* 125:2250–2260, 2015.

Cheng MH, Anderson MS: Monogenic autoimmunity, *Annual Review of Immunology* 30:393–427, 2012.

Chervonsky A: Influence of microbial environment on autoimmunity, *Nature Immunology* 11:28–35, 2010.

Deitiker P, Atassi MZ: Non-MHC genes linked to autoimmune disease, *Critical Reviews of Immunology* 32:193–285, 2012.

Fernando MM, Stevens CR, Walsh EC, et al.: Defining the role of the MHC in autoimmunity: a review and pooled analysis, *PLoS Genetics* 4:e1000024, 2008.

Fourneau JM, Bach JM, van Endert PM, et al.: The elusive case for a role of mimicry in autoimmune diseases, *Molecular Immunology* 40:1095–1102, 2004.

Longman RS, Yang Y, Diehl GE, et al.: Microbiota: host interactions in mucosal homeostasis and systemic autoimmunity, *Cold Spring Harbor Symposium on Quantitative Biology* 78:193–201, 2013.

Marson A, Housley WJ, Hafler DA: Genetic basis of autoimmunity, *Journal of Clinical Investigation* 125:2234–2241, 2015.

Rosenblum MD, Remedios KA, Abbas AK: Mechanisms of human autoimmunity, *Journal of Clinical Investigation* 125:2228–2233, 2015.

Suurmond J, Diamond B: Autoantibodies in systemic autoimmune diseases: specificity and pathogenicity, *Journal of Clinical Investigation* 125:2194–2202, 2015.

Voight BF, Cotsapas C: Human genetics offers an emerging picture of common pathways and mechanisms in autoimmunity, *Current Opinion in Immunology* 24:552–557, 2012.

Zenewicz L, Abraham C, Flavell RA, et al.: Unraveling the genetics of autoimmunity, *Cell* 140:791–797, 2010.

Chapter 10
Immune Responses to Tumors

Boon T, Coulie PG, Van den Eynde BJ, et al.: Human T cell responses against melanoma, *Annual Review of Immunology* 24:175–208, 2006.

Burnet FM: The concept of immunological surveillance, *Progress in Experimental Tumor Research* 13:1–27, 1970.

Coussens LM, Zitvogel L, Palucka AK: Neutralizing tumor-promoting chronic inflammation: a magic bullet? *Science* 339:286–291, 2013.

Gajewski TF, Schreiber H, Fu YX: Innate and adaptive immune cells in the tumor microenvironment, *Nature Immunology* 14:1014–1022, 2013.

Grivennikov SI, Greten FR, Karin M: Immunity, inflammation, and cancer, *Cell* 140:883–899, 2010.

Mantovani A, Allavena P, Sica A, et al.: Cancer-related inflammation, *Nature* 454:436–444, 2008.

Schreiber RD, Old LJ, Smyth MJ: Cancer immunoediting: integrating immunity's roles in cancer suppression and promotion, *Science* 331:1565–1570, 2011.

Tumor Immunotherapy

Kalos M, June CH: Adoptive T cell transfer for cancer immunotherapy in the era of synthetic biology, *Immunity* 39:49–60, 2013.

Mellman I, Coukos G, Dranoff G: Cancer immunotherapy comes of age, *Nature* 480:480–489, 2012.

Palucka K, Banchereau J: Dendritic cell-based therapeutic cancer vaccines, *Immunity* 39:38–48, 2013.

Rosenberg SA, Restifo NP: Adoptive cell transfer as personalized immunotherapy for human cancer, *Science* 348:62–68, 2015.

Schumacher TN, Schreiber RD: Neoantigens in cancer immunotherapy, *Science* 348:69–74, 2015.

Sharma P, Allison JP: Immune checkpoint targeting in cancer therapy: toward combination strategies with curative potential, *Cell* 161:205–214, 2015.

Topalian SL, Drake CG, Pardoll DM: Immune checkpoint blockade: a common denominator approach to cancer therapy, *Cancer Cell* 27:450–461, 2015.

Recognition and Rejection of Allogeneic Transplants

Baldwin WM, Valujskikh A, Fairchild RL: Antibody-mediated rejection: emergence of animal models to answer clinical questions, *American Journal of Transplantation* 10:1135–1142, 2010.

Gras S, Kjer-Nielsen L, Chen Z, et al.: The structural bases of direct T-cell allorecognition: implications for T-cell-mediated transplant rejection, *Immunology and Cell Biology* 89:388–395, 2011.

Lakkis FG, Lechler RI: Origin and biology of the allogeneic response, *Cold Spring Harbor Perspectives in Medicine* 3:1–10, 2013.

LaRosa DF, Rahman AH, Turka LA: The innate immune system in allograft rejection and tolerance, *Journal of Immunology* 178:7503–7509, 2007.

Li XC, Rothstein DM, Sayegh MH: Costimulatory pathways in transplantation: challenges and new developments, *Immunological Reviews* 229:271–293, 2009.

Nagy ZA: Alloreactivity: an old puzzle revisited, *Scandinavian Journal of Immunology* 75:463–470, 2012.

Nankivell BJ, Alexander SI: Rejection of the kidney allograft, *New England Journal of Medicine* 363:1451–1462, 2010.

Thomas KA, Valenzuela NM, Reed EF: The perfect storm: HLA antibodies, complement, FcγRs, and endothelium in transplant rejection, *Trends in Molecular Medicine* S1471–4914, 2015.

Wood KJ, Goto R: Mechanisms of rejection: current perspectives, *Transplantation* 93:1–10, 2012.

Clinical Transplantation

Blazar BR, Murphy WJ, Abedi M: Advances in graft-versus-host disease biology and therapy, *Nature Reviews Immunology* 12:443–458, 2012.

Li HW, Sykes M: Emerging concepts in haematopoietic cell transplantation, *Nature Reviews Immunology* 12:403–416, 2012.

McCall M, Shapiro AM: Update on islet transplantation, *Cold Spring Harbor Perspectives in Medicine* 2:a007823, 2012.

Immunosuppression and Tolerance Induction to Allografts

Chidgey AP, Layton D, Trounson A, et al.: Tolerance strategies for stem-cell-based therapies, *Nature* 453:330–377, 2008.

Halloran PF: Immunosuppressive drugs for kidney transplantation, *New England Journal of Medicine* 351:2715–2729, 2004.

Kinnear G, Jones ND, Wood KJ: Costimulation blockade: current perspectives and implications for therapy, *Transplantation* 95:527–535, 2013.

McDonald-Hyman C, Turka LA, Blazar BR: Advances and challenges in immunotherapy for solid organ and hematopoietic stem cell transplantation, *Science Translational Medicine* 7:280r, 2015.

Chapter 11

Immediate Hypersensitivity

Abraham SN, St John AL: Mast cell-orchestrated immunity to pathogens, *Nature Reviews Immunology* 10:440–452, 2010.

Bossé Y: Genome-wide expression quantitative trait loci analysis in asthma, *Current Opinion in Allergy and Clinical Immunology* 3:443–452, 2013.

Galli SJ, Tsai M: IgE and mast cells in allergic disease, *Nature Medicine* 18:693–704, 2012.

Gurish MF, Austen KF: Developmental origin and functional specialization of mast cell subsets, *Immunity* 37:25–33, 2012.

Holgate ST: Innate and adaptive immune responses in asthma, *Nature Medicine* 18:673–683, 2012.

Lambrecht BN, Hammad H: The immunology of asthma, *Nature Immunology* 16:45–56, 2015.

Licona-Limon P, Kim LK, Flavell RA: TH2, allergy and group 2 innate lymphoid cells, *Nature Immunology* 14:536–542, 2013.

Rothenberg ME, Hogan SP: The eosinophil, *Annual Review of Immunology* 24:147–174, 2006.

Stone KD, Prussin C, Metcalfe DD: IgE, mast cells, basophils, and eosinophils, *Journal of Allergy and Clinical Immunology* 125:S73–S80, 2010.

Voehringer D: Protective and pathological roles of mast cells and basophils, *Nature Reviews Immunology* 13:362–375, 2013.

Wu LC, Zarrin AA: The production and regulation of IgE by the immune system, *Nature Reviews Immunology* 14:247–259, 2014.

Wynn TA: Type 2 cytokines: mechanisms and therapeutic strategies, *Nature Reviews Immunology* 15:271–282, 2015.

Diseases Caused by T Lymphocytes

Weaver CT, Elson CO, Fouser LA, Kolls JK: The Th17 pathway and inflammatory diseases of the intestines, lungs, and skin, *Annual Review of Pathology* 8:477–512, 2013.

Chapter 12

Congenital (Primary) Immunodeficiencies

Bustamante J, Boisson-Dupuis S, Abel L, et al.: Mendelian susceptibility to mycobacterial disease: genetic, immunological, and clinical features of inborn errors of IFN-γ immunity, *Seminars in Immunology* 26:454–470, 2014.

Conley ME, Dobbs AK, Farmer DM, et al.: Primary B cell immunodeficiencies: comparisons and contrasts, *Annual Review of Immunology* 27:199–227, 2009.

Durandy A, Kracker S, Fischer A: Primary antibody deficiencies, *Nature Reviews Immunology* 13:519–533, 2013.

Milner JD, Holland SM: The cup runneth over: lessons from the ever-expanding pool of primary immunodeficiency diseases, *Nature Reviews Immunology* 13:635–668, 2013.

Notarangelo LD: Functional T cell immunodeficiencies (with T cells present), *Annual Review of Immunology* 31:195–225, 2013.

Parvaneh N, Casanova JL, Notarangelo LD, et al.: Primary immunodeficiencies: a rapidly evolving story, *Journal of Allergy and Clinical Immunology* 131:314–323, 2013.

Pieper K, Grimbacher B, Eibel H: B-cell biology and development, *Journal of Allergy and Clinical Immunology* 131:959–971, 2013.

HIV and AIDS

Barouch DH: Challenges in the development of an HIV-1 vaccine, *Nature* 455:613–619, 2008.

Burton DR, Mascola JR: Antibody responses to envelope glycoproteins in HIV-1 infection, *Nature Immunology* 16:571–576, 2015.

Hladik F, McElrath MJ: Setting the stage: host invasion by HIV, *Nature Reviews Immunology* 8:447–457, 2008.

McLaren PJ, Carrington M: The impact of host genetic variation on infection with HIV-1, *Nature Immunology* 16:577–583, 2015.

McMichael AJ, Borrow P, Tomaras GD, et al.: The immune response during acute HIV-1 infection: clues for vaccine development, *Nature Reviews Immunology* 10:11–23, 2010.

Migueles SA, Connors M: Success and failure of the cellular immune response against HIV-1, *Nature Immunology* 16:563–570, 2015.

Moir S, Chun TW, Fauci AS: Pathogenic mechanisms of HIV disease, *Annual Review of Pathology: Mechanisms of Disease* 6:223–248, 2011.

Walker BD, Yu XG: Unraveling the mechanisms of durable control of HIV-1, *Nature Reviews Immunology* 13:487–498, 2013.

Glossary

αβ T cell receptor (αβ TCR) The most common form of TCR, expressed on both CD4$^+$ and CD8$^+$ T cells. The αβ TCR recognizes peptide antigen bound to an MHC molecule. Both α and β chains contain highly variable (V) regions that together form the antigen-binding site as well as constant (C) regions. TCR V and C regions are structurally homologous to the V and C regions of Ig molecules.

ABO blood group antigens Carbohydrate antigens attached mainly to cell surface proteins or lipids that are present on many cell types, including red blood cells. These antigens differ among individuals, depending on inherited alleles encoding the enzymes required for synthesis of the carbohydrate moieties. The ABO antigens act as alloantigens that are responsible for blood transfusion reactions and hyperacute rejection of ABO-mismatched allografts.

Acquired immunodeficiency A deficiency in the immune system that is acquired after birth, usually because of lymphocyte depletion caused by a cancer or drug therapy or infection (e.g., AIDS), and that is not related to a genetic defect. Synonymous with **secondary immunodeficiency.**

Acquired immunodeficiency syndrome (AIDS) A disease caused by human immunodeficiency virus (HIV) infection that is characterized by depletion of CD4$^+$ T cells, leading to a profound defect in cell-mediated immunity. Clinically, AIDS includes opportunistic infections, malignant tumors, wasting, and encephalopathy.

Activation-induced cell death (AICD) Apoptosis of activated lymphocytes, generally used for T cells.

Activation-induced (cytidine) deaminase (AID) An enzyme expressed in B cells that catalyzes the conversion of cytosine into uracil in DNA, which is a step required for somatic hypermutation and affinity maturation of antibodies and for Ig class switching.

Activation protein 1 (AP-1) A family of DNA-binding transcription factors composed of dimers of two proteins that bind to one another through a shared structural motif called a leucine zipper. The best-characterized AP-1 is composed of the proteins Fos and Jun. AP-1 is involved in transcriptional regulation of many different genes that are important in the immune system, such as cytokine genes.

Active immunity The form of adaptive immunity that is induced by exposure to a foreign antigen and activation of lymphocytes and in which the immunized individual plays an active role in responding to the antigen. This type contrasts with passive immunity, in which an individual

receives antibodies or lymphocytes from another individual who was previously actively immunized.

Acute-phase proteins Proteins, mostly synthesized in the liver in response to inflammatory cytokines such as IL-6 and IL-1, whose plasma concentrations increase shortly after infection as part of the systemic inflammatory response syndrome. Examples include C-reactive protein, fibrinogen, and serum amyloid A protein. The acute-phase reactants play various roles in the innate immune response to microbes.

Acute-phase response The increase in plasma concentrations of several proteins, called acute-phase proteins, that occurs as part of the early innate immune response to infections.

Acute rejection A form of graft rejection involving vascular and parenchymal injury mediated by T cells, macrophages, and antibodies that usually occurs days or weeks after transplantation, but may occur later if pharmacologic immunosuppression becomes inadequate.

Adaptive immunity The form of immunity that is mediated by lymphocytes and stimulated by exposure to infectious agents. In contrast to innate immunity, adaptive immunity is characterized by exquisite specificity for distinct macromolecules and by memory, which is the ability to respond more vigorously to repeated exposure to the same microbe. Adaptive immunity is also called specific immunity or acquired immunity.

Adaptor protein Proteins involved in intracellular signal transduction pathways by serving as bridge molecules or scaffolds for the recruitment of other signaling molecules. During lymphocyte antigen receptor or cytokine receptor signaling, adaptor molecules may be phosphorylated on tyrosine residues to enable them to bind other proteins containing Src homology 2 (SH2) domains. Adaptor molecules involved in T cell activation include LAT, SLP-76, and Grb-2.

Addressin Adhesion molecule expressed on endothelial cells in different anatomic sites that directs organ-specific lymphocyte homing. Mucosal addressin cell adhesion molecule 1 (MadCAM-1) is an example of an addressin expressed in Peyer's patches in the intestinal wall that binds to the integrin α4β7 on gut-homing T cells.

Adhesion molecule A cell surface molecule whose function is to promote adhesive interactions with other cells or the extracellular matrix. Leukocytes express various types of adhesion molecules, such as selectins, integrins, and members of the Ig superfamily, and these molecules play crucial roles in cell migration and cellular activation in innate and adaptive immune responses.

Adjuvant A substance, distinct from antigen, that enhances T and B cell activation mainly by promoting the accumulation and activation of antigen-presenting cells (APCs) at the site of antigen exposure. Adjuvants stimulate expression of T cell–activating costimulators and cytokines by APCs and may also prolong the expression of peptide-MHC complexes on the surface of APCs.

Adoptive transfer The process of transferring cells from one individual into another or back into the same individual after in vitro expansion and activation. Adoptive transfer is used in research to define the role of a particular cell population (e.g., T cells) in an immune response. Clinically, adoptive transfer of tumor-reactive T lymphocytes and tumor antigen–presenting dendritic cells is used in experimental cancer therapy, and trials of adoptive transfer of regulatory T cells are ongoing.

Affinity The strength of the binding between a single binding site of a molecule (e.g., an antibody) and a ligand (e.g., an antigen). The affinity of a molecule X for a ligand Y is represented by the dissociation constant (K_d), which is the concentration of Y that is required to occupy the combining sites of half the X molecules present in a solution. A smaller K_d indicates a stronger or higher affinity interaction, and a lower concentration of ligand is needed to occupy the sites.

Affinity maturation The process that leads to increased affinity of antibodies for a particular antigen as a T cell–dependent antibody response progresses. Affinity maturation takes place in germinal centers of lymphoid tissues and is the result of somatic mutation of *Ig* genes, followed by selective survival of the B cells producing the highest affinity antibodies.

Akt (called protein kinase B) An enzyme activated by lymphocyte antigen receptor signaling, which has many roles, including activation of mTOR, thereby regulating cell metabolism, and increasing expression of anti-apoptotic proteins, thus promoting survival of antigen-stimulated lymphocytes.

Allele One of different forms of the same gene present at a particular chromosomal locus. An individual who is heterozygous at a locus has two different alleles, each on a different member of a pair of chromosomes, one inherited from the mother and one from the father. If a particular gene in a population has different alleles, the gene or locus is said to be polymorphic. MHC genes have many alleles (i.e., they are highly polymorphic).

Allelic exclusion The exclusive expression of only one of two inherited alleles encoding Ig heavy and light chains and TCR β chains. Allelic exclusion occurs when the protein product of one productively recombined antigen receptor locus on one chromosome blocks rearrangement of the corresponding locus on the other chromosome. This property ensures that each lymphocyte will express a single antigen receptor and that all antigen receptors expressed by one clone of lymphocytes will have the

identical specificity. Because allelic exclusion does not involve the TCR α chain locus, some T cells do express two different types of TCR.

Allergen An antigen that elicits an immediate hypersensitivity (allergic) reaction. Allergens are proteins or chemicals bound to proteins that induce IgE antibody responses in atopic individuals.

Allergy A disorder caused by an immediate hypersensitivity reaction, often named according to the type of antigen (allergen) that elicits the disease, such as food allergy, bee sting allergy, and penicillin allergy. All of these conditions are the result of IgE production stimulated by IL-4–producing helper T cells, followed by allergen and IgE-dependent mast cell activation.

Alloantibody An antibody specific for an alloantigen (i.e., an antigen present in some individuals of a species but not in others).

Alloantigen A cell or tissue antigen that is present in some individuals of a species but not in others and that is recognized as foreign on an allograft. Alloantigens are usually products of polymorphic genes.

Alloantiserum The alloantibody-containing serum of an individual who has previously been exposed to one or more alloantigens.

Allogeneic graft An organ or tissue graft from a donor who is of the same species but genetically nonidentical to the recipient (also called an allograft).

Alloreactive Reactive to alloantigens; describes T cells or antibodies from one individual that will recognize antigens on cells or tissues of another genetically nonidentical individual.

Allotype The property of a group of antibody molecules defined by the presence of a particular antigenic determinant on the antibodies of some individuals but not others. Antibodies that share such a determinant belong to the same allotype.

Alternative macrophage activation Macrophage activation by IL-4 and IL-13 leading to an antiinflammatory and tissue-reparative phenotype, in contrast to classical macrophage activation by interferon-γ and TLR ligands. Alternatively activated macrophages are also called M2 macrophages.

Alternative pathway of complement activation An antibody-independent pathway of activation of the complement system that occurs when the C3b protein binds to microbial cell surfaces. The alternative pathway is a component of the innate immune system and mediates inflammatory responses to infection as well as direct lysis of microbes.

Anaphylatoxins Complement fragments (mainly C5a and C3a) that are generated during complement activation and promote acute inflammation by stimulating neutrophil chemotaxis and activating mast cells.

Anaphylaxis A severe form of immediate hypersensitivity in which there is systemic mast cell or basophil activation, and the released mediators cause bronchial constriction, tissue edema, and cardiovascular collapse.

Anchor residues The amino acid residues of a peptide whose side chains fit into pockets in the peptide-binding cleft of an MHC molecule. The side chains bind to complementary amino acids in the MHC molecule and therefore serve to anchor the peptide in the cleft of the MHC molecule.

Anergy A state of unresponsiveness to antigenic stimulation. Lymphocyte anergy (also called clonal anergy) is the failure of clones of T or B cells to react to an antigen and is a mechanism of maintaining immunologic tolerance to self. Clinically, anergy describes the lack of T cell–dependent cutaneous delayed-type hypersensitivity reactions to common antigens.

Angiogenesis New blood vessel formation regulated by a variety of protein factors elaborated by cells of the innate and adaptive immune systems and often accompanying chronic inflammation and tissue repair.

Antibody A type of glycoprotein molecule, also called immunoglobulin (Ig), produced by B lymphocytes that binds antigens, often with a high degree of specificity and affinity. The basic structural unit of an antibody is composed of two identical heavy chains and two identical light chains. The N-terminal variable regions of the heavy and light chains form the antigen-binding sites, whereas the C-terminal constant regions of the heavy chains functionally interact with other molecules in the immune system. Every individual has millions of different antibodies, each with a unique antigen-binding site. Secreted antibodies perform various effector functions, including neutralizing antigens, activating complement, and promoting leukocyte-dependent destruction of microbes.

Antibody-dependent cell-mediated cytotoxicity (ADCC) A process by which NK cells are targeted to IgG-coated cells, resulting in lysis of the antibody-coated cells. A specific receptor for the constant region of IgG, called FcγRIII (CD16), is expressed on the NK cell membrane and mediates binding to the IgG.

Antibody feedback The downregulation of antibody production by secreted IgG antibodies that occurs when antigen-antibody complexes simultaneously engage B cell membrane Ig and one type of Fcγ receptor (FcγRIIB). Under these conditions, the cytoplasmic tail of FcγRIIB transduces inhibitory signals inside the B cell.

Antibody repertoire The collection of different antibody specificities expressed in an individual.

Antibody-secreting cell A B lymphocyte that has undergone differentiation and produces the secretory form of Ig. Antibody-secreting cells are generated from naive B cells in response to antigen and reside in the spleen and lymph nodes as well as in the bone marrow. Often used synonymously with plasma cells.

Antigen A molecule that binds to an antibody or a TCR. Antigens that bind to antibodies include all classes of molecules, whereas the antigens for most TCRs are peptide fragments of proteins complexed with MHC molecules.

Antigen presentation The display of peptides bound by MHC molecules on the surface of an APC that permits specific recognition by TCRs and activation of T cells.

Antigen-presenting cell (APC) A cell that displays peptide fragments of protein antigens, in association with MHC

molecules, on its surface and activates antigen-specific T cells. In addition to displaying peptide-MHC complexes, APCs also express costimulatory molecules to optimally activate T lymphocytes.

Antigen processing The intracellular conversion of protein antigens derived from the extracellular space or the cytosol into peptides and loading of these peptides onto MHC molecules for display to T lymphocytes.

Antigenic variation The process by which antigens expressed by microbes may change by various genetic mechanisms and therefore allow the microbe to evade immune responses. One example of antigenic variation is the change in influenza virus surface proteins hemagglutinin and neuraminidase, which necessitates the use of new vaccines each year.

Antiretroviral therapy (ART) Combination chemotherapy for HIV infection, usually consisting of nucleoside reverse transcriptase inhibitors, a viral protease inhibitor, and, more recently, an integrase inhibitor. ART can reduce plasma virus titers to below detectable levels and slow the progression of HIV disease. It is also called *highly active antiretroviral therapy (HAART)*.

Antiserum Serum from an individual previously immunized with an antigen that contains antibody specific for that antigen.

Apoptosis A process of cell death characterized by activation of intracellular caspases, DNA cleavage, nuclear condensation and fragmentation, and plasma membrane blebbing that leads to phagocytosis of cell fragments without inducing an inflammatory response. This type of cell death is important in development of lymphocytes, return to homeostasis after an immune response to an infection, maintenance of tolerance to self antigens, and killing of infected cells by cytotoxic T lymphocytes and natural killer cells.

Arthus reaction A localized form of experimental immune complex–mediated vasculitis induced by injection of an antigen subcutaneously into a previously immunized animal or into an animal that has been given intravenous antibody specific for the antigen. Circulating antibodies bind to the injected antigen and form immune complexes that are deposited in the walls of small arteries at the injection site and give rise to a local cutaneous vasculitis with necrosis.

Asthma See **bronchial asthma.**

Atopy The propensity of an individual to produce IgE antibodies in response to various environmental antigens and to develop strong immediate hypersensitivity (allergic) responses. People who have allergies to environmental antigens, such as pollen or house dust, are said to be atopic.

Attenuated virus vaccine A vaccine composed of a live but nonpathogenic (attenuated) form of a virus. Attenuated viruses carry mutations that interfere with the viral life cycle or pathogenesis. Because live virus vaccines actually infect the recipient cells, they can effectively stimulate immune responses, such as the CTL response, that are optimal for protecting against wild-type viral infection. A commonly used live virus vaccine is the Sabin poliovirus vaccine.

Autoantibody An antibody produced in an individual that is specific for a self antigen. Autoantibodies can cause damage to cells and tissues and are produced in excess in systemic autoimmune diseases, such as systemic lupus erythematosus.

Autocrine factor A molecule that acts on the same cell that produces the factor. For example, IL-2 is an autocrine T cell growth factor that stimulates mitotic activity of the T cell that produces it.

Autoimmune disease A disease caused by a breakdown of self-tolerance such that the adaptive immune system responds to self antigens and mediates cell and tissue damage. Autoimmune diseases can be caused by immune attack against one organ or tissue (e.g., multiple sclerosis, thyroiditis, or type 1 diabetes) or against multiple and systemically distributed antigens (e.g., systemic lupus erythematosus).

Autoimmune regulator (AIRE) A protein that functions to stimulate expression of peripheral tissue protein antigens in thymic medullary epithelial cells. Mutations in the *AIRE* gene in humans and mice lead to an autoimmune disease affecting multiple, mostly endocrine, organs, because of defective expression of tissue antigens in the thymus and failure to delete T cells specific for these antigens.

Autoimmunity The state of adaptive immune system responsiveness to self antigens that occurs when mechanisms of self-tolerance fail.

Autologous graft A tissue or organ graft in which the donor and recipient are the same individual. Autologous bone marrow and skin grafts are performed in clinical medicine.

Autophagy The normal process by which a cell degrades its own components by lysosomal catabolism. Autophagy plays a role in innate immune defense against infections, and polymorphisms of genes that regulate autophagy are linked to risk for some autoimmune diseases.

Avidity The overall strength of interaction between two molecules, such as an antibody and antigen. Avidity depends on both the affinity and the valency of interactions. Therefore, the avidity of a pentameric IgM antibody, with 10 antigen-binding sites, for a multivalent antigen may be much greater than the avidity of a dimeric IgG molecule for the same antigen. Avidity can be used to describe the strength of cell-cell interactions, which are mediated by many binding interactions between cell surface molecules.

B

B lymphocyte The only cell type capable of producing antibody molecules and therefore the mediator of humoral immune responses. B lymphocytes, or B cells, develop in the bone marrow, and mature B cells are found mainly in lymphoid follicles in secondary lymphoid tissues, in bone marrow, and in low numbers in the circulation.

B-1 lymphocytes A subset of B lymphocytes that develop earlier during ontogeny than do conventional B cells, express a limited repertoire of V genes with little junctional diversity, and secrete IgM antibodies that bind T-independent antigens. Many B-1 cells express the CD5 (Ly-1) molecule.

Bare lymphocyte syndrome An immunodeficiency disease characterized by a lack of class II MHC molecule expression that leads to defects in antigen presentation and cell-mediated immunity. The disease is caused by mutations in genes encoding transcription factors that regulate class II MHC gene expression.

Basophil A type of bone marrow–derived circulating granulocyte with structural and functional similarities to mast cells that has granules containing many of the same inflammatory mediators as mast cells and expresses a high-affinity Fc receptor for IgE. Basophils that are recruited into tissue sites where antigen is present may contribute to immediate hypersensitivity reactions.

Bcl-2 family proteins A family of partially homologous cytoplasmic and mitochondrial membrane proteins that regulate apoptosis by influencing mitochondrial outer membrane permeability. Members of this family can be pro-apoptotic (such as Bax, Bad, and Bak) or anti-apoptotic (such as Bcl-2 and Bcl-XL).

Bcl-6 A transcriptional repressor that is required for germinal center B cell development and for Tfh development.

BCR (B cell receptor) The cell surface antigen receptor on B lymphocytes, which is a membrane bound immunoglobulin molecule.

BCR (B cell receptor) complex A multiprotein complex expressed on the surface of B lymphocytes that recognizes antigen and transduces activating signals into the cell. The BCR complex includes membrane Ig, which is responsible for binding antigen, and Igα and Igβ proteins, which initiate signaling events.

β2-Microglobulin The light chain of a class I MHC molecule. β2-Microglobulin is an extracellular protein encoded by a nonpolymorphic gene outside the MHC, is structurally homologous to an Ig domain, and is invariant among all class I molecules.

BLIMP-1 A transcriptional repressor that is required for plasma cell generation.

Bone marrow The tissue within the central cavity of bone that is the site of generation of all circulating blood cells in adults, including immature lymphocytes, and the site of B cell maturation.

Bone marrow transplantation See **hematopoietic stem cell transplantation.**

Bronchial asthma An inflammatory disease usually caused by repeated immediate hypersensitivity reactions in the lung that leads to intermittent and reversible airway obstruction, chronic bronchial inflammation with eosinophils, and bronchial smooth muscle cell hypertrophy and hyperreactivity.

Bruton's tyrosine kinase (Btk) A Tec family tyrosine kinase that is essential for B cell maturation. Mutations in the gene encoding Btk cause X-linked agammaglobulinemia, a disease characterized by failure of B cells to mature beyond the pre–B cell stage.

Burkitt's lymphoma A malignant B cell tumor that is diagnosed by histologic features but almost always carries a reciprocal chromosomal translocation involving *Ig* gene loci and the cellular *MYC* gene on chromosome 8. Many cases of Burkitt's lymphoma in Africa are associated with Epstein-Barr virus infection.

C

C (constant region) gene segments The DNA sequences in the *Ig* and *TCR* gene loci that encode the nonvariable portions of Ig heavy and light chains and TCR α, β, γ, and δ chains.

C1 A serum complement system protein composed of several polypeptide chains that initiates the classical pathway of complement activation by attaching to the Fc portions of IgG or IgM antibody that has bound antigen.

C1 inhibitor (C1 INH) A plasma protein inhibitor of the classical pathway of complement activation. C1 INH is a serine protease inhibitor (serpin) that mimics the normal substrates of the C1r and C1s components of C1. A genetic deficiency in C1 INH causes the disease hereditary angioneurotic edema.

C3 The central and most abundant complement system protein; it is involved in both the classical and alternative pathway cascades. C3 is proteolytically cleaved during complement activation to generate a C3b fragment, which covalently attaches to cell or microbial surfaces, and a C3a fragment, which has various proinflammatory activities.

C3 convertase A multiprotein enzyme complex generated by the early steps of classical, lectin, and alternative pathways of complement activation. C3 convertase cleaves C3, which gives rise to two proteolytic products called C3a and C3b.

C5 convertase A multiprotein enzyme complex generated by C3b binding to C3 convertase. C5 convertase cleaves C5 and initiates the late steps of complement activation leading to formation of the membrane attack complex and lysis of cells.

Calcineurin A cytoplasmic serine/threonine phosphatase that dephosphorylates the transcription factor NFAT, thereby allowing NFAT to enter the nucleus. Calcineurin is activated by calcium signals generated through TCR signaling in response to antigen recognition. The immunosuppressive drugs cyclosporine and FK506 work by blocking calcineurin activity.

Carcinoembryonic antigen (CEA, CD66) A highly glycosylated membrane protein; increased expression of CEA in many carcinomas of the colon, pancreas, stomach, and breast results in a rise in the normal serum levels. The level of serum CEA is used to monitor the persistence or recurrence of metastatic carcinoma after treatment.

Caspases Intracellular proteases with cysteines in their active sites that cleave substrates at the C-terminal sides of aspartic acid residues. Most are components of enzymatic cascades that cause apoptotic death of cells, but caspase-1, which is part of the inflammasome, drives inflammation by processing inactive precursor forms of the cytokines IL-1 and IL-18 into their active forms.

Cathelicidins Polypeptides produced by neutrophils and various barrier epithelia that serve various functions in innate immunity, including direct toxicity to microorganisms, activation of leukocytes, and neutralization of lipopolysaccharide.

Cathepsins Thiol and aspartyl proteases with broad substrate specificities, which are abundant in the endosomes in APCs, and play an important role in generating peptide fragments from exogenous protein antigens that bind to class II MHC molecules.

CD molecules Cell surface molecules expressed on various cell types in the immune system that are designated by the "cluster of differentiation" or CD number. See Appendix III for a list of CD molecules.

Cell-mediated immunity (CMI) The form of adaptive immunity that is mediated by T lymphocytes and serves as the defense mechanism against various types of microbes that are taken up by phagocytes or infect nonphagocytic cells. Cell-mediated immune responses include CD4$^+$ T cell–mediated activation of phagocytes and CD8$^+$ CTL–mediated killing of infected cells.

Central tolerance A form of self-tolerance induced in generative (central) lymphoid organs as a consequence of immature self-reactive lymphocytes recognizing self antigens and subsequently leading to their death or inactivation. Central tolerance prevents the emergence of lymphocytes with high-affinity receptors for the self antigens that are expressed in the bone marrow or thymus.

Centroblasts Rapidly proliferating B cells in the dark zone of germinal centers of secondary lymphoid tissues, which give rise to thousands of progeny, express activation-induced deaminase (AID), and undergo somatic mutation of their *V* genes. Centroblasts become the centrocytes of the light zone of germinal centers.

Centrocytes B cells in the light zone of germinal centers of secondary lymphoid organs, which are the progeny of proliferating centroblasts of the dark zone. Centrocytes that express high-affinity Ig are positively selected to survive and undergo isotype switching and further differentiation into long-lived plasma cells and memory B cells.

Checkpoint blockade A therapeutic strategy to boost host immune responses against tumors by blocking normal inhibitory signals for lymphocytes, thus removing the brakes (checkpoints) on the immune response. Examples in clinical use are blocking antibodies specific for CTLA-4 or PD-1.

Chédiak-Higashi syndrome A rare autosomal recessive immunodeficiency disease caused by a defect in the cytoplasmic granules of various cell types that affects the lysosomes of neutrophils and macrophages as well as the granules of CTLs and NK cells. Patients show reduced resistance to infection with pyogenic bacteria.

Chemokine receptors Cell surface receptors for chemokines that transduce signals stimulating the migration of leukocytes. There are at least 19 *check* different mammalian chemokine receptors, each of which binds a different set of chemokines; all are members of the seven-transmembrane α-helical, G protein–coupled receptor family.

Chemokines A large family of structurally homologous low-molecular-weight cytokines that stimulate leukocyte chemotaxis, regulate the migration of leukocytes from the blood to tissues by activating leukocyte integrins, and maintain the spatial organization of different subsets of lymphocytes and antigen-presenting cells within lymphoid organs.

Chemotaxis Movement of a cell directed by a chemical concentration gradient. The movement of leukocytes within various tissues is often directed by gradients of low-molecular-weight cytokines called chemokines.

Chimeric antigen receptor Chimeric antigen receptors are products of fusion genes typically encoding the extracellular domains of a single chain antibody and the transmembrane and intracellular domains of T cell receptor–associated signaling proteins. When T cells are engineered to express chimeric antigen receptors, these cells can recognize and kill cells that the extracellular domain recognizes. Adoptive transfer of CAR-expressing T cells has been used successfully for the treatment of some types of cancers.

Chromosomal translocation A chromosomal abnormality in which a segment of one chromosome is transferred to another. Many malignant diseases of lymphocytes are associated with chromosomal translocations involving an Ig or TCR locus and a chromosomal segment containing a cellular oncogene.

Chronic granulomatous disease A rare inherited immunodeficiency disease caused by mutations in genes encoding components of the phagocyte oxidase enzyme complex that is needed for microbial killing by polymorphonuclear leukocytes and macrophages. The disease is characterized by recurrent intracellular bacterial and fungal infections, often accompanied by chronic cell-mediated immune responses and the formation of granulomas.

Chronic rejection A form of allograft rejection characterized by fibrosis with loss of normal organ structures occurring during a prolonged period. In many cases, the major pathologic event in chronic rejection is graft arterial occlusion caused by proliferation of intimal smooth muscle cells, which is called graft arteriosclerosis.

c-Kit ligand (stem cell factor) A protein required for hematopoiesis and mast cell development. c-Kit ligand is produced in membrane-bound and soluble forms by stromal cells in the bone marrow and thymus, and it binds to the c-Kit tyrosine kinase membrane receptor on pluripotent stem cells.

Class I major histocompatibility complex (MHC) molecule One of two forms of polymorphic heterodimeric membrane proteins that bind and display peptide fragments of protein antigens on the surface of APCs for recognition by T lymphocytes. Class I MHC molecules usually display peptides derived from proteins in the cytosol of the cell, for recognition by CD8$^+$ T cells.

Class II–associated invariant chain peptide (CLIP) A peptide remnant of the invariant chain that sits in the class II MHC peptide-binding cleft and is removed by action of the HLA-DM molecule before the cleft becomes accessible to peptides produced from extracellular protein antigens.

Class II major histocompatibility complex (MHC) molecule One of two major classes of polymorphic heterodimeric membrane proteins that bind and display peptide fragments of protein antigens on the surface of APCs for recognition by T lymphocytes. Class II MHC molecules usually display peptides derived from extracellular proteins that are internalized into phagocytic or endocytic vesicles, for recognition by CD4$^+$ T cells.

Classical macrophage activation Macrophage activation by interferon-γ, T_H1 cells, and TLR ligands, leading to a proinflammatory and microbicidal phenotype. Classically activated macrophages are also called M1 macrophages.

Classical pathway of complement activation The pathway of activation of the complement system that is initiated by binding of antigen-antibody complexes to the C1 molecule and induces a proteolytic cascade involving multiple other complement proteins. The classical pathway is an effector arm of the humoral immune system that generates inflammatory mediators, opsonins for phagocytosis of antigens, and lytic complexes that destroy cells.

Clonal anergy A state of antigen unresponsiveness of a clone of T lymphocytes experimentally induced by recognition of antigen in the absence of additional signals (costimulatory signals) required for functional activation. Clonal anergy is considered a model for one mechanism of tolerance to self antigens and may be applicable to B lymphocytes as well.

Clonal deletion A mechanism of lymphocyte tolerance in which an immature T cell in the thymus or an immature B cell in the bone marrow undergoes apoptotic death as a consequence of recognizing a self antigen.

Clonal expansion The approximately 1000- to 100,000-fold increase in the number of lymphocytes specific for an antigen that results from antigen stimulation and proliferation of naive T cells. Clonal expansion occurs in lymphoid tissues and is required to generate enough antigen-specific effector lymphocytes from rare naive precursors to eradicate infections.

Clonal selection hypothesis A fundamental tenet of the immune system (no longer a hypothesis) stating that every individual possesses numerous clones of lymphocytes, each of which arises from a single precursor, expresses one antigen receptor, and is capable of recognizing and responding to a distinct antigenic determinant. When an antigen enters, it selects a specific preexisting clone and activates it.

Clone A group of cells derived from a single common precursor. All members of a clone of B or T lymphocytes share the same unique recombined Ig or TCR genes that are different from the rearranged genes in all other clones. Note that the rearranged Ig V genes of cells within a clone of B cells may change in sequence due to somatic hypermutation, which occurs after antigen stimulation of mature B cells.

Collectins A family of proteins, including mannose-binding lectin, that are characterized by a collagen-like domain and a lectin (i.e., carbohydrate-binding) domain. Collectins play a role in the innate immune system by acting as microbial pattern recognition receptors, and they may activate the complement system by binding to C1q.

Colony-stimulating factors (CSFs) Cytokines that promote the expansion and differentiation of bone marrow progenitor cells. CSFs are essential for the maturation of red blood cells, granulocytes, monocytes, and lymphocytes. Examples of CSFs include granulocyte-monocyte colony-stimulating factor (GM-CSF), granulocyte colony-stimulating factor (G-CSF), and IL-3.

Combinatorial diversity The diversity of Ig and TCR specificities generated by the use of many different combinations of different variable, diversity, and joining segments during somatic recombination of DNA in the Ig and TCR loci in developing B and T cells. Combinatorial diversity is one mechanism, which works together with junctional diversity, for the generation of large numbers of different antigen receptor genes from a limited number of DNA gene segments.

Commensal microbes Nonpathogenic microbes that normally live on human skin and mucosal surfaces, which include viruses and bacteria, and contribute to immune homeostasis and serve important metabolic functions.

Complement Serum and cell surface proteins that interact with one another and with other molecules of the immune system to generate important effectors of innate and adaptive immune responses. The classical, alternative, and lectin pathways of the complement system are activated by antigen-antibody complexes, microbial surfaces, and plasma lectins binding to microbes, respectively, and consist of a cascade of proteolytic enzymes that generate inflammatory mediators and opsonins. All three pathways lead to the formation of a common terminal cell lytic complex that is inserted in cell membranes.

Complement receptor type 1 (CR1) A high-affinity receptor for the C3b and C4b fragments of complement. Phagocytes use CR1 to mediate internalization of C3b- or C4b-coated particles. CR1 on erythrocytes serves in the clearance of immune complexes from the circulation. CR1 is also a regulator of complement activation.

Complement receptor type 2 (CR2) A receptor expressed on B cells and follicular dendritic cells that binds proteolytic fragments of the C3 complement protein, including C3d, C3dg, and iC3b. CR2 functions to stimulate humoral immune responses by enhancing B cell activation by antigen and by promoting the trapping of antigen-antibody complexes in germinal centers. CR2 is also the receptor for Epstein-Barr virus.

Complementarity-determining region (CDR) Short segments of Ig and TCR proteins that contain most of the sequence differences between different antibodies or TCRs and make contact with antigen; also called **hypervariable regions.** Three CDRs are present in the variable domain of each antigen receptor polypeptide chain, and six CDRs are present in an intact Ig or TCR molecule. These hypervariable segments assume loop structures that together form a surface complementary to the three-dimensional structure of the bound antigen.

Congenital immunodeficiency A genetic defect in which an inherited deficiency in some aspect of the innate or adaptive immune system leads to an increased susceptibility to infections. Congenital immunodeficiency is frequently manifested early in infancy and childhood but is sometimes clinically detected later in life. Synonymous with *primary immunodeficiency.*

Constant (C) region The portion of Ig or TCR polypeptide chains that does not vary in sequence among different clones and is not involved in antigen binding.

Contact sensitivity An immune reaction to certain chemical agents leading to T cell–mediated delayed-type hypersensitivity reactions upon skin contact. Substances that elicit contact hypersensitivity, including nickel ions, urushiols in poison ivy, and many therapeutic drugs, bind to and modify self proteins on the surfaces of APCs, which are then recognized by CD4+ or CD8+ T cells, or alter MHC molecules directly.

Co-receptor A lymphocyte surface receptor that binds to an antigen complex at the same time that membrane Ig or TCR binds the antigen and delivers signals required for optimal lymphocyte activation. CD4 and CD8 are T cell co-receptors that bind nonpolymorphic parts of an MHC molecule concurrently with the TCR binding to polymorphic residues and the bound peptide. CR2 is a co-receptor on B cells that binds to complement-opsonized antigens at the same time that membrane Ig binds to another part of the antigen.

Costimulator A molecule expressed on the surface of APCs in response to innate immune stimuli, which provides a stimulus (the "second signal"), in addition to antigen (the "first signal"), that is required for the activation of naive T cells. The best-defined costimulators are the B7 molecules (CD80 and CD86) on APCs that bind to the CD28 receptor on T cells.

CpG nucleotides Unmethylated cytidine-guanine sequences found in microbial DNA that stimulate innate immune responses. CpG nucleotides are recognized by Toll-like receptor-9, and they have adjuvant properties in the mammalian immune system.

C-reactive protein (CRP) A member of the pentraxin family of plasma proteins involved in innate immune responses to bacterial infections. CRP is an acute-phase reactant, and it binds to the capsule of pneumococcal bacteria. CRP also binds to C1q and may thereby activate complement or act as an opsonin by interacting with phagocyte C1q receptors.

Cross-matching A screening test performed to minimize the chance of adverse transfusion reactions or graft rejection, in which a patient in need of a blood transfusion or organ allograft is tested for the presence of preformed antibodies against donor cell surface antigens (usually blood group antigens or MHC antigens). The test involves mixing the recipient serum with leukocytes or red blood cells from potential donors and analyzing for agglutination or complement-dependent lysis of the cells.

Cross-presentation A mechanism by which a dendritic cell activates (or primes) a naive CD8+ CTL specific for the antigens of a third cell (e.g., a virus-infected or tumor cell). Cross-presentation occurs, for example, when an infected (often apoptotic) cell is ingested by a dendritic cell and the microbial antigens are processed and presented in association with class I MHC molecules, unlike the general rule for phagocytosed antigens, which are presented in association with class II MHC molecules. The dendritic cell also provides costimulation for the T cells. Also called *cross-priming.*

CTLA-4 An Ig superfamily protein expressed on the surface of activated effector T cells and Treg, which binds B7-1 and B7-2 with high affinity and plays an essential role in inhibiting T cell responses. CTLA-4 is essential for Treg function and T cell tolerance to self antigens. An antibody that inhibits CTLA-4 is used for cancer immunotherapy. The antibody works by blocking the inhibition (checkpoint) in the antitumor immune response ("checkpoint blockade").

C-type lectin A member of a large family of calcium-dependent carbohydrate-binding proteins, many of which play important roles in innate and adaptive immunity. For example, soluble C-type lectins bind to microbial carbohydrate structures and mediate phagocytosis or complement activation (e.g., mannose-binding lectin, dectins, collectins, ficolins).

Cutaneous immune system The components of the innate and adaptive immune system found in the skin that function together in a specialized way to detect and respond to pathogens on or in the skin and to maintain homeostasis with commensal microbes. Components of the cutaneous immune system include keratinocytes, Langerhans cells, dermal dendritic cells, intraepithelial lymphocytes, and dermal lymphocytes.

Cyclosporine A calcineurin inhibitor widely used as an immunosuppressive drug to prevent allograft rejection by blocking T cell activation. Cyclosporine (also called cyclosporin A) binds to a cytosolic protein called cyclophilin, and cyclosporine-cyclophilin complexes bind to and inhibit calcineurin, thereby inhibiting activation and nuclear translocation of the transcription factor NFAT.

Cytokines Proteins that are produced and secreted by many different cell types, and mediate inflammatory and immune reactions. Cytokines are principal mediators of communication between cells of the immune system (see Appendix II).

Cytotoxic (or cytolytic) T lymphocyte (CTL) A type of T lymphocyte whose major effector function is to recognize and kill host cells infected with viruses or other intracellular microbes and to kill tumor cells. CTLs usually express CD8 and recognize microbial peptides displayed by class I MHC molecules. CTL killing of infected or tumor cells involves delivery of the contents of cytoplasmic granules into the cytosol of the cells, leading to apoptotic death.

D

Damage-associated molecular patterns (DAMPs) Endogenous molecules that are produced by or released from damaged and dying cells that bind to pattern recognition receptors and stimulate innate immune responses.

Examples include high-mobility group box 1 (HMGB1) protein, extracellular ATP, and uric acid.

Death receptors Plasma membrane receptors expressed on various cell types that, upon ligand binding, transduce signals that lead to recruitment of the Fas-Associated protein with Death Domain (FADD) adaptor protein, which activates caspase-8, leading to apoptotic cell death. All death receptors, including FAS, TRAIL, and TNFR, belong to the TNF receptor superfamily.

Dectins Pattern recognition receptors expressed on dendritic cells that recognize fungal cell wall carbohydrates (glucans) and induce signaling events that promote cytokine secretion, which induces inflammation and enhances adaptive immune responses.

Defensins Cysteine-rich peptides produced by epithelial barrier cells in the skin, gut, lung, and other tissues and in neutrophil granules that act as broad-spectrum antibiotics to kill a wide variety of bacteria and fungi. The synthesis of defensins is increased in response to stimulation of innate immune system receptors such as Toll-like receptors and inflammatory cytokines such as IL-1 and TNF.

Delayed-type hypersensitivity (DTH) An immune reaction in which T cell–dependent macrophage activation and inflammation cause tissue injury. A DTH reaction to the subcutaneous injection of antigen is often used as an assay for cell-mediated immunity (e.g., the PPD [purified protein derivative] skin test for immunity to *Mycobacterium tuberculosis*).

Dendritic cells Bone marrow–derived cells found in epithelial and lymphoid tissues that are morphologically characterized by thin membranous projections. Many subsets of dendritic cells exist with diverse functions. Classical dendritic cells function as innate sentinel cells and become APCs for naive T lymphocytes upon activation, and they are important for initiation of adaptive immune responses to protein antigen. Immature (resting) classical dendritic cells are important for induction of tolerance to self antigens. Plasmacytoid dendritic cells produce abundant type 1 interferons in response to exposure to viruses.

Desensitization A method of treating immediate hypersensitivity diseases (allergies) that involves repetitive administration of low doses of an antigen to which individuals are allergic. This process often prevents severe allergic reactions on subsequent environmental exposure to the antigen, but the mechanisms are not well understood.

Determinant The specific portion of a macromolecular antigen to which an antibody binds. In the case of a protein antigen recognized by a T cell, the determinant is the peptide portion that binds to an MHC molecule for recognition by the TCR. Synonymous with **epitope.**

Diacylglycerol (DAG) A signaling molecule generated by phospholipase C (PLCγ1)–mediated hydrolysis of the plasma membrane phospholipid phosphatidylinositol 4,5-bisphosphate (PIP2) during antigen activation of lymphocytes. The main function of DAG is to activate an enzyme called protein kinase C that participates in the generation of active transcription factors.

DiGeorge syndrome A selective T cell deficiency caused by a congenital malformation that results in defective development of the thymus, parathyroid glands, and other structures that arise from the third and fourth pharyngeal pouches.

Direct antigen presentation (or direct allorecognition) Presentation of cell surface allogeneic MHC molecules by graft APCs to a graft recipient's T cells that leads to activation of the alloreactive T cells. In direct recognition of allogeneic MHC molecules, a TCR that was selected to recognize a self MHC molecule plus foreign peptide cross-reacts with the allogeneic MHC molecule plus peptide. Direct presentation is partly responsible for strong T cell responses to allografts.

Diversity The existence of a large number of lymphocytes with different antigenic specificities in any individual. Diversity is a fundamental property of the adaptive immune system and is the result of variability in the structures of the antigen-binding sites of lymphocyte receptors for antigens (antibodies and TCRs).

Diversity (D) segments Short coding sequences between the variable (V) and constant (C) gene segments in the Ig heavy chain and TCR β and γ loci that together with J segments are somatically recombined with V segments during lymphocyte development. The resulting recombined VDJ DNA codes for the antigen receptor V regions. Random use of D segments contributes to the diversity of the antigen receptor repertoire.

DNA vaccine A vaccine composed of a bacterial plasmid containing a complementary DNA encoding a protein antigen. DNA vaccines presumably work because professional APCs are transfected in vivo by the plasmid and express immunogenic peptides that elicit specific responses. Furthermore, the plasmid DNA contains CpG nucleotides that act as potent adjuvants.

Double-negative thymocyte A subset of developing T cells in the thymus (thymocytes) that express neither CD4 nor CD8. Most double-negative thymocytes are at an early developmental stage and do not express antigen receptors. They will later express both CD4 and CD8 during the intermediate double-positive stage before further maturation to single-positive T cells expressing only CD4 or CD8.

Double-positive thymocyte A subset of developing T cells in the thymus (thymocytes) that express both CD4 and CD8 and are at an intermediate developmental stage. Double-positive thymocytes also express TCRs and are subject to selection processes, and they mature to single-positive T cells expressing only CD4 or CD8.

E

Effector cells The cells that perform effector functions during an immune response, such as secreting cytokines (e.g., helper T cells), killing microbes (e.g., macrophages), killing microbe-infected host cells (e.g., CTLs), or secreting antibodies (e.g., plasma cells).

Effector phase The phase of an immune response in which a foreign antigen is destroyed or inactivated. For example, in a humoral immune response, the effector phase may be characterized by antibody-dependent complement activation and phagocytosis of antibody- and complement-opsonized bacteria.

Endosome An intracellular membrane-bound vesicle into which extracellular proteins are internalized during antigen processing. Endosomes have an acidic pH and contain proteolytic enzymes that degrade proteins into peptides that bind to class II MHC molecules. A subset of class II MHC–rich endosomes, called MIIC, play a special role in antigen processing and presentation by the class II pathway.

Endotoxin A component of the cell wall of Gram-negative bacteria, also called **lipopolysaccharide** (LPS), that is released from dying bacteria and stimulates innate immune inflammatory responses by binding to TLR4 on many different cell types, including phagocytes, endothelial cells, dendritic cells, and barrier epithelial cells. Endotoxin contains both lipid components and carbohydrate (polysaccharide) moieties.

Envelope glycoprotein (Env) A membrane glycoprotein encoded by a retrovirus that is expressed on the plasma membrane of infected cells and on the host cell–derived membrane coat of viral particles. Env proteins are often required for viral infectivity. The Env proteins of HIV include gp41 and gp120, which bind to CD4 and chemokine receptors, respectively, on human T cells and mediate fusion of the viral and T cell membranes.

Enzyme-linked immunosorbent assay (ELISA) A method of quantifying an antigen immobilized on a solid surface by use of a specific antibody with a covalently coupled enzyme. The amount of antibody that binds the antigen is proportional to the amount of antigen present and is determined by spectrophotometrically measuring the conversion of a clear substrate to a colored product by the coupled enzyme.

Eosinophil A bone marrow–derived granulocyte that is abundant in the inflammatory infiltrates of immediate hypersensitivity late-phase reactions and contributes to many of the pathologic processes in allergic diseases. Eosinophils are important in defense against extracellular parasites, including helminths.

Epitope The specific portion of a macromolecular antigen to which an antibody binds. In the case of a protein antigen recognized by a T cell, an epitope is the peptide portion that binds to an MHC molecule for recognition by the TCR. Synonymous with **determinant.**

Epstein-Barr virus (EBV) A double-stranded DNA virus of the herpesvirus family that is the etiologic agent of infectious mononucleosis and is associated with some B cell malignant tumors and nasopharyngeal carcinoma. EBV infects B lymphocytes and some epithelial cells by specifically binding to CR2 (CD21).

F

Fab (fragment, antigen-binding) A proteolytic fragment, first produced from an IgG antibody molecule, that includes one complete light chain paired with one heavy-chain fragment containing the variable domain and only the first constant domain. All antibodies have Fab regions that retain the ability to monovalently bind an antigen but cannot interact with Fc receptors on cells or with complement. Therefore, Fab preparations are used in research and therapeutic applications when antigen binding is desired without activation of effector functions. (The Fab' fragment retains the hinge region of the heavy chain.)

F(ab')2 region The part of an Ig molecule (first produced by proteolysis of IgG) that includes two complete light chains but only the variable domain, first constant domain, and hinge region of the two heavy chains. $F(ab')_2$ fragments retain the entire bivalent antigen-binding region of an intact Ig molecule but cannot bind complement or Fc receptors. They are used in research and therapeutic applications when antigen binding is desired without antibody effector functions.

Fas (CD95) A death receptor of the TNF receptor family that is expressed on the surface of T cells and many other cell types and initiates a signaling cascade leading to apoptotic death of the cell. The death pathway is initiated when Fas binds to Fas ligand expressed on activated T cells. Fas-mediated killing of lymphocytes is important for the maintenance of self-tolerance. Mutations in the FAS gene cause systemic autoimmune disease (see also **death receptors**).

Fas ligand (CD95 ligand) A membrane protein that is a member of the TNF family of proteins expressed on activated T cells. Fas ligand binds to the death receptor Fas, thereby stimulating a signaling pathway leading to apoptotic cell death of the Fas-expressing cell. Mutations in the Fas ligand gene cause systemic autoimmune disease in mice.

Fc (fragment, crystalline) A proteolytic fragment, first produced from IgG, that contains only the disulfide-linked carboxyl-terminal regions of the two heavy chains. Fc is also used to describe the corresponding region of an intact Ig molecule that mediates effector functions by binding to cell surface receptors or the C1q complement protein. (Fc fragments are so named because they tend to crystallize out of solution.)

Fc receptor A cell surface receptor specific for the carboxyl-terminal constant region of an Ig molecule. Fc receptors typically include signaling components and Ig-binding components. Several types of Fc receptors exist, including those specific for different IgG isotypes, IgE, and IgA. Fc receptors mediate many of the effector functions of antibodies, including phagocytosis of antibody-bound antigens, antigen-induced activation of mast cells, and ADCC. One Fc receptor prolongs the half-life of circulating IgG antibodies by inhibiting their catabolism, and another Fc receptor inhibits B cell activation (the process called antibody feedback).

FcεRI A high-affinity receptor for the carboxyl-terminal constant region of IgE molecules that is expressed on mast cells, basophils, and eosinophils. FcεRI molecules on mast cells are usually occupied by IgE, and antigen-induced cross-linking of these IgE-FcεRI complexes activates the mast cell and initiates immediate hypersensitivity reactions.

Fcγ receptor (FcγR) A specific cell surface receptor for the carboxyl-terminal constant region of IgG molecules. There are several different types of Fcγ receptors, including a high-affinity FcγRI that mediates phagocytosis by macrophages and neutrophils, FcγRIIB that transduces inhibitory signals in B cells, and FcγRIIIA that mediates targeting and activation of NK cells.

Ficolins Hexameric innate immune system plasma proteins, containing collagen-like domains and fibrinogen-like carbohydrate-recognizing domains, that bind to cell wall components of Gram-positive bacteria, opsonizing them and activating complement.

FK506 An immunosuppressive drug (also known as tacrolimus) used to prevent allograft rejection that functions blocking T cell cytokine gene transcription, similar to cyclosporine. FK506 binds to a cytosolic protein called FK506-binding protein, and the resulting complex binds to calcineurin, thereby inhibiting activation and nuclear translocation of the transcription factor NFAT.

Flow cytometry A method of analysis of the phenotype of cell populations requiring a specialized instrument (flow cytometer) that can detect fluorescence on individual cells in a suspension and thereby determine the number of cells expressing the molecule to which a fluorescent probe binds, as well as the relative amount of the molecule expressed. Suspensions of cells are incubated with fluorescently labeled antibodies or other probes, and the amount of probe bound by each cell in the population is measured by passing the cells one at a time through a fluorimeter with a laser-generated incident beam.

Fluorescence-activated cell sorter (FACS) An adaptation of the flow cytometer that is used for the purification of cells from a mixed population according to which and how much fluorescent probe the cells bind. Cells are first stained with a fluorescently labeled probe, such as an antibody specific for a surface antigen of a cell population. The cells are then passed one at a time through a fluorimeter with a laser-generated incident beam and are deflected into different collection tubes by electromagnetic fields whose strength and direction are varied according to the measured intensity of the fluorescence signal.

Follicle See **lymphoid follicle**.

Follicular dendritic cells (FDCs) Cells in lymphoid follicles of secondary lymphoid organs that express complement receptors and Fc receptors and have long cytoplasmic processes that form a meshwork integral to the architecture of the follicles. Follicular dendritic cells display antigens on their surface for B cell recognition and are involved in the selection of B cells expressing high-affinity membrane Ig during the process of affinity maturation. They are nonhematopoietic cells (not of bone marrow origin).

Follicular helper T cell (Tfh) See **T follicular helper (Tfh) cells**.

FoxP3 A forkhead family transcription factor expressed by and required for the development of CD4+ regulatory T cells. Mutations in FoxP3 in mice and humans result in an absence of CD25$^+$ regulatory T cells and multisystem autoimmune disease.

G

G protein–coupled receptor family A diverse family of receptors for hormones, lipid inflammatory mediators, and chemokines that use associated trimeric G proteins for intracellular signaling.

G proteins Proteins that bind guanyl nucleotides and act as exchange molecules by catalyzing the replacement of bound guanosine diphosphate (GDP) by guanosine triphosphate (GTP). G proteins with bound GTP can activate a variety of cellular enzymes in different signaling cascades. Trimeric GTP-binding proteins are associated with the cytoplasmic portions of many cell surface receptors, such as chemokine receptors. Other small soluble G proteins, such as Ras and Rac, are recruited into signaling pathways by adaptor proteins.

γδ T cell receptor (γδ TCR) A form of TCR that is distinct from the more common αβ TCR and is expressed on a subset of T cells found mostly in epithelial barrier tissues. Although the γδ TCR is structurally similar to the αβ TCR, the forms of antigen recognized by γδ TCRs are poorly understood; they do not recognize peptide complexes bound to polymorphic MHC molecules.

GATA-3 A transcription factor that promotes the differentiation of Th2 cells from naive T cells.

Generative lymphoid organ An organ in which lymphocytes develop from immature precursors. The bone marrow and thymus are the major generative lymphoid organs in which B cells and T cells develop, respectively. Also called central or primary lymphoid organ.

Germinal centers Specialized structures in lymphoid organs that develop during T-dependent humoral immune responses, where extensive B cell proliferation, isotype switching, somatic mutation, affinity maturation, memory B cell generation, and induction of long-lived plasma cells take place. Germinal centers appear as lightly stained regions within a lymphoid follicle in spleen, lymph nodes, and mucosal lymphoid tissue.

Germline organization The inherited arrangement of variable, diversity, joining, and constant region gene segments of the antigen receptor loci in nonlymphoid cells or in immature lymphocytes. In developing B or T lymphocytes, the germline organization is modified by somatic recombination to form functional *Ig* or *TCR* genes.

Glomerulonephritis Inflammation of the renal glomeruli, often initiated by immunopathologic mechanisms such as deposition of circulating antigen-antibody complexes in the glomerular basement membrane or binding of antibodies to antigens expressed in the glomerulus. The antibodies can activate complement and phagocytes, and the resulting inflammatory response can lead to renal failure.

Graft A tissue or organ that is removed from one site and placed in another site, usually in a different individual.

Graft arteriosclerosis Occlusion of graft arteries caused by proliferation of intimal smooth muscle cells. This process is evident within 6 months to a year after transplantation and is responsible for chronic rejection of vascularized organ grafts. The mechanism is likely to be a chronic immune response to vessel wall alloantigens. Graft arteriosclerosis is also called accelerated arteriosclerosis.

Graft rejection A specific immune response to an organ or tissue graft that leads to inflammation, damage, and possibly graft failure.

Graft-versus-host disease A disease occurring in hematopoietic stem cell (HSC) transplant recipients that is caused by the reaction of mature T cells in the HSC graft to alloantigens on host cells. The disease most often affects the skin, liver and intestines.

Granulocyte colony-stimulating factor (G-CSF) A cytokine made by activated T cells, macrophages, and endothelial cells at sites of infection that acts on bone marrow to increase the production of and mobilize neutrophils to replace those consumed in inflammatory reactions.

Granulocyte-monocyte colony-stimulating factor (GM-CSF) A cytokine made by activated T cells, macrophages, endothelial cells, and stromal fibroblasts that acts on bone marrow to increase the production of neutrophils and monocytes. GM-CSF is also a macrophage-activating factor and promotes the maturation of dendritic cells.

Granuloma A nodule of inflammatory tissue composed of clusters of activated macrophages and T lymphocytes, usually with associated fibrosis. Granulomatous inflammation is a form of chronic delayed-type hypersensitivity, often in response to persistent microbes, such as *Mycobacterium tuberculosis* and some fungi, or in response to particulate antigens that are not readily phagocytosed.

Granzyme A serine protease enzyme found in the granules of CTLs and NK cells that is released by exocytosis, enters target cells, and proteolytically cleaves and activates caspases, which in turn cleave several substrates and induce target cell apoptosis.

Gut-associated lymphoid tissue (GALT) Collections of lymphocytes and APCs within the mucosa of the gastrointestinal tract where adaptive immune responses to intestinal microbial flora and ingested antigens are initiated (see also **mucosa-associated lymphoid tissues**).

H

H-2 molecule An MHC molecule in the mouse. The mouse MHC was originally called the H-2 locus.

Haplotype The set of MHC alleles inherited from one parent and therefore on one chromosome.

Hapten A small chemical that can bind to an antibody but must be attached to a macromolecule (carrier) to stimulate an adaptive immune response specific for that chemical. For example, immunization with dinitrophenol (DNP) alone will not stimulate an anti-DNP antibody response, but immunization with a protein with covalently attached DNP will. In this case, DNP is the hapten, and the protein is the carrier.

Heavy-chain isotype (class) switching The process by which a B lymphocyte changes the isotype, or class, of the antibodies that it produces from IgM to IgG, IgE, or IgA without changing the antigen specificity of the antibody. Heavy-chain isotype switching is stimulated by cytokines and CD40 ligand expressed by helper T cells and involves recombination of B cell VDJ segments with downstream heavy-chain gene segments.

Helminth A parasitic worm. Helminthic infections often elicit Th2-dependent immune responses characterized by eosinophil-rich inflammatory infiltrates and IgE production.

Helper T cells The class of T lymphocytes whose main functions are to activate macrophages and to promote inflammation in cell-mediated immune responses and to promote B cell antibody production in humoral immune responses. These functions are mediated by secreted cytokines and by T cell CD40 ligand binding to macrophage or B cell CD40. Most helper T cells express the CD4 molecule.

Hematopoiesis The development of mature blood cells, including erythrocytes, leukocytes, and platelets, from pluripotent stem cells in the bone marrow and fetal liver. Hematopoiesis is regulated by several different cytokine growth factors produced by bone marrow stromal cells, T cells, and other cell types.

Hematopoietic stem cell An undifferentiated bone marrow cell that divides continuously and gives rise to additional stem cells and cells of multiple different lineages. A hematopoietic stem cell in the bone marrow will give rise to cells of the lymphoid, myeloid, and erythrocytic lineage.

Hematopoietic stem cell transplantation The transplantation of hematopoietic stem cells taken from the blood or bone marrow; it is performed clinically to treat cancers affecting blood cells (leukemias), immunodeficiency diseases, and diseases of defective hematopoiesis.

High endothelial venules (HEVs) Specialized venules that are the sites of lymphocyte migration from the blood into the stroma of secondary lymphoid tissues. HEVs are lined by plump endothelial cells that protrude into the vessel lumen and express unique adhesion molecules involved in binding naive B and T cells.

Hinge region A region of Ig heavy chains between the first two constant domains that can assume multiple conformations, thereby imparting flexibility in the orientation of the two antigen-binding sites. Because of the hinge region, an antibody molecule can simultaneously bind two epitopes that are anywhere within a range of distances from each other.

Histamine A vasoactive amine stored in the granules of mast cells that is one of the important mediators of immediate hypersensitivity. Histamine binds to specific receptors in various tissues and causes increased vascular permeability and contraction of bronchial and intestinal smooth muscle.

HLA See **human leukocyte antigens.**

HLA-DM A peptide exchange molecule that plays a critical role in the class II MHC pathway of antigen presentation. HLA-DM is found in the specialized MIIC endosomal compartment and facilitates removal of the invariant chain–derived CLIP peptide and the binding of other peptides to class II MHC molecules. HLA-DM is encoded by a gene in the MHC and is structurally similar to class II MHC molecules, but it is not polymorphic.

Homeostasis In the adaptive immune system, the maintenance of a constant number and diverse repertoire of lymphocytes, despite the emergence of new lymphocytes and tremendous expansion of individual clones that may occur during responses to immunogenic antigens. Homeostasis is achieved by several regulated pathways of lymphocyte death and inactivation.

Homing receptor Adhesion molecules expressed on the surface of lymphocytes that are responsible for the different pathways of lymphocyte recirculation and tissue homing. Homing receptors bind to ligands (addressins) expressed on endothelial cells in particular vascular beds.

Human immunodeficiency virus (HIV) The etiologic agent of AIDS. HIV is a retrovirus that infects a variety of cell types, including $CD4^+$ helper T cells, macrophages, and dendritic cells, and causes progressive destruction of the immune system.

Human leukocyte antigens (HLA) MHC molecules expressed on the surface of human cells. Human MHC molecules were first identified as alloantigens on the surface of white blood cells (leukocytes) that bound serum antibodies from individuals previously exposed to other individuals' cells (e.g., mothers or transfusion recipients) (see also **major histocompatibility complex [MHC] molecule**).

Humanized antibody A monoclonal antibody encoded by a recombinant hybrid gene and composed of the antigen-binding sites from a murine monoclonal antibody and the constant region of a human antibody. Humanized antibodies are less likely than mouse monoclonal antibodies to induce an anti-antibody response in humans; they are used clinically in the treatment of inflammatory diseases, tumors, and transplant rejection.

Humoral immunity The type of adaptive immune response mediated by antibodies produced by B lymphocytes. Humoral immunity is the principal defense mechanism against extracellular microbes and their toxins.

Hybridoma A cell line derived by fusion, or somatic cell hybridization, between a normal lymphocyte and an immortalized lymphocyte tumor line. B cell hybridomas created by fusion of normal B cells of defined antigen specificity with a myeloma cell line are used to produce monoclonal antibodies. T cell hybridomas created by fusion of a normal T cell of defined specificity with a T cell tumor line have been used in research.

Hyperacute rejection A form of allograft or xenograft rejection that begins within minutes to hours after transplantation and that is characterized by thrombotic occlusion of the graft vessels. Hyperacute rejection is mediated by preexisting antibodies in the host circulation that bind to donor endothelial antigens, such as blood group antigens or MHC molecules, and activate the complement system.

Hypersensitivity diseases Disorders caused by immune responses. Hypersensitivity diseases include autoimmune diseases, in which immune responses are directed against self antigens, and diseases that result from uncontrolled or excessive responses against foreign antigens, such as microbes and allergens. The tissue damage that occurs in hypersensitivity diseases is due to the same effector mechanisms used by the immune system to protect against microbes.

Hypervariable region (hypervariable loop) Short segments of about 10 amino acid residues within the variable regions of antibody or TCR proteins that form loop structures that contact antigen. Three hypervariable loops, also called CDRs, are present in each antibody heavy chain and light chain and in each TCR chain. Most of the variability between different antibodies or TCRs is located within these loops.

I

Igα and Igβ Proteins that are required for surface expression and signaling functions of membrane Ig on B cells. Igα and Igβ pairs are disulfide linked to each other, noncovalently associated with the cytoplasmic tail of membrane Ig, and form the BCR complex. The cytoplasmic domains of Igα and Igβ contain ITAMs that are involved in early signaling events during antigen-induced B cell activation.

IL-1 receptor antagonist (IL-1RA) A natural inhibitor of IL-1 produced by mononuclear phagocytes that is structurally homologous to IL-1 and binds to the same receptors but is biologically inactive. IL-1RA is used to treat autoinflammatory syndromes caused by dysregulated IL-1 production and also has some efficacy in rheumatoid arthritis.

Immature B lymphocyte A membrane IgM$^+$, IgD$^-$ B cell, recently derived from marrow precursors, that does not proliferate or differentiate in response to antigens but rather may undergo apoptotic death or become functionally unresponsive. Many immature B cells leave the bone marrow and complete their maturation in the spleen.

Immediate hypersensitivity The type of immune reaction responsible for allergic diseases, which is dependent on antigen-mediated activation of IgE-coated tissue mast cells. The mast cells release mediators that cause increased vascular permeability, vasodilation, bronchial and visceral smooth muscle contraction, and local inflammation.

Immune complex A multimolecular complex of antibody molecules with bound antigen. Because each antibody molecule has a minimum of two antigen-binding sites and many antigens are multivalent, immune complexes can vary greatly in size. Immune complexes activate effector mechanisms of humoral immunity, such as the classical complement pathway and Fc receptor–mediated phagocyte activation. Deposition of circulating immune complexes in blood vessel walls or renal glomeruli can lead to inflammation and disease.

Immune complex disease An inflammatory disease caused by the deposition of antigen-antibody complexes in blood vessel walls, resulting in local complement activation and phagocyte recruitment. Immune complexes may form because of overproduction of antibodies against microbial antigens or as a result of autoantibody production in the setting of an autoimmune disease such as systemic lupus erythematosus. Immune complex deposition in the specialized capillary basement membranes of renal glomeruli can cause glomerulonephritis and impair renal function. Systemic deposition of immune complexes in arterial walls can cause vasculitis, with thrombosis and ischemic damage to various organs.

Immune-mediated inflammatory disease A general term for disorders in which immune responses, either to self or foreign antigens, and chronic inflammation are major components.

Immune response A collective and coordinated response to the introduction of foreign substances in an individual mediated by the cells and molecules of the immune system.

Immune response (Ir) genes Originally defined as genes in inbred strains of guinea pigs and mice that were inherited in a dominant Mendelian manner and that controlled the ability of the animals to make antibodies against simple synthetic polypeptides. We now know that *Ir* genes are the polymorphic genes that encode class II MHC molecules, which display peptides to T lymphocytes and are therefore required for T cell activation and helper T cell–dependent B cell (antibody) responses to protein antigens.

Immune surveillance The concept that a physiologic function of the immune system is to recognize and destroy clones of transformed cells before they grow into tumors and to kill tumors after they are formed. The term *immune surveillance* is sometimes used in a general sense to describe the function of T lymphocytes to detect and destroy any cell, not necessarily a tumor cell, that is expressing foreign (e.g., microbial) antigens.

Immune system The molecules, cells, tissues, and organs that collectively function to provide immunity, or protection, against foreign organisms.

Immunity Protection against disease, usually infectious disease, mediated by the cells and tissues that are collectively called the immune system. In a broader sense, immunity refers to the ability to respond to foreign substances, including microbes and noninfectious molecules.

Immunodeficiency See **acquired immunodeficiency** and **congenital immunodeficiency.**

Immunodominant epitope The epitope of a protein antigen that elicits most of the response in an individual immunized with the native protein. Immunodominant epitopes correspond to the peptides of the protein that are proteolytically generated within APCs and bind most avidly to MHC molecules and are most likely to stimulate T cells.

Immunofluorescence A technique in which a molecule is detected by the use of an antibody labeled with a fluorescent probe. For example, in immunofluorescence microscopy, cells that express a particular surface antigen can be stained with a fluorescein-conjugated antibody specific for the antigen and then visualized with a fluorescent microscope.

Immunogen An antigen that induces an immune response. Not all antigens are immunogens. For example, small chemicals (haptens) can bind to antibodies but will not stimulate an immune response unless they are linked to macromolecules (carriers).

Immunoglobulin (Ig) Synonymous with antibody (see **antibody**).

Immunoglobulin domain A three-dimensional globular structural motif found in many proteins in the immune system, including Igs, TCRs, and MHC molecules. Ig domains are about 110 amino acid residues in length, include an internal disulfide bond, and contain two layers of β-pleated sheets, each layer composed of three to five strands of antiparallel polypeptide chain. Ig domains are classified as V-like or C-like on the basis of closest homology to either the Ig V or C domains.

Immunoglobulin heavy chain One of two types of polypeptide chains in an antibody molecule. The basic structural unit of an antibody includes two identical disulfide-linked heavy chains and two identical light chains. Each heavy chain is composed of a variable (V) domain and three or four constant (C) domains. The different antibody isotypes, including IgM, IgD, IgG, IgA, and IgE, are distinguished by structural differences in their heavy chain constant regions. The heavy chain constant regions also mediate effector functions, such as complement activation or engagement of phagocytes.

Immunoglobulin light chain One of two types of polypeptide chains in an antibody molecule. The basic structural unit of an antibody includes two identical light chains, each disulfide linked to one of two identical heavy chains. Each light chain is composed of one variable (V) domain and one constant (C) domain. There are two light chain isotypes, called κ and λ, both functionally identical. About 60% of human antibodies have κ light chains, and 40% have λ light chains.

Immunoglobulin superfamily A large family of proteins that contain a globular structural motif called an Ig domain, or Ig fold, originally described in antibodies. Many proteins of importance in the immune system, including antibodies, TCRs, MHC molecules, CD4, and CD8, are members of this superfamily.

Immunohistochemistry A technique to detect the presence of an antigen in histologic tissue sections by use of an enzyme-coupled antibody that is specific for the antigen. The enzyme converts a colorless substrate to a colored insoluble substance that precipitates at the site where the antibody and, thus, the antigen are localized. The positions of the colored precipitate and the antigen in the tissue section are observed by conventional light microscopy. Immunohistochemistry is a routine technique in diagnostic pathology and various fields of research.

Immunologic tolerance See **tolerance**.

Immunologically privileged site A site in the body that is inaccessible to or constitutively suppresses immune responses. The anterior chamber of the eye, the testes, and the brain are examples of immunologically privileged sites.

Immunoreceptor tyrosine-based activation motif (ITAM) A conserved protein motif composed of two copies of the sequence tyrosine-x-x-leucine (where x is an unspecified amino acid) found in the cytoplasmic tails of various membrane proteins in the immune system that are involved in signal transduction. ITAMs are present in the ζ and CD3 proteins of the TCR complex, in Igα and Igβ proteins in the BCR complex, and in several Ig Fc receptors. When these receptors bind their ligands, the tyrosine residues of the ITAMs become phosphorylated and form docking sites for other molecules involved in propagating cell-activating signal transduction pathways.

Immunoreceptor tyrosine-based inhibition motif (ITIM) A six–amino acid (isoleucine-x-tyrosine-x-x-leucine) motif found in the cytoplasmic tails of various inhibitory receptors in the immune system, including FcγRIIB on B cells and killer cell Ig-like receptors (KIRs) on NK cells. When these receptors bind their ligands, the ITIMs become phosphorylated on their tyrosine residues and form a docking site for protein tyrosine phosphatases, which in turn function to inhibit other signal transduction pathways.

Immunosuppression Inhibition of one or more components of the adaptive or innate immune system as a result of an underlying disease or intentionally induced by drugs for the purpose of preventing or treating graft rejection or autoimmune disease. A commonly used immunosuppressive drug is cyclosporine, which blocks T cell cytokine production.

Immunotherapy The treatment of a disease with therapeutic agents that promote or inhibit immune responses. Cancer immunotherapy, for example, involves promotion of active immune responses to tumor antigens or administration of antitumor antibodies or T cells to establish passive immunity.

Immunotoxins Reagents that may be used in the treatment of cancer and consist of covalent conjugates of a potent cellular toxin, such as ricin or diphtheria toxin, with antibodies specific for antigens expressed on the surface of tumor cells. It is hoped that such reagents can specifically target and kill tumor cells without damaging normal cells, but safe and effective immunotoxins have yet to be developed.

Indirect antigen presentation (or indirect allorecognition) In transplantation immunology, a pathway of presentation of donor (allogeneic) MHC molecules by recipient APCs that involves the same mechanisms used to present microbial proteins. The allogeneic MHC proteins are processed by recipient dendritic cells, and peptides derived from the allogeneic MHC molecules are presented, in association with recipient (self) MHC molecules, to host T cells. In contrast to indirect antigen presentation, direct antigen presentation involves recipient T cell recognition of unprocessed allogeneic MHC molecules on the surface of graft cells.

Inflammasome A multiprotein complex in the cytosol of mononuclear phagocytes, dendritic cells, and other cell types that proteolytically generates the active form of IL-1β from the inactive pro-IL-1β precursor. The formation of the inflammasome complex, which includes NLRP3 (a NOD-like pattern recognition receptor), an adaptor protein, and the enzyme caspase-1, is stimulated by a variety of microbial products, cell damage–associated molecules, and crystals.

Inflammation A complex reaction of vascularized tissue to infection or cell injury that involves extravascular accumulation of plasma proteins and leukocytes. Acute inflammation is a common result of innate immune responses, and local adaptive immune responses can also promote inflammation. Although inflammation serves a protective function in controlling infections and promoting tissue repair, it can also cause tissue damage and disease.

Inflammatory bowel disease (IBD) A group of disorders, including ulcerative colitis and Crohn's disease, characterized by chronic inflammation in the gastrointestinal tract. The etiology of IBD is not known, but some evidence indicates that it is caused by inadequate regulation of T cell responses, probably against intestinal commensal bacteria. IBD develops in gene knockout mice lacking IL-2, IL-10, or the TCR α chain.

Innate immunity Protection against infection that relies on mechanisms that exist before infection, are capable of a rapid response to microbes, and react in essentially the same way to repeated infections. The innate immune system includes epithelial barriers, phagocytic cells (neutrophils, macrophages), NK cells and other innate lymphoid cells, the complement system, and cytokines, largely made by dendritic cells and mononuclear phagocytes, that regulate and coordinate many activities of the cells of innate immunity.

Innate lymphoid cells Cells of the innate immune system derived from the common lymphoid precursor but of a distinct lineage from lymphocytes and are grouped into Groups 1, 2, and 3. They secrete cytokines that are also typical of CD4+ Th1, Th2, and Th17 cells, respectively.

Inositol 1,4,5-triphosphate (IP3) A molecule derived from the hydrolysis of the membrane phospholipid phosphatidylinositol 4,5-bisphosphate (PIP2) in response to lymphocyte antigen receptor signaling that binds to IP3 receptors on the endoplasmic reticulum (ER) membrane and stimulates release of Ca^{2+} from the ER, thereby raising the cytosolic Ca^{2+} concentration.

Integrins Heterodimeric cell surface proteins whose major functions are to mediate the adhesion of cells to other cells or to extracellular matrix. Integrins are important for T cell interactions with APCs and for migration of leukocytes from blood into tissues. The ligand-binding activity of leukocyte integrins depends on signals induced by chemokines binding to chemokine receptors. Two integrins important in the immune system are VLA-4 (very late antigen 4) and LFA-1 (leukocyte function-associated antigen 1).

Interferon regulatory factors (IRFs) A family of inducibly activated transcription factors that are important in expression of inflammatory and antiviral genes. For example, IRF3 is activated by TLR signals and regulates expression of type I interferons, which are cytokines that protect cells from viral infection.

Interferons A subgroup of cytokines originally named for their ability to interfere with viral infections but that have other important immunomodulatory functions. Type I interferons include interferon-α and interferon-β, whose main function is to prevent viral replication in cells; type II interferon, more commonly called interferon-γ, activates macrophages and various other cell types.

Interleukins Molecularly defined cytokines that are named with a numerical suffix roughly sequentially in order of discovery or characterization (e.g., interleukin-1, interleukin-2). Some cytokines were originally named for their biologic activities and do not have an interleukin designation.

Intracellular bacterium A bacterium that survives or replicates within cells, usually in endosomes. The principal defense against intracellular bacteria, such as *Mycobacterium tuberculosis*, is T cell–mediated immunity.

Intraepithelial lymphocytes T lymphocytes present in the epidermis of the skin and in mucosal epithelia that typically express a limited diversity of antigen receptors. Some of these lymphocytes, called invariant NKT cells, may recognize microbial products, such as glycolipids, associated with nonpolymorphic class I MHC–like molecules. Others, called γδ T cells, recognize various nonpeptide antigens, not bound to MHC molecules. Intraepithelial T lymphocytes may be considered effector cells of innate immunity and function in host defense by secreting cytokines and activating phagocytes and by killing infected cells.

Invariant chain (Ii) A nonpolymorphic protein that binds to newly synthesized class II MHC molecules in the endoplasmic reticulum. The invariant chain prevents loading of the class II MHC peptide-binding cleft with peptides present in the endoplasmic reticulum, and such peptides are left to associate with class I molecules. The invariant chain also promotes folding and assembly of class II molecules and directs newly formed class II molecules to the specialized endosomal MIIC compartment, where peptide loading takes place.

Isotype One of five types of antibodies, determined by which of five different forms of heavy chain is present. Antibody isotypes include IgM, IgD, IgG, IgA, and IgE, and each isotype performs a different set of effector functions. Additional structural variations characterize distinct subtypes of IgG and IgA.

J

JAK-STAT signaling pathway A signaling pathway initiated by cytokine binding to type I and type II cytokine receptors. This pathway sequentially involves activation of receptor-associated Janus kinase (JAK) tyrosine kinases, JAK-mediated tyrosine phosphorylation of the cytoplasmic tails of cytokine receptors, docking of signal transducers and activators of transcription (STATs) to the phosphorylated receptor chains, JAK-mediated tyrosine phosphorylation of the associated STATs, dimerization and nuclear translocation of the STATs, and STAT binding to regulatory regions of target genes, causing transcriptional activation of those genes.

Janus kinases (JAKs) A family of tyrosine kinases that associate with the cytoplasmic tails of several different cytokine receptors, including the receptors for IL-2, IL-3, IL-4, IFN-γ, IL-12, and others. In response to cytokine binding and receptor dimerization, JAKs phosphorylate the cytokine receptors to permit the binding of STATs, and then the JAKs phosphorylate and thereby activate the STATs. Different JAKs associate with different cytokine receptors.

Joining (J) chain A polypeptide that links IgA or IgM molecules to form multimers (e.g., dimeric IgA and pentameric IgM).

Joining (J) segments Short coding sequences between the variable (V) and constant (C) gene segments in all Ig and TCR loci, which together with D segments are somatically recombined with V segments during lymphocyte development. The resulting recombined VDJ DNA codes for the carboxyl-terminal ends of the antigen receptor V regions, including the third hypervariable (CDR) regions. Random use of different J segments contributes to the diversity of the antigen receptor repertoire.

Junctional diversity The diversity in antibody and TCR repertoires that is attributed to the random addition or removal of nucleotide sequences at junctions between V, D, and J gene segments.

K

Killer cell Ig-like receptors (KIRs) Ig superfamily receptors expressed by NK cells that recognize different alleles of HLA-A, HLA-B, and HLA-C molecules. Some KIRs have signaling components with ITIMs in their cytoplasmic tails, and these deliver inhibitory signals to inactivate the NK cells. Some members of the KIR family have short cytoplasmic tails without ITIMs but associate with other ITAM-containing polypeptides and function as activating receptors.

Knockout mouse A mouse with a targeted disruption of one or more genes that is created by homologous recombination techniques. Knockout mice lacking functional genes encoding cytokines, cell surface receptors, signaling molecules, and transcription factors have provided extensive information about the roles of these molecules in the immune system.

L

Lamina propria A layer of loose connective tissue underlying epithelium in mucosal tissues such as the intestines and airways, where dendritic cells, mast cells, lymphocytes, and macrophages mediate immune responses to invading pathogens.

Langerhans cells Immature dendritic cells found as a meshwork in the epidermal layer of the skin whose major function is to trap microbes and antigens that enter through the skin and transport the antigens to draining lymph nodes. During their migration to the lymph nodes, Langerhans cells differentiate into mature dendritic cells, which can efficiently present antigen to naive T cells.

Large granular lymphocyte Another name for an NK cell based on the morphologic appearance of this cell type in the blood.

Late-phase reaction A component of the immediate hypersensitivity reaction that ensues 2 to 4 hours after mast cell degranulation and that is characterized by an inflammatory infiltrate of eosinophils, basophils, neutrophils, and lymphocytes. Repeated bouts of this late-phase inflammatory reaction can cause tissue damage.

Lck A Src family nonreceptor tyrosine kinase that noncovalently associates with the cytoplasmic tails of CD4 and CD8 molecules in T cells and is involved in the early signaling events of antigen-induced T cell activation. Lck mediates tyrosine phosphorylation of the cytoplasmic tails of CD3 and ζ proteins of the TCR complex.

Lectin pathway of complement activation A pathway of complement activation triggered by the binding of microbial polysaccharides to circulating lectins such as MBL. MBL is structurally similar to C1q and activates the C1r-C1s enzyme complex (like C1q) or activates another serine esterase, called mannose-binding protein–associated serine esterase. The remaining steps of the lectin pathway, beginning with cleavage of C4, are the same as the classical pathway.

Leukemia A malignant disease of bone marrow precursors of blood cells in which large numbers of leukemic cells usually occupy the bone marrow and often circulate in the bloodstream. Lymphocytic leukemias are derived from B or T cell precursors, myelogenous leukemias are derived from granulocyte or monocyte precursors, and erythroid leukemias are derived from red blood cell precursors.

Leukocyte adhesion deficiency (LAD) One of a rare group of immunodeficiency diseases with infectious complications that is caused by defective expression of the leukocyte adhesion molecules required for tissue recruitment of phagocytes and lymphocytes. LAD-1 is due to mutations in the gene encoding the CD18 protein, which is part of β_2 integrins. LAD-2 is caused by mutations in a gene that encodes a fucose transporter involved in the synthesis of leukocyte ligands for endothelial selectins.

Leukotrienes A class of arachidonic acid–derived lipid inflammatory mediators produced by the lipoxygenase pathway in many cell types. Mast cells make abundant leukotriene C_4 (LTC_4) and its degradation products LTD_4 and LTE_4, which bind to specific receptors on smooth muscle cells and cause prolonged bronchoconstriction. Leukotrienes contribute to the pathologic processes of bronchial asthma. Collectively, LTC_4, LTD_4, and LTE_4 constitute what was once called slow-reacting substance of anaphylaxis.

Lipopolysaccharide Synonymous with **endotoxin.**

Lymph node Small, nodular, encapsulated lymphocyte-rich organs situated along lymphatic channels throughout the body where adaptive immune responses to lymph-borne antigens are initiated. Lymph nodes have a specialized anatomic architecture that regulates the interactions of B cells, T cells, dendritic cells, and antigens to maximize the induction of protective immune responses.

Lymphatic system A system of vessels throughout the body that collects tissue fluid called lymph, originally derived from the blood, and returns it through the thoracic duct to the circulation. Lymph nodes are interspersed along these vessels and trap and retain antigens present in the lymph.

Lymphocyte homing The directed migration of subsets of circulating lymphocytes into particular tissue sites. Lymphocyte homing is regulated by the selective expression of endothelial adhesion molecules and chemokines in different tissues. For example, some lymphocytes preferentially home to the intestinal mucosa in response to the chemokine CCL25 and the endothelial adhesion molecule Mad-CAM, both expressed in the gut, which bind respectively to the CCR9 chemokine receptor and the $\alpha_4\beta_1$ integrin on gut-homing lymphocytes.

Lymphocyte maturation The process by which pluripotent bone marrow stem cells develop into mature, antigen receptor–expressing naive B or T lymphocytes that populate peripheral lymphoid tissues. This process takes place in the specialized environments of the bone marrow (for B cells) and the thymus (for T cells). Synonymous with *lymphocyte development.*

Lymphocyte migration The movement of lymphocytes from the bloodstream into peripheral tissues.

Lymphocyte recirculation The continuous movement of naive lymphocytes from the bloodstream to secondary lymphoid organs, and back into the blood.

Lymphocyte repertoire The complete collection of antigen receptors and therefore antigen specificities expressed by the B and T lymphocytes of an individual.

Lymphoid follicle A B cell–rich region of a lymph node or the spleen that is the site of antigen-induced B cell proliferation and differentiation. In T cell–dependent B cell responses to protein antigens, a germinal center forms within the follicles.

Lymphokine An old name for a cytokine (soluble protein mediator of immune responses) produced by lymphocytes.

Lymphoma A malignant tumor of B or T lymphocytes usually arising in and spreading between lymphoid tissues but that may spread to other tissues. Lymphomas often express phenotypic characteristics of the normal lymphocytes from which they were derived.

Lymphotoxin (LT, TNF-β) A cytokine produced by T cells that is homologous with and binds to the same receptors as TNF. Like TNF, LT has proinflammatory effects, including endothelial and neutrophil activation. LT is also critical for the normal development of lymphoid organs.

Lysosome A membrane-bound, acidic organelle abundant in phagocytic cells that contains proteolytic enzymes that degrade proteins derived both from the extracellular environment and from within the cell. Lysosomes are involved in the class II MHC pathway of antigen processing.

M

M cells Specialized gastrointestinal mucosal epithelial cells overlying Peyer's patches in the gut that play a role in delivery of antigens to Peyer's patches.

M1 macrophages See **classical macrophage activation.**

M2 macrophages See **alternative macrophage activation.**

Macrophage A tissue-based phagocytic cell derived from fetal hematopoietic organs or blood monocytes that plays important roles in innate and adaptive immune responses. Macrophages are activated by microbial products such as endotoxin and by T cell cytokines such as IFN-γ. Activated macrophages phagocytose and kill microorganisms, secrete proinflammatory cytokines, and present antigens to helper T cells. Macrophages in different tissues are given different names and may serve special functions; these cells include microglia in the central nervous system, Kupffer cells in the liver, alveolar macrophages in the lung, and osteoclasts in bone.

Major histocompatibility complex (MHC) A large genetic locus (on human chromosome 6 and mouse chromosome 17) that includes the highly polymorphic genes encoding the peptide-binding molecules recognized by T lymphocytes. The MHC locus also includes genes encoding cytokines, molecules involved in antigen processing, and complement proteins.

Major histocompatibility complex (MHC) molecule A heterodimeric membrane protein encoded in the MHC locus that serves as a peptide display molecule for recognition by T lymphocytes. Two structurally distinct types of MHC molecules exist. Class I MHC molecules are present on most nucleated cells, bind peptides derived from cytosolic proteins, and are recognized by CD8$^+$ T cells. Class II MHC molecules are restricted largely to dendritic cells, macrophages, and B lymphocytes; bind peptides derived from endocytosed proteins; and are recognized by CD4$^+$ T cells.

Mannose-binding lectin (MBL) A plasma protein that binds to mannose residues on bacterial cell walls and acts as an opsonin by promoting phagocytosis of the bacterium by macrophages. Macrophages express a surface receptor for C1q that can also bind MBL and mediate uptake of the opsonized organisms.

Mannose receptor A carbohydrate-binding receptor (lectin) expressed by macrophages that binds mannose and fucose residues on microbial cell walls and mediates phagocytosis of the organisms.

Marginal zone A peripheral region of splenic lymphoid follicles containing macrophages that are particularly efficient at trapping polysaccharide antigens. Such antigens may persist for prolonged periods on the surfaces of marginal zone macrophages, where they are recognized by specific B cells, or they may be transported into follicles.

Marginal zone B lymphocytes A subset of B lymphocytes, found exclusively in the marginal zone of the spleen, that respond rapidly to blood-borne microbial antigens by producing IgM antibodies with limited diversity.

Mast cell The major effector cell of immediate hypersensitivity (allergic) reactions. Mast cells are derived from the marrow, reside in most tissues adjacent to blood vessels, express a high-affinity Fc receptor for IgE, and contain numerous mediator-filled granules. Antigen-induced cross-linking of IgE bound to the mast cell Fc receptors causes release of their granule contents as well as new synthesis and secretion of other mediators, leading to an immediate hypersensitivity reaction.

Mature B cell IgM+ IgD+, functionally competent naive B cells that represent the final stage of B cell maturation and that populate peripheral lymphoid organs.

Membrane attack complex (MAC) A lytic complex of the terminal components of the complement cascade, including multiple copies of C9, which forms in the membranes of target cells. The MAC causes lethal ionic and osmotic changes in cells.

Memory The property of the adaptive immune system to respond more rapidly, with greater magnitude, and more effectively to a repeated exposure to an antigen compared with the response to the first exposure.

Memory lymphocytes Memory B and T cells are produced by antigen stimulation of naive lymphocytes and survive in a functionally quiescent state for many years after the antigen is eliminated. Memory lymphocytes mediate rapid and enhanced (i.e., memory or recall) responses to second and subsequent exposures to antigens.

MHC restriction The characteristic of T lymphocytes that they recognize a foreign peptide antigen only when it is bound to a particular allelic form of an MHC molecule.

Mitogen-activated protein (MAP) kinase cascade A signal transduction cascade initiated by the active form of the Ras protein and involving the sequential activation of three serine/threonine kinases, the last one being MAP kinase. MAP kinase in turn phosphorylates and activates other enzymes and transcription factors. The MAP kinase pathway is one of several signal pathways activated by antigen binding to the TCR and BCR.

Mixed leukocyte reaction (MLR) An in vitro reaction of alloreactive T cells from one individual against MHC antigens on blood cells from another individual. The MLR involves proliferation of and cytokine secretion by both CD4+ and CD8+ T cells.

Molecular mimicry A postulated mechanism of autoimmunity triggered by infection with a microbe containing antigens that cross-react with self antigens. Immune responses to the microbe result in reactions against self tissues.

Monoclonal antibody An antibody that is specific for one antigen and is produced by a B cell hybridoma (a cell line derived by the fusion of a single normal B cell and an immortal B cell tumor line). Monoclonal antibodies are widely used in research, clinical diagnosis, and therapy.

Monocyte A type of bone marrow–derived circulating blood cell that is the precursor to tissue macrophages. Monocytes are actively recruited into inflammatory sites, where they differentiate into macrophages.

Mononuclear phagocytes Cells with a common lineage whose primary function is phagocytosis. These cells function as antigen-presenting cells in the recognition and activation phases of adaptive immune responses and as effector cells in innate and adaptive immunity. Mononuclear phagocytes circulate in the blood in an incompletely differentiated form called monocytes, and once they settle in tissues, they mature into macrophages.

Mucosa-associated lymphoid tissue (MALT) Collections of lymphocytes, dendritic cells, and other cell types within the mucosa of the gastrointestinal and respiratory tracts that are sites of adaptive immune responses to antigens. Mucosa-associated lymphoid tissues contain intraepithelial lymphocytes, mainly T cells, and organized collections of lymphocytes, often rich in B cells, below mucosal epithelia, such as Peyer's patches in the gut or pharyngeal tonsils.

Mucosal immune system A part of the immune system that responds to and protects against microbes that enter the body through mucosal surfaces, such as the gastrointestinal and respiratory tracts, but also maintains tolerance to commensal organisms that live on the outside of the mucosal epithelium. The mucosal immune system is composed of organized mucosa-associated lymphoid tissues, such as Peyer's patches, as well as diffusely distributed cells within the lamina propria.

Multiple myeloma A malignant tumor of antibody-producing B cells that often secretes Igs or parts of Ig molecules. The monoclonal antibodies produced by multiple myelomas were critical for early biochemical analyses of antibody structure.

Multivalency See **polyvalency.**

Mycobacterium A genus of aerobic bacteria, many species of which can survive within phagocytes and cause disease. The principal host defense against mycobacteria such as *Mycobacterium tuberculosis* is cell-mediated immunity.

N

N nucleotides The name given to nucleotides randomly added to the junctions between V, D, and J gene segments in *Ig* or *TCR* genes during lymphocyte development. The addition of up to 20 of these nucleotides, which is mediated by the enzyme terminal deoxyribonucleotidyl transferase, contributes to the diversity of the antibody and TCR repertoires.

Naive lymphocyte A mature B or T lymphocyte that has not previously encountered antigen. When naive lymphocytes are stimulated by antigen, they differentiate into effector lymphocytes, such as antibody-secreting B cells or helper T cells and CTLs. Naive lymphocytes have surface markers and recirculation patterns that are distinct from those of previously activated lymphocytes. ("Naive" also refers to an unimmunized individual.)

Natural antibodies IgM antibodies, largely produced by B-1 cells, specific for bacteria that are common in the environment and gastrointestinal tract. Normal individuals contain natural antibodies without any evidence of infection, and these antibodies serve as a preformed defense mechanism against microbes that succeed in penetrating epithelial barriers. Some of these antibodies cross-react with ABO blood group antigens and are responsible for transfusion reactions.

Natural killer (NK) cells A subset of innate lymphoid cells that function in innate immune responses to kill microbe-infected cells by direct lytic mechanisms and by secreting IFN-γ. NK cells do not express clonally distributed antigen receptors like Ig receptors or TCRs, and their activation is regulated by a combination of cell surface stimulatory and inhibitory receptors, the latter recognizing self MHC molecules.

Natural killer T cells (NKT cells) A numerically small subset of lymphocytes that express T cell receptors and some surface molecules characteristic of NK cells. Some NKT cells, called invariant NKT (iNKT), express αβ T cell antigen receptors with very little diversity, recognize lipid antigens presented by CD1 molecules, and perform various effector functions typical of helper T cells.

Negative selection The process by which developing lymphocytes that express self-reactive antigen receptors are eliminated, thereby contributing to the maintenance of self-tolerance. Negative selection of developing T lymphocytes (thymocytes) is best understood and involves high-avidity binding of a thymocyte to self MHC molecules with bound peptides on thymic APCs, leading to apoptotic death of the thymocyte.

Neonatal Fc receptor (FcRn) An IgG-specific Fc receptor that mediates the transport of maternal IgG across the placenta and the neonatal intestinal epithelium and, in adults, promotes the long half-life of IgG molecules in the blood by protecting them from catabolism by phagocytes or endothelial cells.

Neonatal immunity Passive humoral immunity to infections in mammals in the first months of life, before full development of the immune system. Neonatal immunity is mediated by maternally produced antibodies transported across the placenta into the fetal circulation before birth or derived from ingested milk and transported across the gut epithelium.

Neutrophil (also polymorphonuclear leukocyte, PMN) A phagocytic cell characterized by a segmented lobular nucleus and cytoplasmic granules filled with degradative enzymes. PMNs are the most abundant type of circulating white blood cells and are the major cell type mediating acute inflammatory responses to bacterial infections.

Nitric oxide A molecule with a broad range of activities that in macrophages functions as a potent microbicidal agent to kill ingested organisms.

Nitric oxide synthase A member of a family of enzymes that synthesize the vasoactive and microbicidal compound nitric oxide from arginine. Macrophages express an inducible form of this enzyme on activation by various microbial or cytokine stimuli.

NOD-like receptors (NLRs) A family of cytosolic multidomain proteins that sense cytoplasmic PAMPs and DAMPs and recruit other proteins to form signaling complexes that promote inflammation.

Nuclear factor κB (NF-κB) A family of transcription factors composed of homodimers or heterodimers of proteins homologous to the c-Rel protein. NF-κB proteins are required for the inducible transcription of many genes important in both innate and adaptive immune responses.

Nuclear factor of activated T cells (NFAT) A transcription factor required for the expression of IL-2, IL-4, TNF, and other cytokine genes. The four different NFATs are each encoded by separate genes; NFATp and NFATc are found in T cells. Cytoplasmic NFAT is activated by calcium/calmodulin-dependent, calcineurin-mediated dephosphorylation that permits NFAT to translocate into the nucleus and bind to consensus binding sequences in the regulatory regions of IL-2, IL-4, and other cytokine genes, usually in association with other transcription factors such as AP-1.

Nude mouse A strain of mice that lacks development of the thymus, and therefore T lymphocytes, as well as hair follicles. Nude mice have been used experimentally to define the role of T lymphocytes in immunity and disease.

O

Oncofetal antigen Proteins that are expressed at high levels on some types of cancer cells and in normal developing fetal (but not adult) tissues. Antibodies specific for these proteins are often used in histopathologic identification of tumors or to monitor the progression of tumor growth in patients. CEA (CD66) and α-fetoprotein are two oncofetal antigens commonly expressed by certain carcinomas.

Opsonin A molecule that becomes attached to the surface of a microbe and can be recognized by surface receptors of neutrophils and macrophages and that increases the efficiency of phagocytosis of the microbe. Opsonins include IgG antibodies, which are recognized by the Fcγ receptor on phagocytes, and fragments of complement proteins, which are recognized by CR1 (CD35) and by the leukocyte integrin Mac-1.

Opsonization The process of attaching opsonins, such as IgG or complement fragments, to microbial surfaces to target the microbes for phagocytosis.

Oral tolerance The suppression of systemic humoral and cell-mediated immune responses to an antigen after the oral administration of that antigen as a result of anergy of antigen-specific T cells or the production of immunosuppressive cytokines such as transforming growth factor-β. Oral tolerance is a possible mechanism for prevention of immune responses to food antigens and to bacteria that normally reside as commensals in the intestinal lumen.

P

P nucleotides Short inverted repeat nucleotide sequences in the VDJ junctions of rearranged *Ig* and *TCR* genes that are generated by RAG-1– and RAG-2–mediated asymmetric cleavage of hairpin DNA intermediates during somatic recombination events. P nucleotides contribute to the junctional diversity of antigen receptors.

Passive immunity The form of immunity to an antigen that is established in one individual by transfer of antibodies or lymphocytes from another individual who is immune to that antigen. The recipient of such a transfer can become immune to the antigen without ever having been exposed to or having responded to the antigen. An example of passive immunity is the transfer of human sera containing antibodies specific for certain microbial toxins or snake venom to a previously unimmunized individual.

Pathogen-associated molecular patterns (PAMPs) Structures produced by microorganisms but not mammalian (host) cells, which are recognized by and stimulate the innate immune system. Examples include bacterial lipopolysaccharide and viral double-stranded RNA.

Pathogenicity The ability of a microorganism to cause disease. Multiple mechanisms may contribute to pathogenicity, including production of toxins, stimulation of host inflammatory responses, and perturbation of host cell metabolism.

Pattern recognition receptors Signaling receptors of the innate immune system that recognize PAMPs and DAMPs, and thereby activate innate immune responses. Examples include Toll-like receptors (TLRs) and Nod-like receptors (NLRs).

PD-1 An inhibitory receptor homologous to CD28 that is expressed on activated T cells and binds to its ligands PD-L1 or PD-L2, members of the B7 protein family expressed on various cell types. PD-1 is upregulated on T cells in the setting of chronic infection or tumors, and blockade of PD-1 with monoclonal antibodies enhances antitumor immune responses (checkpoint blockade).

Pentraxins A family of plasma proteins that contain five identical globular subunits; includes the acute-phase reactant C-reactive protein.

Peptide-binding cleft The portion of an MHC molecule that binds peptides for display to T cells. The cleft is composed of paired α helices resting on a floor made up of an eight-stranded β-pleated sheet. The polymorphic residues, which are the amino acids that vary among different MHC alleles, are located in and around this cleft. Also called the peptide-binding groove.

Perforin A protein present in the granules of CTLs and NK cells. When perforin is released from the granules of activated CTLs or NK cells, it promotes entry of granzymes into the target cell, leading to apoptotic death of the cell.

Periarteriolar lymphoid sheath (PALS) A cuff of lymphocytes surrounding small arterioles in the spleen, adjacent to lymphoid follicles. A PALS contains mainly T lymphocytes, about two thirds of which are CD4+ and one third CD8+. In humoral immune responses to protein antigens, B lymphocytes are activated at the interface between the PALS and follicles and then migrate into the follicles to form germinal centers.

Peripheral lymphoid organs and tissues Organized collections of lymphocytes and accessory cells, including the spleen, lymph nodes, and mucosa-associated lymphoid tissues, in which adaptive immune responses are initiated. Also called secondary lymphoid organs and tissues.

Peripheral tolerance Unresponsiveness to self antigens that are present in peripheral tissues. Peripheral tolerance is induced by the recognition of antigens without adequate levels of the costimulators required for lymphocyte activation.

Peyer's patches Organized lymphoid tissue in the lamina propria of the small intestine in which immune responses to intestinal pathogens and other ingested antigens may be initiated. Peyer's patches are composed mostly of B cells, with smaller numbers of T cells and accessory cells, all arranged in follicles similar to those found in lymph nodes, often with germinal centers.

Phagocytosis The process by which certain cells of the innate immune system, including macrophages and neutrophils, engulf large particles (>0.5 μm in diameter) such as intact microbes. The cell surrounds the particle with extensions of its plasma membrane by an energy- and cytoskeleton-dependent process; this process results in the formation of an intracellular vesicle called a phagosome, which contains the ingested particle.

Phagosome A membrane-bound intracellular vesicle that contains microbes or particulate material from the extracellular environment. Phagosomes are formed during the process of phagocytosis. They fuse with other vesicular structures such as lysosomes, leading to enzymatic degradation of the ingested material.

Phosphatase (protein phosphatase) An enzyme that removes phosphate groups from the side chains of certain amino acid residues of proteins. Protein phosphatases in lymphocytes, such as CD45 or calcineurin, regulate the activity of various signal transduction molecules and transcription factors. Some protein phosphatases may be specific for phosphotyrosine residues and others for phosphoserine and phosphothreonine residues.

Phosphatidylinositol-3 (PI-3) kinase An enzyme involved in lymphocyte antigen receptor signaling that phosphorylates the membrane phospholipid PIP2 to generate PIP3. PIP3 is required for the activation of a number of other enzymes, including the serine-threonine kinase called protein kinase B, or Akt.

Phosphatidylinositol 4,5-bisphosphate (PIP2) A plasma membrane inositol phospholipid that is hydrolyzed by phospholipase-Cγ during lymphocyte antigen receptor signaling, generating downstream singling molecules inositol 1,4,5-triphosphate (IP3), and diacylglcerol (DAG) .

Phospholipase Cγ (PLCγ) An enzyme that catalyzes hydrolysis of the plasma membrane phospholipid PIP2 to generate two signaling molecules, IP3 and DAG. PLCγ becomes activated in lymphocytes by antigen binding to the antigen receptor.

Phytohemagglutinin (PHA) A carbohydrate-binding protein, or lectin, that is produced by plants that cross-links human T cell surface molecules, including the T cell receptor, thereby inducing polyclonal activation and agglutination of T cells. PHA is frequently used in experimental immunology to study T cell activation. In clinical medicine, PHA is used to assess whether a patient's T cells are functional or to induce T cell mitosis for the purpose of generating karyotypic data.

Plasmablast Circulating antibody-secreting cells that may be precursors to the plasma cells that reside in the bone marrow and other tissues.

Plasma cell A terminally differentiated antibody-secreting B lymphocyte with a characteristic histologic appearance, including an oval shape, eccentric nucleus, and perinuclear halo.

Polyclonal activators Agents that are capable of activating many clones of lymphocytes, regardless of their antigen specificities. Examples of polyclonal activators include anti-IgM antibodies for B cells and anti-CD3 antibodies, bacterial superantigens, and PHA for T cells.

Poly-Ig receptor An Fc receptor expressed by mucosal epithelial cells that mediates the transport of IgA and IgM through the epithelial cells into the intestinal lumen.

Polymorphism The existence of two or more alternative forms, or variants, of a gene that are present at stable frequencies in a population. Each common variant of a polymorphic gene is called an allele, and one individual may carry two different alleles of a gene, each inherited from a different parent. The MHC genes are the most polymorphic genes in the mammalian genome, some of which have thousands of alleles.

Polyvalency The presence of multiple identical copies of an epitope on a single antigen molecule, cell surface, or particle. Polyvalent antigens, such as bacterial capsular polysaccharides, are often capable of activating B lymphocytes independent of helper T cells. Used synonymously with multivalency.

Positive selection The process by which developing T cells in the thymus (thymocytes) whose TCRs bind to self MHC molecules are rescued from programmed cell death, whereas thymocytes whose receptors do not recognize self MHC molecules die by default. Positive selection ensures that mature T cells are self MHC restricted and that CD8$^+$ T cells are specific for complexes of peptides with class I MHC molecules and CD4$^+$ T cells for complexes of peptides with class II MHC molecules.

Pre-B cell A developing B cell present only in hematopoietic tissues that is at a maturational stage characterized by expression of cytoplasmic Ig μ heavy chains and surrogate light chains but not Ig light chains. Pre–B cell receptors composed of μ chains and surrogate light chains deliver signals that stimulate further maturation of the pre–B cell into an immature B cell.

Pre–B cell receptor A receptor expressed on developing B lymphocytes at the pre–B cell stage that is composed of Ig μ heavy chains and invariant surrogate light chains. The pre–B cell receptor associates with the Igα and Igβ signal transduction proteins to form the pre–B cell receptor complex. Pre–B cell receptors are required for stimulating the proliferation and continued maturation of the developing B cell, serving as a checkpoint for productive μ heavy chain VDJ rearrangement. It is not known whether the pre–B cell receptor binds a specific ligand.

Pre–T cell A developing T lymphocyte in the thymus at a maturational stage characterized by expression of the TCR β chain but not the α chain or CD4 or CD8. In pre-T cells, the TCR β chain is found on the cell surface as part of the pre–T cell receptor.

Pre–T cell receptor A receptor expressed on the surface of pre–T cells that is composed of the TCR β chain and an invariant pre-Tα protein. This receptor associates with CD3 and ζ molecules to form the pre–T cell receptor complex.

The function of this complex is similar to that of the pre–B cell receptor in B cell development—namely, the delivery of signals that stimulate further proliferation, antigen receptor gene rearrangements, and other maturational events. It is not known whether the pre–T cell receptor binds a specific ligand.

Pre-Tα An invariant transmembrane protein with a single extracellular Ig-like domain that associates with the TCR β chain in pre–T cells to form the pre–T cell receptor.

Primary immune response An adaptive immune response that occurs after the first exposure of an individual to a foreign antigen. Primary responses are characterized by relatively slow kinetics and small magnitude compared with the responses after a second or subsequent exposure.

Primary immunodeficiency See **congenital immunodeficiency**.

Pro–B cell A developing B cell in the bone marrow that is the earliest cell committed to the B lymphocyte lineage. Pro–B cells do not produce Ig, but they can be distinguished from other immature cells by the expression of B lineage–restricted surface molecules such as CD19 and CD10.

Pro–T cell A developing T cell in the thymic cortex that is a recent arrival from the bone marrow and does not express TCRs, CD3, ζ chains, or CD4 or CD8 molecules. Pro–T cells are also called double-negative thymocytes.

Programmed cell death See **apoptosis**.

Prostaglandins A class of lipid inflammatory mediators that are derived from arachidonic acid in many cell types through the cyclooxygenase pathway and that have vasodilator, bronchoconstrictor, and chemotactic activities. Prostaglandins made by mast cells are important mediators of allergic reactions.

Proteasome A large multiprotein enzyme complex with a broad range of proteolytic activity that is found in the cytoplasm of most cells and generates from cytosolic proteins the peptides that bind to class I MHC molecules. Proteins are targeted for proteasomal degradation by covalent linkage of ubiquitin molecules.

Protein kinase C (PKC) Any of several isoforms of an enzyme that mediates the phosphorylation of serine and threonine residues in many different protein substrates and thereby serves to propagate various signal transduction pathways leading to transcription factor activation. In T and B lymphocytes, PKC is activated by DAG, which is generated in response to antigen receptor ligation.

Protein tyrosine kinases (PTKs) Enzymes that mediate the phosphorylation of tyrosine residues in proteins and thereby promote phosphotyrosine-dependent protein-protein interactions. PTKs are involved in numerous signal transduction pathways in cells of the immune system.

Protozoa Single-celled eukaryotic organisms, many of which are human parasites and cause diseases. Examples of pathogenic protozoa include *Entamoeba histolytica*, which causes amebic dysentery; *Plasmodium*, which causes malaria; and *Leishmania*, which causes leishmaniasis. Protozoa stimulate both innate and adaptive immune responses. It has proved difficult to develop effective vaccines against many of these organisms.

Provirus A DNA copy of the genome of a retrovirus that is integrated into the host cell genome and from which viral genes are transcribed and the viral genome is reproduced. HIV proviruses can remain inactive for long periods and thereby represent a latent form of HIV infection that is not accessible to immune defense.

Purified antigen (subunit) vaccine A vaccine composed of purified antigens or subunits of microbes. Examples of this type of vaccine include diphtheria and tetanus toxoids, pneumococcus and *Haemophilus influenzae* polysaccharide vaccines, and purified polypeptide vaccines against hepatitis B and influenza virus. Purified antigen vaccines may stimulate antibody and helper T cell responses, but they typically do not generate CTL responses.

Pyogenic bacteria Bacteria, such as Gram-positive staphylococci and streptococci, that induce inflammatory responses rich in polymorphonuclear leukocytes (giving rise to pus). Antibody responses to these bacteria greatly enhance the efficacy of innate immune effector mechanisms to clear infections.

R

Rapamycin An immunosuppressive drug (also called sirolimus) used clinically to prevent allograft rejection. Rapamycin inhibits the activation of a protein called molecular target of rapamycin (mTOR), which is a key signaling molecule in a variety of metabolic and cell growth pathways, including the pathway required for interleukin-2–mediated T cell proliferation.

Ras A member of a family of 21-kD guanine nucleotide–binding proteins with intrinsic GTPase activity that are involved in many different signal transduction pathways in diverse cell types. Mutated *ras* genes are associated with neoplastic transformation. In T cell activation, Ras is recruited to the plasma membrane by tyrosine-phosphorylated adaptor proteins, where it is activated by GDP-GTP exchange factors. GTP·Ras then initiates the MAP kinase cascade, which leads to expression of the *fos* gene and assembly of the AP-1 transcription factor.

Reactive oxygen species (ROS) Highly reactive metabolites of oxygen, including superoxide anion, hydroxyl radical, and hydrogen peroxide, that are produced by activated phagocytes. Reactive oxygen species are used by the phagocytes to form oxyhalides that damage ingested bacteria. They may also be released from cells and promote inflammatory responses or cause tissue damage.

Receptor editing A process by which some immature B cells that recognize self antigens in the bone marrow may be induced to change their Ig specificities. Receptor editing involves reactivation of the *RAG* genes, additional light-chain VJ recombinations, and new Ig light-chain production, which allows the cell to express a different Ig receptor that is not self-reactive.

Recombination-activating genes 1 and 2 (*RAG1* and *RAG2*) The genes encoding RAG-1 and RAG-2 proteins,

which make up the V(D)J recombinase and are expressed in developing B and T cells. RAG proteins bind to recombination signal sequences and are critical for DNA recombination events that form functional *Ig* and *TCR* genes. Therefore, RAG proteins are required for expression of antigen receptors and for the maturation of B and T lymphocytes.

Recombination signal sequences Specific DNA sequences found adjacent to the V, D, and J segments in antigen receptor loci and are recognized by the RAG-1/RAG-2 complex during V(D)J recombination. The recognition sequences consist of a highly conserved stretch of 7 nucleotides, called the heptamer, located adjacent to the V, D, or J coding sequence, followed by a spacer of exactly 12 or 23 nonconserved nucleotides and a highly conserved stretch of 9 nucleotides, called the nonamer.

Red pulp A compartment of the spleen composed of vascular sinusoids, scattered among which are large numbers of erythrocytes, macrophages, dendritic cells, sparse lymphocytes, and plasma cells. Red pulp macrophages clear the blood of microbes, other foreign particles, and damaged red blood cells.

Regulatory T cells A population of T cells that inhibits the activation of other T cells and is necessary to maintain peripheral tolerance to self antigens. Most regulatory T cells are CD4+ and express the α chain of the IL-2 receptor (CD25), CTLA-4, and the transcription factor FoxP3.

Respiratory burst The process by which reactive oxygen intermediates such as superoxide anion, hydroxyl radical, and hydrogen peroxide are produced in macrophages and polymorphonuclear leukocytes. The respiratory burst is mediated by the enzyme phagocyte oxidase and is usually triggered by inflammatory mediators, such as the cytokines IFN-γ and TNF or by bacterial products, such as LPS.

Reverse transcriptase An enzyme encoded by retroviruses, such as HIV, that synthesizes a DNA copy of the viral genome from the RNA genomic template. Purified reverse transcriptase is used widely in molecular biology research for purposes of cloning complementary DNAs encoding a gene of interest from messenger RNA. Reverse transcriptase inhibitors are used as drugs to treat HIV-1 infection.

Rh blood group antigens A complex system of protein alloantigens expressed on red blood cell membranes that are the cause of transfusion reactions and hemolytic disease of the newborn. The most clinically important Rh antigen is designated D.

Rheumatoid arthritis An autoimmune disease characterized primarily by inflammatory damage to joints and sometimes inflammation of blood vessels, lungs, and other tissues. CD4+ T cells, activated B lymphocytes, and plasma cells are found in the inflamed joint lining (synovium), and numerous proinflammatory cytokines, including IL-1 and TNF, are present in the synovial (joint) fluid.

RIG-like receptors (RLRs) Cytosolic receptors of the innate immune system that recognize viral RNA and induce production of type I interferons. The two best-characterized

RLRs are RIG-I (retinoic acid–inducible gene I) and MDA5 (melanoma differentiation-associated gene 5).

RORγT (retinoid-related orphan receptor γ T) A transcription factor expressed in and required for differentiation of Th17 cells and Group 3 innate lymphoid cells.

S

Scavenger receptors A family of cell surface receptors expressed on macrophages, originally defined as receptors that mediate endocytosis of oxidized or acetylated low-density lipoprotein particles but that also bind and mediate the phagocytosis of a variety of microbes.

SCID mouse A mouse strain in which B and T cells are absent because of an early block in maturation from bone marrow precursors. SCID mice carry a mutation in a component of the enzyme DNA-dependent protein kinase, which is required for double-stranded DNA break repair. Deficiency of this enzyme results in abnormal joining of *Ig* and *TCR* gene segments during recombination and therefore failure to express antigen receptors.

Secondary immune response An adaptive immune response that occurs on second exposure to an antigen. A secondary response is characterized by more rapid kinetics and greater magnitude relative to the primary immune response, which occurs on first exposure.

Secondary immunodeficiency See **acquired immunodeficiency.**

Secretory component The proteolytically cleaved portion of the extracellular domain of the poly-Ig receptor that remains bound to an IgA molecule in mucosal secretions.

Selectin Any one of three separate but closely related carbohydrate-binding proteins that mediate adhesion of leukocytes to endothelial cells. Each of the selectin molecules is a single-chain transmembrane glycoprotein with a similar modular structure, including an extracellular calcium-dependent lectin domain. The selectins include L-selectin (CD62L), expressed on leukocytes; P-selectin (CD62P), expressed on platelets and activated endothelium; and E-selectin (CD62E), expressed on activated endothelium.

Self MHC restriction The limitation (or restriction) of T cells to recognize antigens displayed by MHC molecules that the T cell encountered during maturation in the thymus (and thus sees as self).

Self-tolerance Unresponsiveness of the adaptive immune system to self antigens, largely as a result of inactivation or death of self-reactive lymphocytes induced by exposure to these antigens. Self-tolerance is a cardinal feature of the normal immune system, and failure of self-tolerance leads to autoimmune diseases.

Septic shock A severe complication of bacterial infections that spread to the bloodstream (sepsis) and is characterized by vascular collapse, disseminated intravascular coagulation, and metabolic disturbances. This syndrome is due to the effects of bacterial cell wall components, such as LPS or peptidoglycan, that bind to TLRs on various cell types and induce expression of inflammatory cytokines, including TNF and IL-12.

Serology The study of blood (serum) antibodies and their reactions with antigens. The term *serology* is often used to refer to the diagnosis of infectious diseases by detection of microbe-specific antibodies in the serum.

Serotype An antigenically distinct subset of a species of an infectious organism that is distinguished from other subsets by serologic (i.e., serum antibody) tests. Humoral immune responses to one serotype of microbes (e.g., influenza virus) may not be protective against another serotype.

Serum The cell-free fluid that remains when blood or plasma forms a clot. Blood antibodies are found in the serum fraction.

Serum amyloid A (SAA) An acute-phase protein whose serum concentration rises significantly in the setting of infection and inflammation, mainly because of IL-1– and TNF-induced synthesis by the liver. SAA activates leukocyte chemotaxis, phagocytosis, and adhesion to endothelial cells.

Serum sickness A disease caused by the injection of large doses of a protein antigen into the blood and characterized by the deposition of antigen-antibody (immune) complexes in blood vessel walls, especially in the kidneys and joints. Immune complex deposition leads to complement fixation and leukocyte recruitment and subsequently to glomerulonephritis and arthritis. Serum sickness was originally described as a disorder that occurred in patients receiving injections of serum containing antitoxin antibodies to prevent diphtheria.

Severe combined immunodeficiency (SCID) Immunodeficiency diseases in which both B and T lymphocytes do not develop or do not function properly, and therefore both humoral immunity and cell-mediated immunity are impaired. Children with SCID usually have infections during the first year of life and succumb to these infections unless the immunodeficiency is treated. SCID has several different genetic causes.

Single-positive thymocyte A maturing T cell precursor in the thymus that expresses CD4 or CD8 molecules but not both. Single-positive thymocytes are found mainly in the medulla and have matured from the double-positive stage, during which thymocytes express both CD4 and CD8 molecules.

Signal transducer and activator of transcription (STAT) A member of a family of proteins that function as transcription factors in response to binding of cytokines to type I and type II cytokine receptors. STATs are present as inactive monomers in the cytosol of cells and are recruited to the cytoplasmic tails of cross-linked cytokine receptors, where they are tyrosine phosphorylated by JAKs. The phosphorylated STAT proteins dimerize and move to the nucleus, where they bind to specific sequences in the promoter regions of various genes and stimulate their transcription. Different STATs are activated by different cytokines.

Smallpox A disease caused by variola virus. Smallpox was the first infectious disease shown to be preventable by vaccination and the first disease to be completely eradicated by a worldwide vaccination program.

Somatic hypermutation High-frequency point mutations in Ig heavy and light chains that occur in germinal center B cells in response to signals from Tfh cells. Mutations that result in increased affinity of antibodies for antigen impart a selective survival advantage to the B cells producing those antibodies and lead to affinity maturation of a humoral immune response.

Somatic recombination The process of DNA recombination by which the functional genes encoding the variable regions of antigen receptors are formed during lymphocyte development. A limited set of inherited, or germline, DNA sequences that are initially separated from one another are brought together by enzymatic deletion of intervening sequences and religation. This process occurs only in developing B or T lymphocytes and is mediated by RAG-1 and RAG-2 proteins. This process is also called V(D)J recombination or somatic rearrangement.

Specificity A cardinal feature of the adaptive immune system—namely, that immune responses are directed toward and able to distinguish between distinct antigens or small parts of macromolecular antigens. This fine specificity is attributed to lymphocyte antigen receptors that may bind to one molecule but not to another, even closely related, molecule.

Spleen A secondary lymphoid organ in the left upper quadrant of the abdomen. The spleen is the major site of adaptive immune responses to blood-borne antigens. The red pulp of the spleen is composed of blood-filled vascular sinusoids lined by active phagocytes that ingest opsonized antigens and damaged red blood cells. The white pulp of the spleen contains lymphocytes and lymphoid follicles where B cells are activated.

Stem cell An undifferentiated cell that divides continuously and gives rise to additional stem cells and to cells of multiple different lineages. For example, all blood cells arise from a common hematopoietic stem cell.

Superantigens Proteins that bind to and activate all of the T cells in an individual that express a particular set or family of Vβ *TCR* genes. Superantigens are presented to T cells by binding to nonpolymorphic regions of class II MHC molecules on APCs, and they interact with conserved regions of TCR Vβ domains. Several staphylococcal enterotoxins are superantigens. Their importance lies in their ability to activate many T cells, which results in large amounts of cytokine production and a clinical syndrome that is similar to septic shock.

Surrogate light chains Two nonvariable proteins that associate with Ig μ heavy chains in pre–B cells to form the pre–B cell receptor. The two surrogate light chain proteins include the V pre–B protein, which is homologous to a light-chain V domain, and λ5, which is covalently attached to the μ heavy chain by a disulfide bond.

Switch recombination The molecular mechanism underlying Ig isotype switching in which a rearranged VDJ gene segment in an antibody-producing B cell recombines with a downstream C gene and the intervening C gene or genes are deleted. DNA recombination events in switch recombination are triggered by CD40 and cytokines and involve nucleotide sequences called switch regions located in the introns at the 5′ end of each C_H locus.

Syk A cytoplasmic protein tyrosine kinase, similar to ZAP-70 in T cells, that is critical for early signaling steps in antigen-induced B cell activation. Syk binds to phosphorylated tyrosines in the cytoplasmic tails of the Igα and Igβ chains of the BCR complex and in turn phosphorylates adaptor proteins that recruit other components of the signaling cascade.

Syngeneic Genetically identical. All animals of an inbred strain and monozygotic twins are syngeneic.

Syngeneic graft A graft from a donor who is genetically identical to the recipient. Syngeneic grafts are not rejected.

Synthetic vaccine Vaccines composed of recombinant DNA–derived antigens. Synthetic vaccines for hepatitis B virus and herpes simplex virus are now in use.

Systemic inflammatory response syndrome (SIRS) The systemic changes observed in patients who have disseminated bacterial infections. In its mild form, SIRS consists of neutrophilia, fever, and a rise in acute-phase reactants in the plasma. These changes are stimulated by bacterial products such as LPS and are mediated by cytokines of the innate immune system. In severe cases, SIRS may include disseminated intravascular coagulation, adult respiratory distress syndrome, and septic shock.

Systemic lupus erythematosus (SLE) A chronic systemic autoimmune disease that affects predominantly women and is characterized by rashes, arthritis, glomerulonephritis, hemolytic anemia, thrombocytopenia, and central nervous system involvement. Many different autoantibodies are found in patients with SLE, particularly anti-DNA antibodies. Many of the manifestations of SLE are due to the formation of immune complexes composed of autoantibodies and their specific antigens, with deposition of these complexes in small blood vessels in various tissues. The underlying mechanism for the breakdown of self-tolerance in SLE is not understood.

T

T cell receptor (TCR) The clonally distributed antigen receptor on CD4+ and CD8+ T lymphocytes that recognizes complexes of foreign peptides bound to self MHC molecules on the surface of APCs. The most common form of TCR is composed of a heterodimer of two disulfide-linked transmembrane polypeptide chains, designated α and β, each containing one N-terminal Ig-like variable (V) domain, one Ig-like constant (C) domain, a hydrophobic transmembrane region, and a short cytoplasmic region. (Another less common type of TCR, composed of γ and δ chains, is found on a small subset of T cells and recognizes different forms of antigen.)

T follicular helper (Tfh) cells A heterogeneous subset of CD4+ helper T cells present in lymphoid follicles that are critical to providing signals to B cells in the germinal center reaction that stimulate somatic hypermutation, isotype switching, and the generation of memory B cells and long-lived plasma cells. Tfh cells express CXCR5, ICOS, IL-21, and Bcl-6.

T lymphocyte The key component of cell-mediated immune responses in the adaptive immune system. T lymphocytes mature in the thymus, circulate in the blood, populate secondary lymphoid tissues, and are recruited to peripheral sites of antigen exposure. They express antigen receptors (TCRs) that recognize peptide fragments of foreign proteins bound to self MHC molecules. Functional subsets of T lymphocytes include $CD4^+$ helper T cells and $CD8^+$ CTLs.

T-bet A T-box family transcription factor that promotes the differentiation of T_H1 cells from naive T cells.

T-dependent antigen An antigen that requires helper T cells to stimulate B cells to mount an antibody response. T-dependent antigens are protein antigens that contain some epitopes recognized by T cells and other epitopes recognized by B cells. Helper T cells produce cytokines and cell surface molecules that stimulate B cell growth and differentiation into antibody-secreting cells. Humoral immune responses to T-dependent antigens are characterized by isotype switching, affinity maturation, and memory.

T-independent antigen Nonprotein antigens, such as polysaccharides and lipids, that can stimulate antibody responses without a requirement for antigen-specific helper T lymphocytes. T-independent antigens usually contain multiple identical epitopes that can cross-link membrane Ig on B cells and thereby activate the cells. Humoral immune responses to T-independent antigens show relatively little heavy-chain isotype switching or affinity maturation, two processes that require signals from helper T cells.

Tertiary lymphoid organ A collection of lymphocytes and antigen-presenting cells organized into B cell follicles and T cell zones that develop in sites of chronic immune-mediated inflammation, such as the joint synovium of rheumatoid arthritis patients.

Th1 cells A subset of $CD4^+$ helper T cells that secrete a particular set of cytokines, including IFN-γ, and whose principal function is to stimulate phagocyte-mediated defense against infections, especially with intracellular microbes.

Th2 cells A functional subset of $CD4^+$ helper T cells that secrete a particular set of cytokines, including IL-4, IL-5, and IL-3, and whose principal function is to stimulate IgE and eosinophil/mast cell–mediated immune reactions.

Th17 cells A functional subset of $CD4^+$ helper T cells that secrete a particular set of inflammatory cytokines, including IL-17 and IL-22, that are protective against bacterial and fungal infections and also mediate inflammatory reactions in autoimmune and other inflammatory diseases.

Thymic epithelial cells Epithelial cells abundant in the cortical and medullary stroma of the thymus that play a critical role in T cell development. In the process of positive selection, maturing T cells that weakly recognize self peptides bound to MHC molecules on the surface of thymic epithelial cells are rescued from programmed cell death.

Thymocyte A precursor of a mature T lymphocyte present in the thymus.

Thymus A bilobed organ situated in the anterior mediastinum that is the site of maturation of T lymphocytes from bone marrow–derived precursors. Thymic tissue is divided into an outer cortex and an inner medulla and contains stromal thymic epithelial cells, macrophages, dendritic cells, and numerous T cell precursors (thymocytes) at various stages of maturation.

Tissue typing The determination of the particular MHC alleles expressed by an individual for the purpose of matching allograft donors and recipients. Tissue typing, also called HLA typing, is usually done by molecular (PCR-based) sequencing of HLA alleles or by serologic methods (lysis of an individual's cells by panels of anti-HLA antibodies).

Tolerance Unresponsiveness of the adaptive immune system to antigens, as a result of inactivation or death of antigen-specific lymphocytes, induced by exposure to the antigens. Tolerance to self antigens is a normal feature of the adaptive immune system, but tolerance to foreign antigens may be induced under certain conditions of antigen exposure.

Tolerogen An antigen that induces immunologic tolerance, in contrast to an immunogen, which induces an immune response. Many antigens can be either tolerogens or immunogens, depending on how they are administered. Tolerogenic forms of antigens include large doses of the proteins administered without adjuvants and orally administered antigens.

Toll-like receptors A family of pattern recognition receptors of the innate immune system that are expressed on the surface and in endosomes of many cell types and that recognize microbial structures, such as endotoxin and viral RNA, and transduce signals that lead to the expression of inflammatory and antiviral genes.

Transfusion Transplantation of circulating blood cells, platelets, or plasma from one individual to another. Transfusions are performed to treat blood loss from hemorrhage or to treat a deficiency in one or more blood cell types resulting from inadequate production or excess destruction.

Transfusion reactions An immunologic reaction against transfused blood products, usually mediated by preformed antibodies in the recipient that bind to donor blood cell antigens, such as ABO blood group antigens or histocompatibility antigens. Transfusion reactions can lead to intravascular lysis of red blood cells and, in severe cases, kidney damage, fever, shock, and disseminated intravascular coagulation.

Transplantation The process of transferring cells, tissues, or organs (i.e., grafts) from one individual to another or from one site to another in the same individual. Transplantation is used to treat a variety of diseases in which there is a functional disorder of a tissue or organ. The major barrier to successful transplantation between individuals is immunologic reaction (rejection) to the transplanted graft.

Transporter associated with antigen processing (TAP) An adenosine triphosphate (ATP)-dependent peptide transporter that mediates the active transport of peptides from the cytosol to the site of assembly of class I MHC molecules inside the endoplasmic reticulum. TAP is a heterodimeric molecule composed of TAP-1 and TAP-2 polypeptides, both encoded by genes in the MHC. Because peptides are required for stable assembly of class I MHC molecules, TAP-deficient animals express few cell surface class I MHC molecules, which results in diminished development and activation of $CD8^+$ T cells.

Tumor immunity Protection against the development or progression of tumors by the immune system. Although immune responses to naturally occurring tumors can frequently be demonstrated, tumors often escape these responses. New therapies that target T cell inhibitory molecules, such as PD-1, are proving effective in enhancing effective T cell mediated antitumor immunity.

Tumor-infiltrating lymphocytes (TILs) Lymphocytes isolated from the inflammatory infiltrates present in and around surgical resection samples of solid tumors that are enriched with tumor-specific CTLs and NK cells. In an experimental mode of cancer treatment, TILs are grown in vitro in the presence of high doses of IL-2 and are then adoptively transferred back into patients with the tumor.

Tumor necrosis factor receptor superfamily (TNFRSF) A large family of structurally homologous transmembrane proteins that bind TNFSF proteins and generate signals that regulate proliferation, differentiation, apoptosis, and inflammatory gene expression.

Tumor necrosis factor superfamily (TNFSF) A large family of structurally homologous transmembrane proteins that regulate diverse functions in responding cells, including proliferation, differentiation, apoptosis, and inflammatory gene expression. TNFSF members typically form homotrimers, either within the plasma membrane or after proteolytic release from the membrane, and bind to homotrimeric TNF receptor superfamily (TNFRSF) molecules, which then initiate a variety of signaling pathways.

Type 1 diabetes mellitus A disease characterized by a lack of insulin that leads to various metabolic and vascular abnormalities. The insulin deficiency results from autoimmune destruction of the insulin-producing β cells of the islets of Langerhans in the pancreas, usually during childhood. $CD4^+$ and $CD8^+$ T cells, antibodies, and cytokines have been implicated in the islet cell damage. Also called insulin-dependent diabetes mellitus.

U

Ubiquitination Covalent linkage of one or several copies of a small polypeptide called ubiquitin to a protein. Ubiquitination frequently serves to target proteins for proteolytic degradation by lysosomes or by proteasomes, the latter a critical step in the class I MHC pathway of antigen processing and presentation.

Urticaria Localized transient swelling and redness of the skin caused by leakage of fluid and plasma proteins from small vessels into the dermis during an immediate hypersensitivity reaction.

V

V gene segments A DNA sequence that encodes the variable domain of an Ig heavy chain or light chain or a TCR α, β, γ, or δ chain. Each antigen receptor locus contains many different V gene segments, any one of which may recombine with downstream D or J segments during lymphocyte maturation to form functional antigen receptor genes.

V(D)J recombinase The complex of RAG1 and RAG2 proteins that catalyzes lymphocyte antigen receptor gene recombination.

Vaccine A preparation of microbial antigen, often combined with adjuvants, that is administered to individuals to induce protective immunity against microbial infections. The antigen may be in the form of live but avirulent (attenuated) microorganisms, killed microorganisms, purified macromolecular components of a microorganism, or a plasmid that contains a complementary DNA encoding a microbial antigen.

Variable region The extracellular, N-terminal region of an Ig heavy or light chain or a TCR α, β, γ, or δ chain that contains variable amino acid sequences that differ between every clone of lymphocytes and that are responsible for the specificity for antigen. The antigen-binding variable sequences are localized to extended loop structures or hypervariable segments.

Virus A primitive obligate intracellular parasitic organism or infectious particle that consists of a simple nucleic acid genome packaged in a protein capsid, sometimes surrounded by a membrane envelope. Many pathogenic animal viruses cause a wide range of diseases. Humoral immune responses to viruses can be effective in blocking infection of cells, and NK cells and CTLs are necessary to kill cells already infected.

Vasoactive amines Low-molecular-weight nonlipid compounds, such as histamine, that all have an amine group, are stored in and released from the cytoplasmic granules of mast cells, and mediate many of the biologic effects of immediate hypersensitivity (allergic) reactions. (Biogenic amines are sometimes called vasoactive amines.)

W

Wheal-and-flare reaction Local swelling and redness in the skin at a site of an immediate hypersensitivity reaction. The wheal reflects increased vascular permeability, and the flare results from increased local blood flow, both changes resulting from mediators such as histamine released from activated dermal mast cells.

White pulp The part of the spleen that is composed predominantly of lymphocytes, arranged in periarteriolar lymphoid sheaths, and follicles and other leukocytes. The remainder of the spleen contains sinusoids lined with phagocytic cells and filled with blood, called the red pulp.

Wiskott-Aldrich syndrome An X-linked disease characterized by eczema, thrombocytopenia (reduced blood platelets), and immunodeficiency manifested as susceptibility to bacterial infections. The defective gene encodes a cytosolic protein involved in signaling cascades and regulation of the actin cytoskeleton.

X

Xenoantigen An antigen on a graft from another species.

Xenograft (xenogeneic graft) An organ or tissue graft derived from a species different from the recipient. Transplantation of xenogeneic grafts (e.g., from a pig) to humans is not yet practical because of special problems related to immunologic rejection.

Xenotransplantation The transplantation of a living tissue or organ from one species to another. Successful xenotransplantation into humans to treat diseases has not been achieved.

X-linked agammaglobulinemia An immunodeficiency disease, also called Bruton's agammaglobulinemia, characterized by a block in early B cell maturation and an absence of serum Ig. Patients suffer from pyogenic bacterial infections. The disease is caused by mutations or deletions in the gene encoding Btk, an enzyme involved in signal transduction in developing B cells.

X-linked hyper-IgM syndrome A rare immunodeficiency disease caused by mutations in the CD40 ligand gene and characterized by failure of B cell heavy-chain isotype switching and cell-mediated immunity. Patients suffer from both pyogenic bacterial and protozoal infections.

Z

ζ Chain A transmembrane protein expressed in T cells as part of the TCR complex that contains ITAMs in its cytoplasmic tail and binds the ZAP-70 protein tyrosine kinase during T cell activation.

Zeta-associated protein of 70 kD (ZAP-70) A cytoplasmic protein tyrosine kinase, similar to Syk in B cells, that is critical for early signaling steps in antigen-induced T cell activation. ZAP-70 binds to phosphorylated tyrosines in the cytoplasmic tails of the ζ chain and CD3 chains of the TCR complex and in turn phosphorylates adaptor proteins that recruit other components of the signaling cascade.

Cytokines

Cytokine and Subunits	Principal Cell Source	Cytokine Receptor and Subunits*	Principal Cellular Targets and Biologic Effects
Type I Cytokine Family Members			
Interleukin-2 (IL-2)	T cells	CD25 (IL-2Rα) CD122 (IL-2Rβ) CD132 (γc)	T cells: proliferation and differentiation into effector and memory cells; promotes regulatory T cell development, survival, and function NK cells: proliferation, activation
Interleukin-3 (IL-3)	T cells	CD123 (IL-3R) CD131 (βc)	Immature hematopoietic progenitors: induced maturation of all hematopoietic lineages
Interleukin-4 (IL-4)	CD4+ T cells (Th2), mast cells	CD124 (IL-4R) CD132 (γc)	B cells: isotype switching to IgE T cells: Th2 differentiation, proliferation Macrophages: alternative activation and inhibition of IFN-γ–mediated classical activation
Interleukin-5 (IL-5)	CD4+ T cells (Th2), group 2 ILCs	CD125 (IL-5R) CD131 (βc)	Eosinophils: activation, increased generation
Interleukin-6 (IL-6)	Macrophages, endothelial cells, T cells	CD126 (IL-6R) CD130 (gp130)	Liver: synthesis of acute-phase protein B cells: proliferation of antibody-producing cells T cells: Th17 differentiation
Interleukin-7 (IL-7)	Fibroblasts, bone marrow stromal cells	CD127 (IL-7R) CD132 (γc)	Immature lymphoid progenitors: proliferation of early T and B cell progenitors T lymphocytes: survival of naive and memory cells
Interleukin-9 (IL-9)	CD4+ T cells	CD129 (IL-9R) CD132 (γc)	Mast cells, B cells, T cells, and tissue cells: survival and activation
Interleukin-11 (IL-11)	Bone marrow stromal cells	IL-11Rα CD130 (gp130)	Production of platelets
Interleukin-12 (IL-12): IL-12A (p35) IL-12B (p40)	Macrophages, dendritic cells	CD212 (IL-12Rβ1) IL-12Rβ2	T cells: Th1 differentiation NK cells and T cells: IFN-γ synthesis, increased cytotoxic activity
Interleukin-13 (IL-13)	CD4+ T cells (Th2), NKT cells, group 2 ILCs, mast cells	CD213a1 (IL-13Rα1) CD213a2 (IL-13Rα2) CD132 (γc)	B cells: isotype switching to IgE Epithelial cells: increased mucus production Macrophages: alternative activation
Interleukin-15 (IL-15)	Macrophages, other cell types	IL-15Rα CD122 (IL-2Rβ) CD132 (γc)	NK cells: proliferation T cells: survival and proliferation of memory CD8+ cells

Continued

303

Cytokine and Subunits	Principal Cell Source	Cytokine Receptor and Subunits*	Principal Cellular Targets and Biologic Effects
Interleukin-17A (IL-17A) Interleukin-17F (IL-17F)	CD4+ T cells (Th17), group 3 ILCs	CD217 (IL-17RA) IL-17RC	Endothelial cells: increased chemokine production Macrophages: increased chemokine and cytokine production Epithelial cells: GM-CSF and G-CSF production
Interleukin-21 (IL-21)	Th2 cells, Th17cells, Tfh cells	CD360 (IL-21R) CD132 (γc)	B cells: activation, proliferation, differentiation Tfh cells: development Th17 cells: increased generation NK cells: functional maturation
Interleukin-23 (IL-23): IL-23A (p19) IL-12B (p40)	Macrophages, dendritic cells	IL-23R CD212 (IL-12Rβ1)	T cells: differentiation and expansion of Th17 cells
Interleukin-25 (IL-25; IL-17E)	T cells, mast cells, eosinophils, macrophages, mucosal epithelial cells	IL-17RB	T cells and group 2 ILCs: production of IL-5, IL-13
Interleukin-27 (IL-27): IL-27 (p28) EBI3 (IL-27B)	Macrophages, dendritic cells	IL-27Rα CD130 (gp130)	T cells: enhances Th1 differentiation inhibition of Th17 differentiation
Stem cell factor (c-Kit ligand)	Bone marrow stromal cells	CD117 (KIT)	Pluripotent hematopoietic stem cells: induced maturation of all hematopoietic lineages
Granulocyte-monocyte CSF (GM-CSF)	T cells, macrophages, endothelial cells, fibroblasts	CD116 (GM-CSFRα) CD131 (βc)	Immature and committed progenitors: induced maturation of granulocytes and monocytes Macrophage activation
Monocyte CSF (M-CSF, CSF1)	Macrophages, endothelial cells, bone marrow cells, fibroblasts	CD115 (CSF1R)	Committed hematopoietic progenitors: induced maturation of monocytes
Granulocyte CSF (G-CSF, CSF3)	Macrophages, fibroblasts, endothelial cells	CD114 (CSF3R)	Committed hematopoietic progenitors: induced maturation of granulocytes
Type II Cytokine Family Members			
IFN-α (multiple proteins)	Plasmacytoid dendritic cells, macrophages	IFNAR1 CD118 (IFNAR2)	All cells: antiviral state, increased class I MHC expression NK cells: activation
IFN-β	Fibroblasts, plasmacytoid dendritic cells	IFNAR1 CD118 (IFNAR2)	All cells: antiviral state, increased class I MHC expression NK cells: activation
Interferon-γ (IFN-γ)	T cells (Th1, CD8+ T cells), NK cells and group 1 ILCs	CD119 (IFNGR1) IFNGR2	Macrophages: classical activation (increased microbicidal functions) B cells: isotype switching to opsonizing and complement-fixing IgG subclasses (established in mice) T cells: Th1 differentiation Various cells: increased expression of class I and class II MHC molecules, increased antigen processing and presentation to T cells

Cytokine and Subunits	Principal Cell Source	Cytokine Receptor and Subunits*	Principal Cellular Targets and Biologic Effects
Interleukin-10 (IL-10)	Macrophages, T cells (mainly regulatory T cells)	CD210 (IL-10Rα) IL-10Rβ	Macrophages, dendritic cells: inhibition of expression of IL-12, costimulators, and class II MHC
Interleukin-22 (IL-22)	Th17 cells	IL-22Rα1 IL-10Rβ2 or IL-22α2 IL-10Rβ2	Epithelial cells: production of defensins, increased barrier function Hepatocytes: survival Adipocytes: lipolysis
Interferon-λs (type III interferons)	Dendritic cells	IFNLR1 (IL-28R) CD210B (IL-10Rβ2)	Epithelial cells: antiviral state
Leukemia inhibitory factor (LIF)	Embryonic trophectoderm Bone marrow stromal cells	CD118 (LIFR) CD130 (gp130)	Stem cells: block in differentiation
Oncostatin M	Bone marrow stromal cells	OSMR CD130 (gp130)	Endothelial cells: regulation of hematopoietic cytokine production
TNF Superfamily Cytokines†			
Tumor necrosis factor (TNF, TNFSF1)	Macrophages, NK cells, T cells	CD120a (TNFRSF1) or CD120b (TNFRSF2)	Endothelial cells: activation (inflammation, coagulation) Neutrophils: activation Hypothalamus: fever Muscle, fat: catabolism (cachexia)
Lymphotoxin-α (LTα, TNFSF1)	T cells, B cells	CD120a (TNFRSF1) or CD120b (TNFRSF2)	Same as TNF
Lymphotoxin-αβ (LTαβ)	T cells, NK cells, follicular B cells, lymphoid inducer cells	LTβR	Lymphoid tissue stromal cells and follicular dendritic cells: chemokine expression and lymphoid organogenesis
BAFF (CD257, TNFSF13B)	Dendritic cells, monocytes, follicular dendritic cells, B cells	BAFF-R (TNFRSF13C) or TACI (TNFRSF13B) or BCMA (TNFRSF17)	B cells: survival, proliferation
APRIL (CD256, TNFSF13)	T cells, dendritic cells, monocytes, follicular dendritic cells	TACI (TNFRSF13B) or BCMA (TNFRSF17)	B cells: survival, proliferation
Osteoprotegrin (OPG, TNFRSF11B)	Osteoblasts	RANKL	Osteoclast precursor cells: inhibits osteoclast differentiation
IL-1 Family Cytokines			
Interleukin-1α (IL-1α)	Macrophages, dendritic cells, fibroblasts, endothelial cells, keratinocytes	CD121a (IL-1R1) IL-1RAP or CD121b (IL-1R2)	Endothelial cells: activation (inflammation, coagulation) Hypothalamus: fever Liver: synthesis of acute-phase proteins
Interleukin-1β (IL-1β)	Macrophages, dendritic cells, fibroblasts, endothelial cells, keratinocytes	CD121a (IL-1R1) IL-1RAP or CD121b (IL-1R2)	Endothelial cells: activation (inflammation, coagulation) Hypothalamus: fever Liver: synthesis of acute-phase proteins T cells: Th17 differentiation
Interleukin-1 receptor antagonist (IL-1RA)	Macrophages	CD121a (IL-1R1) IL-1RAP	Various cells: competitive antagonist of IL-1

Continued

Cytokine and Subunits	Principal Cell Source	Cytokine Receptor and Subunits*	Principal Cellular Targets and Biologic Effects
Interleukin-18 (IL-18)	Monocytes, macrophages, dendritic cells, Kupffer cells, keratinocytes, chondrocytes, synovial fibroblasts, osteoblasts	CD218a (IL-18R) CD218b (IL-18Rβ)	NK cells and T cells: IFN-γ synthesis Monocytes: expression of GM-CSF, TNF, IL-1β Neutrophils: activation, cytokine release
Interleukin-33 (IL-33)	Endothelial cells, smooth muscle cells, keratinocytes, fibroblasts	ST2 (IL1RL1) IL-1 Receptor Accessory Protein (IL1RAP)	T cells: Th2 development ILCs: activation of group 2 ILCs
Other Cytokines			
Transforming growth factor–β (TGF-β)	T cells (mainly Tregs), macrophages, other cell types	TGF-β R1 TGF-β R2 TGF-β R3	T cells: inhibition of proliferation and effector functions; differentiation of Th17 and Treg B cells: inhibition of proliferation; IgA production Macrophages: inhibition of activation; stimulation of angiogenic factors Fibroblasts: increased collagen synthesis

APRIL, A proliferation-inducing ligand; *BAFF*, B cell–activating factor belonging to the TNF family; *BCMA*, B cell maturation protein; *CSF*, colony-stimulating factor; *IFN*, interferon; *ILC*, innate lymphoid cell; *MHC*, major histocompatibility complex; *NK cell*, natural killer cell; *OSMR*, oncostatin M receptor; *RANK*, receptor activator for nuclear factor κB ligand; *RANKL*, RANK ligand; *TACI*, transmembrane activator and calcium modulator and cyclophilin ligand interactor; *TNF*, tumor necrosis factor; *TNFSF*, TNF superfamily; *TNFRSF*, TNF receptor superfamily.

*Most cytokine receptors are dimers or trimers composed of different polypeptide chains, some of which are shared between receptors for different cytokines. The set of polypeptides that compose a functional receptor (cytokine binding plus signaling) for each cytokine are listed. The functions of each subunit polypeptide are not listed.

†All TNF superfamily (TNFSF) members are expressed as cell surface transmembrane proteins, but only the ones that are active as proteolytically released soluble cytokines are listed in the table. Other TNFSF members that function predominantly in the membrane-bound form and are not, strictly speaking, cytokines are not listed in the table. These membrane-bound proteins and the TNFRSF receptors they bind to include OX40L (CD252, TNFSF4):OX40 (CD134, TNFRSF4); CD40L (CD154, TNFSF5):CD40 (TNFRSF5); FasL (CD178, TNFSF6):Fas (CD95, TNFRSF6); CD70 (TNFSF7):CD27 (TNFRSF27); CD153 (TNFSF8):CD30 (TNFRSF8); TRAIL (CD253, TNFSF10):TRAIL-R (TNFRSF10A-D); RANKL (TNFSF11):RANK (TNFRSF11); TWEAK (CD257, TNFSF12):TWEAKR (CD266, TNFRSF12); LIGHT (CD258, TNFSF14):HVEM (TNFRSF14); GITRL (TNFSF18):GITR (TNFRSF18); 4-IBBL:4-IBB (CD137).

Principal Features of Selected CD Molecules

The following list includes selected CD molecules that are referred to in the text. Many cytokines and cytokine receptors have been assigned CD numbers, but we refer to these by the more descriptive cytokine designation. A complete and up-to-date listing of CD molecules may be found at http://www.hcdm.org.

CD Number (Other Names)	Molecular Structure, Family	Main Cellular Expression	Known or Proposed Function(s)
CD1a-d	49 kD; class I MHC-like Ig superfamily; β2-microglobulin associated	Thymocytes, dendritic cells (including Langerhans cells)	Presentation of nonpeptide (lipid and glycolipid) antigens to some T cells
CD1e	28 kD; class I MHC-like; β2-microglobulin associated	Dendritic cells	Same as CD1a
CD2 (LFA-2)	50 kD; Ig superfamily	T cells, NK cells	Adhesion molecule (binds CD58); T cell activation; CTL- and NK cell–mediated lysis
CD3γ	25-28 kD; associated with CD3δ and CD3ε in TCR complex; Ig superfamily; ITAM in cytoplasmic tail	T cells	Cell surface expression of and signal transduction by the T cell antigen receptor
CD3δ	20 kD; associated with CD3γ and CD3ε in TCR complex; Ig superfamily; ITAM in cytoplasmic tail	T cells	Cell surface expression of and signal transduction by the T cell antigen receptor
CD3ε	20 kD; associated with CD3δ and CD3γ in TCR complex; Ig superfamily; ITAM in cytoplasmic tail	T cells	Cell surface expression of and signal transduction by the T cell antigen receptor
CD4	55 kD; Ig superfamily	Class II MHC–restricted T cells; some dendritic cells and macrophages	Coreceptor in class II MHC-restricted antigen-induced T cell activation (binds to class II MHC molecules); thymocyte development; receptor for HIV
CD5	67 kD; scavenger receptor family	T cells; B-1 B cell subset	Signaling molecule; binds CD72
CD8α	34 kD; expressed as a homodimer or heterodimer with CD8β	Class I MHC–restricted T cells; subset of dendritic cells	Coreceptor in class I MHC-restricted antigen-induced T cell activation (binds to class I MHC molecules); thymocyte development
CD8β	34 kD; expressed as a heterodimer with CD8α Ig superfamily	Class I MHC–restricted T cells	Same as CD8α

Continued

CD Number (Other Names)	Molecular Structure, Family	Main Cellular Expression	Known or Proposed Function(s)
CD10	100 kD; type II membrane protein	Immature and some mature B cells; lymphoid progenitors, granulocytes	Metalloproteinase; unknown function in the immune system
CD11a (LFA-1 α chain)	180 kD; noncovalently linked to CD18 to form LFA-1 integrin	Leukocytes	Cell-cell adhesion; binds to ICAM-1 (CD54), ICAM-2 (CD102), and ICAM-3 (CD50)
CD11b (Mac-1; CR3)	165 kD; noncovalently linked to CD18 to form Mac-1 integrin	Granulocytes, monocytes, macrophages, dendritic cells, NK cells	Phagocytosis of iC3b-coated particles; neutrophil and monocyte adhesion to endothelium (binds CD54) and extracellular matrix proteins
CD11c (p150,95; CR4α chain)	145 kD; noncovalently linked to CD18 to form p150,95 integrin	Monocytes, macrophages, granulocytes, NK cells	Similar functions as CD11b
CD14	53 kD; GPI linked	Dendritic cells, monocytes, macrophages, granulocytes	Binds complex of LPS and LPS-binding protein and displays LPS to TLR4; required for LPS-induced macrophage activation
CD16a (FcγRIIIA)	50-70 kD; transmembrane protein; Ig superfamily	NK cells, macrophages	Binds Fc region of IgG; phagocytosis and antibody-dependent cellular cytotoxicity
CD16b (FcγRIIIB)	50-70 kD; GPI linked; Ig superfamily	Neutrophils	Binds Fc region of IgG; role immune complex–mediated neutrophil activation
CD18	95 kD; noncovalently linked to CD11a, CD11b, or CD11c to form γ_2 integrins	Leukocytes	See CD11a, CD11b, CD11c
CD19	95 kD; Ig superfamily	Most B cells	B cell activation; forms a coreceptor complex with CD21 and CD81 that delivers signals that synergize with signals from B cell antigen receptor complex
CD20	35-37 kD; tetraspan (TM4SF) family	B cells	? Role in B cell activation or regulation; calcium ion channel
CD21 (CR2; C3d receptor)	145 kD; regulators of complement activation	Mature B cells, follicular dendritic cells	Receptor for complement fragment C3d; forms a coreceptor complex with CD19 and CD81 that delivers activating signals in B cells; receptor for Epstein-Barr virus
CD22	130-140 kD; Ig superfamily; sialoadhesin family; ITIM in cytoplasmic tail	B cells	Regulation of B cell activation; adhesion molecule
CD23 (FcεRIIB)	45 kD; C-type lectin	Activated B cells, monocytes, macrophages	Low-affinity Fcε receptor, induced by IL-4; function is not clear
CD25 (IL-2 receptor α chain)	55 kD; noncovalently associated with IL-2Rβ (CD122) and IL-2Rγ (CD132) chains to form a high-affinity IL-2 receptor	Activated T and B cells, regulatory T cells (Treg)	Binds IL-2 and promotes responses to low concentrations of IL-2

CD Number (Other Names)	Molecular Structure, Family	Main Cellular Expression	Known or Proposed Function(s)
CD28	Homodimer of 44-kD chains; Ig superfamily	T cells (all CD4+ and >50% of CD8+ cells in humans; all mature T cells in mice)	T cell receptor for costimulatory molecules CD80 (B7-1) and CD86 (B7-2)
CD29	130 kD; noncovalently linked to CD49a-d chains to form VLA (β1) integrins	T cells, B cells, monocytes, granulocytes	Leukocyte adhesion to extracellular matrix proteins and endothelium (see CD49)
CD30 (TNFRSF8)	120 kD; TNFR superfamily	Activated T and B cells; NK cells, monocytes, Reed-Sternberg cells in Hodgkin's disease	Not established
CD31 (platelet/ endothelial cell adhesion molecule 1 [PECAM-1])	130-140 kD; Ig superfamily	Platelets, monocytes, granulocytes, B cells, endothelial cells	Adhesion molecule involved in leukocyte transmigration through endothelium
CD32 (FcγRII)	40 kD; Ig superfamily; ITIM in cytoplasmic tail; A, B, and C forms are products of different but homologous genes	B cells, macrophages, dendritic cells, granulocytes	Fc receptor for aggregated IgG; acts as inhibitory receptor that blocks activation of B cells and other cells
CD34	105-120 kD; sialomucin	Precursors of hematopoietic cells; endothelial cells in high endothelial venules	? Role in cell-cell adhesion
CD35 (type 1 complement receptor, CR1)	190-285 kD (four products of polymorphic alleles); regulator of complement activation family	Granulocytes, monocytes, erythrocytes, B cells, follicular dendritic cells, some T cells	Binds C3b and C4b; promotes phagocytosis of C3b- or C4b-coated particles and immune complexes; regulates complement activation
CD36	85-90 kD	Platelets, monocytes, macrophages, endothelial cells	Scavenger receptor for oxidized low-density lipoprotein; platelet adhesion; phagocytosis of apoptotic cells
CD40	Homodimer of 44- to 48-kD chains; TNFR superfamily	B cells, macrophages, dendritic cells, endothelial cells	Binds CD154 (CD40 ligand); role in helper T cell–mediated activation of B cells, macrophages, and dendritic cells
CD43	95-135 kD; sialomucin	Leukocytes (except circulating B cells)	? Role in cell-cell adhesion
CD44	80->100 kD, highly glycosylated	Leukocytes, erythrocytes	Binds hyaluronan; involved in leukocyte adhesion to endothelial cells and extracellular matrix
CD45 (leukocyte common antigen [LCA])	Multiple isoforms, 180-220 kD (see CD45R); protein tyrosine phosphatase receptor family; fibronectin type III family	Hematopoietic cells	Tyrosine phosphatase that regulates T and B cell activation
CD45R	CD45RO: 180 kD CD45RA: 220 kD CD45RB: 190-, 205-, and 220-kD isoforms	CD45RO: memory T cells; subset of B cells, monocytes, macrophages CD45RA: naive T cells, B cells, monocytes CD45RB: B cells, subset of T cells	See CD45

Continued

CD Number (Other Names)	Molecular Structure, Family	Main Cellular Expression	Known or Proposed Function(s)
CD46 (membrane cofactor protein [MCP])	52-58 kD; regulators of complement activation family	Leukocytes, epithelial cells, fibroblasts	Regulation of complement activation
CD47	47-52 kD; Ig superfamily	All hematopoietic cells, epithelial cells, endothelial cells, fibroblasts	Leukocyte adhesion, migration, activation; "Don't eat me" signal to phagocytes
CD49d	150 kD; noncovalently linked to CD29 to form VLA-4 ($\alpha4\beta1$ integrin)	T cells, monocytes, B cells, NK cells, eosinophils, dendritic cells, thymocytes	Leukocyte adhesion to endothelium and extracellular matrix; binds to VCAM-1 and MadCAM-1; binds fibronectin and collagens
CD54 (ICAM-1)	75-114 kD; Ig superfamily	T cells, B cells, monocytes, endothelial cells (cytokine inducible)	Cell-cell adhesion; ligand for CD11aCD18 (LFA-1) and CD11bCD18 (Mac-1); receptor for rhinovirus
CD55 (decay-accelerating factor [DAF])	55-70 kD; GPI linked; regulators of complement activation family	Broad	Regulation of complement activation
CD58 (leukocyte function–associated antigen 3 [LFA-3])	55-70 kD; GPI-linked or integral membrane protein	Broad	Leukocyte adhesion; binds CD2
CD59	18-20 kD; GPI linked	Broad	Binds C9; inhibits formation of complement membrane attack complex
CD62E (E-selectin)	115 kD; selectin family	Endothelial cells	Leukocyte-endothelial adhesion
CD62L (L-selectin)	74-95 kD; selectin family	B cells, T cells, monocytes, granulocytes, some NK cells	Leukocyte-endothelial adhesion; homing of naive T cells to peripheral lymph nodes
CD62P (P-selectin)	140 kD; selectin family	Platelets, endothelial cells (present in granules, translocated to cell surface on activation)	Leukocyte adhesion to endothelium, platelets; binds CD162 (PSGL-1)
CD64 (FcγRI)	72 kD; Ig superfamily; noncovalently associated with the FcR common γ chain	Monocytes, macrophages, activated neutrophils	High-affinity Fcγ receptor; role in phagocytosis, ADCC, macrophage activation
CD66e (carcinoembryonic antigen [CEA])	180-220 kD; Ig superfamily; CEA family	Colonic and other epithelial cells	? Adhesion; clinical marker of carcinoma burden
CD69	23 kD; C-type lectin	Activated B cells, T cells, NK cells, neutrophils	Binds to and impairs surface expression of S1PR1, thereby promoting retention of recently activated lymphocytes in lymphoid organs
CD74 (Class II MHC invariant chain [I$_i$])	33-, 35-, and 41-kD isoforms	B cells, dendritic cells, monocytes, macrophages; other class II MHC–expressing cells	Binds to and directs intracellular sorting of newly synthesized class II MHC molecules
CD79a (Igα)	33, 45 kD; forms dimer with CD79b; Ig superfamily; ITAM in cytoplasmic tail	Mature B cells	Required for cell surface expression of and signal transduction by the B cell antigen receptor complex

CD Number (Other Names)	Molecular Structure, Family	Main Cellular Expression	Known or Proposed Function(s)
CD79b (Igβ)	37-39 kD; forms dimer with CD79α; Ig superfamily; ITAM in cytoplasmic tail	Mature B cells	Required for cell surface expression of and signal transduction by the B cell antigen receptor complex
CD80 (B7-1)	60 kD; Ig superfamily	Dendritic cells, activated B cells and macrophages	Costimulator for T lymphocyte activation; ligand for CD28 and CD152 (CTLA-4)
CD81 (target for antiproliferative antigen 1 [TAPA-1])	26 kD; tetraspan (TM4SF)	T cells, B cells, NK cells, dendritic cells, thymocytes, endothelial cells	B cell activation; forms a co-receptor complex with CD19 and CD21 that delivers signals that synergize with signals from the B cell antigen receptor complex
CD86 (B7-2)	80 kD; Ig superfamily	B cells, monocytes; dendritic cells; some T cells	Costimulator for T lymphocyte activation; ligand for CD28 and CD152 (CTLA-4)
CD88 (C5a receptor)	43 kD; G protein–coupled, 7 membrane–spanning receptor family	Granulocytes, monocytes, dendritic cells, mast cells	Receptor for C5a complement fragment; role in complement-induced inflammation
CD89 (Fcα receptor [FcαR])	55-75 kD; Ig superfamily; noncovalently associated with the common FcR γ chain	Granulocytes, monocytes, macrophages, T cell subset, B cell subset	Binds IgA; mediates IgA-dependent cellular cytotoxicity
CD90 (Thy-1)	25-35 kD; GPI linked; Ig superfamily	Thymocytes, peripheral T cells (mice), CD34+ hematopoietic progenitor cells, neurons	Marker for T cells; unknown function
CD94	43 kD; C-type lectin; on NK cells, covalently assembles with other C-type lectin molecules (NKG2)	NK cells; subset of CD8+ T cells	CD94/NKG2 complex functions as an NK cell inhibitory receptor; binds HLA-E class I MHC molecules
CD95 (Fas)	Homotrimer of 45-kD chains; TNFR superfamily	Broad	Binds Fas ligand; delivers signals leading to apoptotic death
CD102 (ICAM-2)	55-65 kD; Ig superfamily	Endothelial cells, lymphocytes, monocytes, platelets	Ligand for CD11aCD18 (LFA-1); cell-cell adhesion
CD103 (αE integrin subunit)	Dimer of 150- and 25-kD subunits; noncovalently linked to β7 integrin subunit to form αEβ7 integrin	Intraepithelial lymphocytes, other cell types	Role in T cell homing to and retention in mucosa; binds E-cadherin
CD106 (vascular cell adhesion molecule 1 [VCAM-1])	100-110 kD; Ig superfamily	Endothelial cells, macrophages, follicular dendritic cells, marrow stromal cells	Adhesion of cells to endothelium; receptor for CD49dCD29 (VLA-4) integrin; role in lymphocyte trafficking, activation
CD134 (OX40, TNFRSF4)	29 kD; TNFR superfamily	Activated T cells	Receptor for T cell CD252; T cell costimulation
CD150 (signaling lymphocyte activation molecule [SLAM])	37 kD; Ig superfamily	Thymocytes, activated lymphocytes, dendritic cells, endothelial cells	Regulation of B cell–T cell interactions and lymphocyte activation

Continued

CD Number (Other Names)	Molecular Structure, Family	Main Cellular Expression	Known or Proposed Function(s)
CD152 (cytotoxic T lympho-cyte–associ-ated protein 4 [CTLA-4])	33, 50 kD; Ig superfamily	Activated T lymphocytes, regulatory T cells	Mediates suppressive function of regulatory T cells; inhibits T cell responses; binds CD80 (B7-1) and CD86 (B7-2) on antigen-presenting cells
CD154 (CD40 ligand [CD40L])	Homotrimer of 32- to 39-kD chains; TNFR superfamily	Activated CD4+ T cells	Activation of B cells, macrophages, and endothelial cells; ligand for CD40
CD158 (killer Ig-like receptor [KIR])	50, 58 kD; Ig superfamily; killer Ig-like receptor (KIR) family; ITIMs or ITAMs in cytoplasmic tail	NK cells, T cell subset	Inhibition or activation of NK cells on interaction with appropriate class I HLA molecules
CD159a (NKG2A)	43 kD; C-type lectin; forms heterodimer with CD94	NK cells, T cell subset	Inhibition or activation of NK cells on interaction with class I HLA molecules
CD159c (NKG2C)	40 kD; C-type lectin; forms heterodimer with CD94	NK cells	Activation of NK cells on interaction with the appropriate class I HLA molecules
CD162 (P-selectin glycoprotein ligand 1 [PSGL-1])	Homodimer of 120-kD chains; sialomucin	T cells, monocytes, granulocytes, some B cells	Ligand for selectins (CD62P, CD62L); adhesion of leukocytes to endothelium
CD178 (Fas ligand [FasL])	Homotrimer of 31-kD subunits; TNF superfamily	Activated T cells	Ligand for CD95 (Fas); triggers apoptotic death
CD206 (mannose receptor)	166 kD; C-type lectin	Macrophages	Binds high-mannose–containing glycoproteins on pathogens; mediates macrophage endocytosis of glycoproteins and phagocytosis of bacteria, fungi, and other pathogens
CD244 (2B4)	41 kD; Ig superfamily; CD2/CD48/CD58 family; SLAM family	NK cells, CD8 T cells, γδ T cells	Receptor for CD148; modulates NK cell cytolytic activity
CD247 (TCR ζ chain)	18 kD; ITAMs in cytoplasmic tail	T cells; NK cells	Signaling chain of TCR- and NK cell–activating receptors
CD252 (OX40 ligand)	21 kD; TNF superfamily	Dendritic cells, macrophages, B cells	Ligand for CD134 (OX40,TNFRSF4); costimulates T cells
CD267 (TACI)	31 kD; TNFR superfamily	B cells	Receptor for cytokines BAFF and APRIL; mediates B cell survival
CD268 (BAFF receptor)	19 kD; TNFR superfamily	B cells	Receptor for BAFF; mediates B cell survival
CD269 (BCMA [B cell maturation antigen])	20 kD; TNFR superfamily	B cells	Receptor for BAFF and APRIL; mediates B cell survival
CD273 (PD-L2)	25 kD; Ig superfamily; structurally homologous to B7	Dendritic cells, monocytes, macrophages	Ligand for PD-1; inhibits T cell activation
CD274 (PD-L1)	33 kD; Ig superfamily; structurally homologous to B7	Leukocytes, other cells	Ligand for PD-1; inhibits T cell activation

CD Number (Other Names)	Molecular Structure, Family	Main Cellular Expression	Known or Proposed Function(s)
CD275 (ICOS ligand)	60 kD; Ig superfamily; structurally homologous to B7	B cells, dendritic cells, monocytes	Binds ICOS (CD278); T cell costimulation
CD278 (ICOS [inducible costimulator])	55-60 kD; Ig superfamily; structurally homologous to CD28	Activated T cells	Binds ICOS-L (CD275); T cell costimulation
CD279 (PD1)	55 kD; Ig superfamily; structurally homologous to CD28	Activated T and B cells	Binds PD-L1 and PD-L2; inhibits T cell activation
CD314 (NKG2D)	42 kD; C-type lectin	NK cells, activated CD8+ T cells, NK-T cells, some myeloid cells	Binds MHC class I, and the class I-like molecules MIC-A, MIC-B, Rae1, and ULBP4; role in NK cell and CTL activation
CD357 (GITR)	26 kD; TNFR superfamily	CD4+ and CD8+ T cells, Treg	? Role in T cell tolerance/Treg function
CD363 (S1PR1 [type 1 sphingosine-1-phosphate receptor 1])	42.8 kD; G protein–coupled, 7 membrane–spanning receptor family	Lymphocytes, endothelial cells	Binds sphingosine 1-phosphate and mediates chemotaxis of lymphocytes out of lymphoid organs

ADCC, Antibody-dependent cell-mediated cytotoxicity; *APRIL*, a proliferation-inducing ligand; *BAFF*, B cell–activating factor belonging to the TNF family; *CTL*, cytotoxic T lymphocyte; *gp*, glycoprotein; *GPI*, glycophosphatidylinositol; *ICAM*, intercellular adhesion molecule; *Ig*, immunoglobulin; *IL*, interleukin; *ITAM*, immunoreceptor tyrosine-based activation motif; *ITIM*, immunoreceptor tyrosine-based inhibition motif; *LFA*, lymphocyte function–associated antigen; *LPS*, lipopolysaccharide; *MadCAM*, mucosal addressin cell adhesion molecule; *MHC*, major histocompatibility complex; *NK cells*, natural killer cells; *PAMPs*, pathogen-associated molecular patterns; *TACI*, transmembrane activator and CAML interactor; *TCR*, T cell receptor; *TNF*, tumor necrosis factor; *TNFR*, TNF receptor; *VCAM*, vascular cell adhesion molecule; *VLA*, very late activation.

*The lowercase letters affixed to some CD numbers refer to CD molecules that are encoded by multiple genes or that belong to families of structurally related proteins.

Clinical Cases

This appendix presents five clinical cases illustrating various diseases involving the immune system. These cases are not meant to teach clinical skills but rather to show how the basic science of immunology contributes to our understanding of human diseases. Each case illustrates typical ways in which a disease manifests, what tests are used in diagnosis, and common modes of treatment. The appendix was compiled with the assistance of Dr. Richard Mitchell and Dr. Jon Aster, Department of Pathology, Brigham and Women's Hospital, Boston; Dr. Robin Colgrove, Harvard Medical School, Boston; Dr. George Tsokos, Department of Medicine, Beth Israel-Deaconess Hospital, Boston; Dr. David Erle and Dr. Laurence Cheng, Department of Medicine, University of California San Francisco; Dr. James Faix, Department of Pathology, Stanford University School of Medicine, Palo Alto.

CASE 1: LYMPHOMA

E.B. was a 58-year-old chemical engineer who had been well all his life. One morning, he noticed a lump in his left groin while showering. It was not tender, and the overlying skin appeared normal. After a few weeks, he began to worry about it because it did not go away, and he finally made an appointment with a physician after 2 months. On physical examination, the physician noted a subcutaneous firm, movable nodule, about 3 cm in diameter, in the left inguinal region. The physician asked E.B. if he had recently noticed any infections of his left foot or leg; E.B. had not. E.B. did complain that he had been waking up frequently at night drenched in perspiration. The physician also found some slightly enlarged lymph nodes in E.B.'s right neck. Otherwise, the physical examination findings were normal. The physician explained that the inguinal mass probably was a lymph node that was enlarged as a result of a reaction to some infection. However, he drew some blood for tests and referred E.B. to a surgeon, who performed a fine-needle aspiration of cells from the lymph node. Examination of smears prepared from aspirated cells revealed mainly small, irregular lymphocytes. Flow cytometric evaluation of these cells showed a 10-fold excess of cells expressing λ immunoglobulin (Ig) light chain compared with cells expressing κ Ig light chain.

Because of the suspicion of B cell lymphoma, a malignant tumor of cells of the B lymphocyte lineage, the surgeon elected to remove the entire lymph node. Histologic examination revealed an expansion of the node by follicular structures composed of mainly small to intermediate-sized lymphocytes with irregular or "cleaved" nuclear contours mixed with smaller numbers of large lymphocytes with prominent nucleoli (Fig. A-1). Flow cytometric analysis of these cells showed a predominant population of B cells expressing IgM, λ light chain, CD10, and CD20, and immunohistochemical stains performed on slides showed strong cytoplasmic staining for BCL-2. On this basis, the diagnosis of follicular lymphoma of low histologic grade was made.

1. Why does the presence of a B cell population in which a large majority of the cells express λ light chain indicate a neoplasm rather than a response to an infection?
2. If the lymph node cells were analyzed by PCR to assess Ig heavy-chain rearrangements, what abnormal finding would you expect?
3. Normal follicular center B cells fail to express the BCL-2 protein. Why might the tumor cells express BCL-2?

315

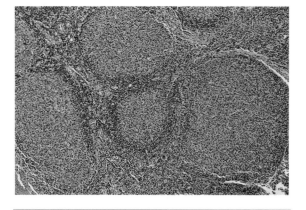

FIGURE A-1 Lymph node biopsy with follicular lymphoma. The microscopic appearance of the patient's inguinal lymph node is shown. The follicular structures are abnormal, composed of a monotonous collection of neoplastic cells. By contrast, a lymph node with reactive hyperplasia would have follicles with germinal center formation, containing a heterogeneous mixture of cells.

E.B.'s blood tests indicated that he was anemic (low red blood cell count). He underwent staging tests to determine the extent of his lymphoma. Positron emission tomography (PET) and computed tomography (CT) scanning showed enlarged hilar and mediastinal lymph nodes, an enlarged spleen, and lesions in the liver. A bone marrow biopsy showed presence of lymphoma as well. E.B. was treated with injections of a mouse/human chimeric monoclonal IgG antibody called rituximab, which is specific for human CD20. Imaging studies performed 6 months after the rituximab treatment was begun showed regression in the size of lesions, and E.B. felt well enough to continue working.

4. By what mechanisms would the anti-CD20 antibody help this patient?

5. What are the advantages of using a "humanized" antibody, such as rituximab, as a drug instead of a mouse antibody?

Answers to Questions for Case 1

1. Each clone of B cells has a unique rearrangement of its Ig heavy-chain and light-chain genes, which encode a unique Ig protein composed of two identical heavy chains and two identical κ or λ light chains (see Chapter 4). In an infection, many different clones of lymphocytes are activated. More than one clone may be specific for the same microbial antigen, and different clones may be responding to different antigens produced by the microbe. Furthermore, even in a lymph node draining a site of infection, there are many clones of normal B cells not specific for the microbe. Thus, immune reactions in a lymph node draining a site of infection contain polyclonal mixtures of B cells that on average include about equal numbers of cells expressing either κ or λ light chains, which can be stained with specific antibodies. B cell tumors such as follicular lymphoma arise from a single transformed cell, the progeny of which share the same set of rearranged Ig genes and express the same immunoglobulin as the cell of origin. Because E.B.'s lymph node was filled with B cells all derived from a single clone, the cells produce and all stain positive for the same Ig light chain, in this case λ light chain, indicating that this is a monoclonal proliferation, which only occurs in tumors.

2. As explained above, B cell lymphomas are monoclonal, being composed of cells that all contain the same Ig heavy-chain and light-chain gene rearrangements. In addition to staining for light-chain expression, reactive polyclonal proliferations and monoclonal B cell tumors can be reliably distinguished by the use of polymerase chain reaction (PCR) amplification of rearranged Ig heavy-chain (IgH) gene segments. This method uses consensus PCR primers that hybridize with virtually all IgH variable (V) gene segments and joining (J) gene segments. These primers are used in the PCR to amplify essentially all the heavy-chain gene rearrangements in a sample (e.g., DNA prepared from enlarged lymph node). The size of the amplified products is then analyzed by capillary electrophoresis, which can separate PCR products that differ in size by as little as a single nucleotide. When the V, D, and J segments of IgH genes (as well as other antigen

receptor genes) are joined during antigen receptor rearrangement in pre-B cells, the rearranged segments are of differing length due to the action of enzymes that remove nucleotides (nucleases) and add bases (a specialized DNA polymerase called terminal deoxyribonucleotide transferase [TdT]). Within a normal population of B cells, many PCR products of different sizes are generated, and these appear as a broad distribution of fragments of differing size. In the case of a B cell lymphoma, all the B cells have the same VDJ rearrangement, and the PCR product is of one size, appearing as a single, sharp peak.

3. Many lymphomas have characteristic underlying acquired mutations that dysregulate specific oncogenes. More than 90% of follicular lymphomas have an acquired chromosomal 14;18 translocation that fuses the coding sequence of BCL-2, a gene encoding a protein that inhibits programmed cell death (apoptosis), to enhancer elements within the Ig heavy chain locus. As a result, BCL-2 is overexpressed in follicular lymphoma cells. Parenthetically, in most instances the chromosomal breakpoint in the IgH gene involved in the translocation is located precisely at the point where RAG proteins normally cut the DNA of B cells that are undergoing Ig gene rearrangement, suggesting that the translocation stems from a mistake that occurs during normal antigen receptor gene rearrangement. Clinically, the presence of a BCL-2/IgH fusion gene, the consequence of the t(14;18), may be determined by fluorescent in situ hybridization using probes of different colors that are specific for IgH and BCL-2. These probes are hybridized to nuclei isolated from tissues involved by follicular lymphoma, and spatial superimposition of the probes indicates the existence of an IgH/BCL-2 fusion gene. Alternatively, it is possible to perform PCR on DNA isolated from the tumor with primer pairs in which one primer is specific for IgH and the other specific for BCL-2. These primers will only produce a product when the IgH and BCL-2 genes are joined to one another, which is taken as indirect evidence of a t(14;18).

4. CD20 is expressed on most mature B cells and is also uniformly expressed by all the tumor cells in follicular lymphomas. Injected rituximab (rituxan) will therefore bind to the lymphoma cells and facilitate their destruction, likely through similar mechanisms by which antibodies normally destroy microbes. These mechanisms involve binding of the Fc portion of rituximab to different proteins in the patient, including Fc receptors on macrophages leading to phagocytic clearance of the lymphoma cells, and binding of the Fc portion to complement proteins leading to complement-mediated killing of the lymphoma cells (see Chapter 8). Many normal B cells will also be destroyed by rituximab, although antibody-secreting plasma cells, which do not express CD20, are not affected.

5. Monoclonal antibodies (mAbs) derived from nonhuman B cells (e.g., mouse) will appear foreign to the human immune system. When injected multiple times with these mAbs, humans will mount humoral immune responses and produce antibodies specific for the injected foreign mAb. These anti-antibody responses will promote clearance of the mAb from the circulation and therefore reduce the therapeutic benefits of the mAb. Furthermore, the Fc regions of human IgG bind better than mouse IgG to human Fc receptors and complement proteins, both of which are important for the effectiveness of mAb drugs (see Answer 3). For these reasons, most recently developed mAbs used as drugs have been genetically engineered to contain mainly or all human Ig amino acid sequences, or mAbs are being produced from genes encoding human Igs. Patients will generally not react against these drugs, just as they do not respond to their own antibodies. Rituximab is a chimeric mAb, with the CD20-binding variable regions originating from mouse IgG, while the remainder of the antibody including the Fc region originates from human IgG. The small amount of mouse sequences in rituximab do not appear to induce anti-antibody responses in patients, perhaps because potentially responding B cells are destroyed by the drug.

CASE 2: HEART TRANSPLANTATION COMPLICATED BY ALLOGRAFT REJECTION

C.M., a computer software salesman, was 48 years old when he came to his primary care physician because of fatigue and shortness of breath. He had not seen a doctor on a regular basis before this visit and felt well until 1 year ago, when he began experiencing difficulty climbing stairs or playing basketball with his children. Over the past 6 months he has had trouble breathing when he lies down in bed. He did not remember ever experiencing significant chest pain and had no family history of heart disease. He did recall that about 18 months ago he had to take 2 days off from work because of a severe flulike illness.

On examination, he had a pulse of 105 beats per minute, a respiratory rate of 32 breaths per minute, a blood pressure of 100/60 mm Hg, and was afebrile. His physician heard rales (evidence of abnormal fluid accumulation) in the bases of both lungs. His feet and ankles were swollen. A chest x-ray showed pulmonary edema and pleural effusions and a significantly enlarged left ventricle. These findings were consistent with right and left ventricular congestive heart failure, which is a reduced capacity of the heart to pump normal volumes of blood, resulting in fluid accumulation in various tissues. C.M. was admitted to the cardiology service of the University Hospital. On the basis of further tests, including coronary angiography and echocardiography, C.M. was given the diagnosis of dilated cardiomyopathy (a progressive and fatal form of heart failure in which the heart chambers become dilated and inefficient at pumping blood). His physicians told him he would benefit from aggressive medical management, including drugs that enhance heart muscle contraction, reduce the workload of the heart, and enhance excretion of accumulated fluid, but if his underlying heart disease continued to progress, the best long-term option would be to receive a heart transplant. Unfortunately, despite optimal medical management, his symptoms of congestive heart failure continued to worsen until he was no longer able to manage even routine activities of daily living, and he was listed for heart transplantation.

A panel-reactive antibody (PRA) test was performed on C.M.'s serum to determine whether he had been previously sensitized to alloantigens. This test showed the patient had no circulating antibodies against human leukocyte antigens (HLA), and no further immunologic testing was performed. Two weeks later in a nearby city, a donor heart was removed from a victim of a construction site accident. The donor had the same ABO blood group type as C.M. The transplant surgery, performed 4 hours after the donor heart was removed, went well, and the allograft was functioning properly postoperatively.

1. What problems might arise if the transplant recipient and the donor have different blood types or if the recipient has high levels of anti-HLA antibodies?

C.M. was placed on immunosuppressive therapy the day after transplantation, which included daily doses of tacrolimus (FK506), mycophenolic acid, and prednisone. Endomyocardial biopsy was performed 1 week after surgery and showed no evidence of myocardial injury or inflammatory cells. He was sent home 10 days after surgery, and within a month he was able to do light exercise without problems. A routinely scheduled endomyocardial biopsy performed within the first 3 months after transplantation was normal, but a biopsy performed 14 weeks after surgery showed the presence of numerous lymphocytes within the myocardium and a few apoptotic muscle fibers (Fig. A-2). The findings were interpreted as evidence of acute allograft rejection.

2. What was the patient's immune system responding to, and what were the effector mechanisms in the acute rejection episode?

C.M.'s serum creatinine level, an indicator of renal function, was high (2.2 mg/dL; normal, <1.5 mg/dL). His physicians therefore did not want to increase his tacrolimus dose because this drug can be toxic to the kidneys. He was given three additional doses of a steroid drug over 18 hours, and a repeat endomyocardial biopsy

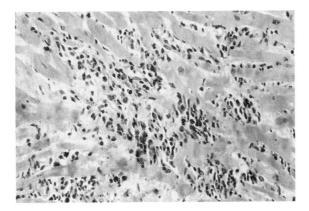

FIGURE A-2 Endomyocardial biopsy showing acute cellular rejection. The heart muscle is infiltrated by lymphocytes, and necrotic muscle fibers are present. (Courtesy Dr. Richard Mitchell, Department of Pathology, Brigham and Women's Hospital, Boston.)

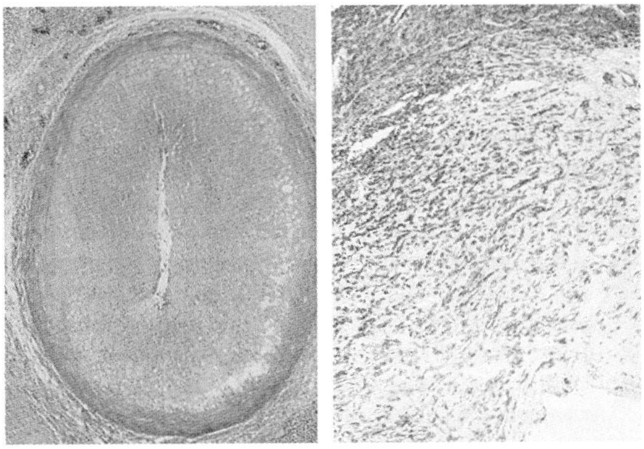

FIGURE A-3 Coronary artery with transplant-associated arteriosclerosis. This histologic section was taken from a coronary artery of a cardiac allograft that was removed from a patient 5 years after transplantation because of graft failure. The lumen is greatly narrowed by the presence of intimal smooth muscle cells. (Courtesy Dr. Richard Mitchell, Department of Pathology, Brigham and Women's Hospital, Boston.)

1 week later showed only a few scattered macrophages and a small focus of healing tissue. C.M. went home feeling well, and he was able to live a relatively normal life, taking tacrolimus, mycophenolic acid, and prednisone daily.

3. What is the goal of the immunosuppressive drug therapy?

Coronary angiograms performed yearly since the transplant showed a gradual narrowing of the lumens of the coronary arteries. In the sixth year after transplantation, C.M. began experiencing shortness of breath after mild exercise and showed left ventricular dilation on radiographic examination. An intravascular ultrasound examination demonstrated significant thickening of the walls and narrowing of the lumen of the coronary arteries (Fig. A-3). An endomyocardial biopsy showed areas of microscopic subendocardial infarction, as well as evidence of sublethal ischemia (myocyte vacuolization), C.M. and his physicians are now considering the possibility of a second cardiac transplant.

4. What process has led to failure of the graft after 6 years?

Answers to Questions for Case 2

1. If the recipient and the heart donor had different blood types, or if the recipient had high levels of anti-HLA antibodies, hyperacute rejection might occur after transplantation (see Chapter 10). People with type A, B, or O blood groups have circulating IgM antibodies against the antigens they do not possess (B, A, or both, respectively). People who have received previous blood transfusions or transplants, or were previously pregnant, may have circulating anti-HLA antibodies. Blood group antigens and HLA antigens are present on endothelial cells. If the antibodies are already present in the recipient at the time of transplantation, they can bind to the antigens on graft endothelial cells, causing complement activation, leukocyte recruitment, and thrombosis. As a result, the graft blood supply becomes impaired, and the organ can rapidly undergo ischemic necrosis. The PRA test typically is performed to determine whether a patient needing a transplant has preexisting antibodies specific for a broad panel of HLA antigens. The test is performed by mixing the patient's serum with a collection of HLA-coated microbeads; antibody binding is detected by flow cytometry of the beads, after addition of fluorescence-labeled antibodies directed against human immunoglobulin. The results are expressed as a percentage (0% to 100%) of the various HLA-coated beads that have bound to the patient's serum antibodies. The higher the PRA value obtained, the greater the chance that the recipient will have an antibody that can potentially react with a graft and cause hyperacute rejection.

2. In the acute rejection episode, the patient's immune system is responding to alloantigens in the graft. These antigens are likely to include donor major histocompatibility complex (MHC) molecules encoded by alleles not shared by the recipient, as well as unshared allelic variants of other proteins (minor histocompatibility antigens). These alloantigens may be expressed on the donor endothelial cells, leukocytes, and parenchymal cells within the donor heart. The effector mechanisms in the acute rejection episode include both cell-mediated and humoral immune responses. Recipient CD4$^+$ T cells secrete cytokines that promote macrophage activation and inflammation and can cause myocyte or endothelial cell injury and dysfunction, and CD8$^+$ cytotoxic T lymphocytes can directly kill graft cells. Recipient antibodies, produced in response to graft antigens, bind to graft cells, leading to complement activation and leukocyte recruitment.

3. The goal of immunosuppressive drug therapy is to suppress the recipient's immune response to alloantigens present in the graft, thereby preventing rejection. The drugs work by depleting T cells (anti-thymocyte globulin), and by blocking T cell activation (FK506, cyclosporine and rapamycin), lymphocyte proliferation (mycophenolic acid), and inflammatory cytokine production (prednisone). An attempt is made to preserve some immune function to combat infections.

4. The graft has failed as a consequence of thickening of the walls and narrowing of the lumens of the graft arteries (see Chapter 10). This vascular change, called graft arteriosclerosis or transplant-associated arteriosclerosis, diffusely involves the coronary vasculature and leads to downstream ischemic damage to the heart; it is the most frequent reason for long-term graft failure. It may be caused by a T cell–mediated inflammatory reaction directed against vessel wall alloantigens, which subsequently smolders as a chronic macrophage-mediated injury that results in cytokine-stimulated smooth muscle cell migration into the intima, with smooth muscle cell proliferation and increased matrix synthesis.

CASE 3: ALLERGIC ASTHMA

Ten-year-old I.E. was brought to her pediatrician's office in November because of frequent coughing for the past 2 days, wheezing, and a feeling of tightness in her chest. Her symptoms had been especially severe at night. In addition to her routine checkups, she had visited the physician in the past for occasional ear and upper respiratory tract infections but had not previously experienced wheezing or chest tightness. She had eczema, but otherwise, she was in good health and was developmentally normal. Her immunizations were up to date. She lived at home with her mother, father, two sisters aged 12 and 4, and a pet cat. Both of her parents smoked cigarettes, and her father suffered from hay fever.

At the time of her physical examination, I.E. had a temperature of 37° C (98.6° F), blood pressure of 105/65 mm Hg, and a respiratory rate of 28 breaths per minute. She did not appear short of breath. There were no signs of ear infection or pharyngitis. Auscultation of the chest revealed diffuse wheezing in both lungs. There was no evidence of pneumonia. The physician made a presumptive diagnosis of bronchospasm and referred I.E. to a pediatric allergist-immunologist. In the meantime, she was given a prescription for a short-acting β2-adrenergic agonist bronchodilator inhaler and was instructed to administer the drug every 6 hours to relieve symptoms. This drug binds to β2-adrenergic receptors on bronchial smooth muscle cells and causes them to relax, resulting in dilation of the bronchioles. The family was also prescribed a spacer and taught to administer the inhaler using the spacer device to optimize delivery of the medication.

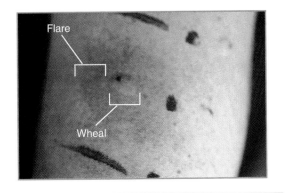

FIGURE A-4 Positive result on prick skin testing for environmental antigens. Small amounts of the antigens are applied into the superficial layers of the skin using a short needle to prick the skin. If mast cells are present with bound IgE specific for the test antigen, the antigen will cross-link the Fc receptors to which the IgE is bound. This induces degranulation of the mast cells and the release of mediators that cause the wheal and flare reaction.

1. Asthma is often an *atopic* disease, particularly in patients beyond 6 to 8 years of age. What are the different ways in which atopy may manifest clinically?

One week later, I.E. was seen again by the allergist. He auscultated her lungs and confirmed the presence of wheezing. I.E. was instructed to blow into a spirometer, and the physician determined that her forced expiratory volume in 1 second (FEV1) was 65% of normal, indicating airway obstruction. The physician then administered a nebulized bronchodilator, and 10 minutes later performed the test again. The repeat FEV1 was 85% of normal, indicating reversibility of the airway obstruction. Blood was drawn and sent for total and differential blood cell count and determination of IgE levels. In addition, a skin test was performed to determine hypersensitivity to various antigens and showed a positive result for cat dander and house dust (Fig. A-4). The patient was instructed to begin using an inhaled corticosteroid and to use her bronchodilator only as needed for respiratory symptoms. Her parents were instructed to make a return appointment 2 weeks later for reevaluation of I.E. and discussion of blood test results.

2. What is the immunologic basis for a positive skin test?

At I.E.'s return appointment 2 weeks later, laboratory tests revealed that she had a serum IgE level of 1200 IU/mL (normal range, 0-180) and a total white blood cell count of 7000/mm³ (normal, 4300-10,800/mm³), with an absolute eosinophil count of 700/mm³ (normal, <500). When she returned to the allergist's office 1 week later, her respiratory status on physical examination was significantly improved, with no audible wheezing. I.E.'s FEV1 had improved to 90% of predicted. The family was told that I.E. had reversible airway obstruction, possibly triggered by a viral illness and possibly related to cat and dust allergies. The physician advised that the cat should at least be kept out of I.E.'s bedroom. The mother was told that smoking in the house probably was contributing to I.E.'s symptoms. The physician recommended that I.E. continue to use the short-acting inhaler for acute episodes of wheezing or shortness of breath. She was asked to return in 3 months, or sooner if she used the inhaler more than twice per month, particularly for nighttime symptoms.

3. What is the mechanism for the increased IgE levels seen in patients who have allergic symptoms?

The family cat was given to a neighbor, and I.E. did well on the therapy for about 6 months, experiencing only mild wheezing a few times. The next spring, she began to have more frequent episodes of coughing and wheezing. During a soccer game one Saturday, she became very short of breath, and her parents brought her to the emergency department (ED) of the local hospital. After confirming that she was wheezing and showed signs of accessory respiratory muscle use, the ED physician treated her with a nebulized β2-agonist bronchodilator and an oral corticosteroid. After 6 hours, her symptoms resolved, and she was sent home. The following week, I.E. was brought to her allergist, who increased her maintenance dose of the inhaled corticosteroid. She has subsequently been well, with occasional mild attacks that are cleared by the bronchodilator inhaler.

4. What are the therapeutic approaches to allergic asthma?

Answers to Questions for Case 3

1. Atopic reactions to essentially harmless antigens are mediated by IgE on mast cells but may manifest in a variety of ways (see Chapter 11). The signs and symptoms usually reflect the site of entry of the allergen. Hay fever (allergic rhinitis) and asthma usually are responses to inhaled allergens, whereas urticaria and eczema more often occur with skin exposure or ingestion. Food allergies may also cause gastrointestinal symptoms. The most dramatic presentation of allergies to insect venom, foods, or drugs is anaphylaxis, a reaction characterized by systemic vasodilation, increased vascular permeability, and airway obstruction (laryngeal edema or bronchoconstriction). Without intervention, patients with anaphylaxis may progress to asphyxia and cardiovascular collapse. The most effective treatment for anaphylaxis is the administration of epinephrine through intramuscular injection. Epinephrine constricts blood vessels and reverses the fall in blood pressure as well as increased vascular permeability.

2. Immediate release of histamine from triggered mast cells produces a central wheal of edema (from leakage of plasma) and the surrounding flare of vascular congestion (from vessel dilation). The allergy skin test should not be confused with the skin test used to assess prior sensitization to certain infectious agents, such as *Mycobacterium tuberculosis*. A positive tuberculosis skin test is an example of a delayed-type hypersensitivity (DTH) reaction, mediated by antigen-stimulated helper T cells, which release cytokines such as interferon-γ, leading to macrophage activation and inflammation (see Chapter 6). Serum IgE tests are also routinely performed and give complementary information to traditional allergy prick skin testing.

3. For unknown reasons, patients with atopy mount helper T cell responses of the Th2 type to a variety of essentially harmless protein antigens, and the Th2 cells produce interleukin-4 (IL-4), IL-5, and IL-13. IL-4 induces IgE synthesis by B cells, IL-5 activates eosinophils, and IL-13 stimulates mucus production (see Chapters 6 and 11). Atopy appears to run in families, and genetic susceptibility is clearly involved. Attention has been focused especially on genes on the long arm of chromosome 5 (5q) that encode several Th2 cytokines; on 11q, where the gene for the α chain of the IgE receptor is located; and on genes on chromosomes 2 and 9, which encode the IL-33 receptor (ST2) and IL-33, respectively. IL-33 is a cytokine secreted by epithelial cells that is believed to activate group 2 innate lymphoid cells (ILC2), which may play a role in inducing strong Th2 responses.

4. A major therapeutic approach for allergies is prevention by avoidance of precipitating allergens, identified through either allergy skin testing or serum IgE measurement. Although pharmacologic therapy previously has been focused on treating the symptoms of bronchoconstriction by elevating intracellular cyclic adenosine monophosphate (cAMP) levels (using β2-adrenergic agents and inhibitors of cAMP degradation), the balance of therapy has shifted to the use of antiinflammatory agents. These include corticosteroids (which block cytokine release) and receptor antagonists for lipid mediators (e.g., leukotrienes). A newer treatment that is also approved for asthma is anti-IgE antibody.

CASE 4: SYSTEMIC LUPUS ERYTHEMATOSUS

N.Z., a 25-year-old woman, presented to her primary care physician with complaints of joint pain involving her wrists, fingers, and ankles. When seen in the physician's office, N.Z. had normal body temperature, heart rate, blood pressure, and respiratory rate. There was a noticeable red rash on her cheeks, most marked around her nose, sparing the nasolabial folds, and on questioning she said the redness worsened after being in the sun for 1 or 2 hours. The joints of her hands and her wrists were swollen and tender. The other physical examination findings were unremarkable.

Her physician took a blood sample for various tests. Her hematocrit was 35% (normal, 37% to

48%). The total white blood cell count was 9800/mm³ (within normal range), with a normal differential count. The erythrocyte sedimentation rate (ESR) was 40 mm per hour (normal, 1-20). Her serum antinuclear antibody (ANA) test was positive at 1:256 dilution (normally, negative at 1:8 dilution). Other laboratory findings were unremarkable. On the basis of these findings, a diagnosis of systemic lupus erythematosus (SLE) was made. N.Z.'s physician prescribed oral prednisone, a corticosteroid, and with this treatment, her joint pain subsided.

1. What is the significance of the positive result for the ANA test?

Three months later, N.Z. began feeling unusually tired and thought she had the flu. For about a week she had noticed that her ankles were swollen, and she had difficulty putting on her shoes. She returned to her primary care physician. Her ankles and feet showed severe edema (swollen as a result of extra fluid in the tissue). Her abdomen appeared slightly distended, with a mild shifting dullness to percussion (a sign of an abnormally large amount of fluid in the peritoneal cavity). Her physician ordered several laboratory tests. Her ANA test result was still positive, with a titer of 1:256, and her ESR

was 120 mm/hour. Serum albumin was 0.8 g/dL (normal, 3.5-5.0). Measurement of serum complement proteins revealed a C3 of 42 mg/dL (normal, 80-180) and a C4 of 5 mg/dL (normal, 15-45). Urinalysis showed 4+ proteinuria, both red and white blood cells, and numerous hyaline and granular casts. A 24-hour urine sample contained 4 g of protein.

2. What is the likely reason for the decreased complement levels and the abnormalities in blood and urinary proteins?

Because of the abnormal urinalysis findings, the physician recommended a renal biopsy, which was performed 1 week later. The biopsy specimen was examined by routine histologic methods, immunofluorescence, and electron microscopy (Fig. A-5).

3. What is the explanation for the pathologic changes seen in the kidney?

The physician made the diagnosis of proliferative lupus glomerulonephritis, prescribed a higher dose of prednisone, and recommended treatment with a cytotoxic drug (mycophenolate). N.Z.'s proteinuria and edema subsided over a 2-week period, and serum C3 levels returned to normal. Her corticosteroid dose was tapered to a lower amount. Over the next few years, she

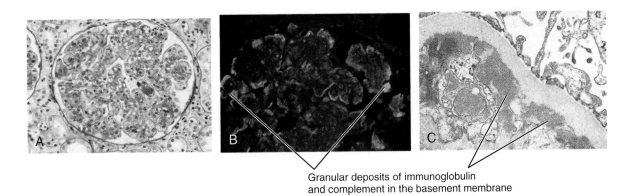

Granular deposits of immunoglobulin
and complement in the basement membrane

FIGURE A-5 Glomerulonephritis with immune complex deposition in systemic lupus erythematosus. **A,** Light micrograph of a renal biopsy specimen in which neutrophilic infiltration in a glomerulus can be seen. **B,** Immunofluorescence micrograph showing granular deposits of immunoglobulin G (IgG) along the basement membrane. (In this technique, called immunofluorescence microscopy, a frozen section of the kidney is incubated with a fluorescein-conjugated antibody against IgG, and the site of deposition of the IgG is defined by determining where the fluorescence is located.) **C,** Electron micrograph of the same tissue revealing immune complex deposition. (Courtesy Dr. Helmut Rennke, Department of Pathology, Brigham and Women's Hospital, Boston.)

has had intermittent flare-ups of her disease, with joint pain and tissue swelling and laboratory tests indicating depressed C3 levels and proteinuria. These have been effectively managed with corticosteroids, and N.Z. has been able to lead an active life.

Answers to Questions for Case 4

1. A positive ANA test reveals the presence of serum antibodies that bind to components of cellular nuclei. The test is performed by placing different dilutions of the patient's serum on top of a monolayer of human cells on a glass slide. A second fluorescently labeled anti-Ig antibody is then added, and the cells are examined with a fluorescent microscope to detect if any serum antibodies bound to the nuclei. The ANA titer is the maximum dilution of the serum that still produces detectable nuclear staining. Patients with SLE usually (98%) have ANAs, which may be specific for histones, other nuclear proteins, or double-stranded DNA. These are autoantibodies, and their production is evidence of autoimmunity. Autoantibodies may also be produced against various cell membrane protein antigens. Autoantibodies may be present for 5 years or more before the diagnosis of SLE. Titers of autoantibodies do not reflect disease activity and should not be used to adjust treatment.

2. Some of the autoantibodies form circulating immune complexes by binding to antigens in the blood. Nuclear antigens may be increased in the circulation of patients with SLE because of increased apoptosis of several cell types (e.g., white blood cells, keratinocytes) and defective clearance of apoptotic cells. When these immune complexes deposit in the basement membranes of vessel walls, they may activate the classical pathway of complement, leading to inflammation and depletion of complement proteins through consumption. Inflammation caused by the immune complexes in the kidney leads to leakage of protein and red blood cells into the urine. The loss of protein in the urine results in reduced plasma albumin, reduction of osmotic pressure of the plasma, and fluid loss into the tissues. This explains the edema of the feet and abdominal distention.

3. The pathologic changes in the kidney result from the deposition of circulating immune complexes in the basement membranes of renal glomeruli. In addition, autoantibodies may bind directly to tissue antigens and form in situ immune complexes. These deposits can be seen by immunofluorescence (indicating type of antibody deposited) and electron microscopy (showing exact localization). The immune complexes activate complement, and leukocytes are recruited by complement by-products (C3a, C5a) and by binding of leukocyte Fc receptors to the IgG molecules in the complexes. These leukocytes become activated, and they produce reactive oxygen species and lysosomal enzymes that damage the glomerular basement membrane. These findings are characteristic of immune complex–mediated tissue injury, and complexes may deposit in joints and small blood vessels anywhere in the body, as well as in the kidney. SLE is a prototype of an immune complex disease (see Chapter 11).

CASE 5: HUMAN IMMUNODEFICIENCY VIRUS INFECTION: ACQUIRED IMMUNODEFICIENCY SYNDROME

On first presentation to a clinic physician, J.C. was a 28-year-old assistant carpenter with 3 weeks of low-grade fevers, sore throat, and lymphadenopathy. Physical examination revealed "track marks," and when asked, the patient stated that 2 months earlier, he had begun using heroin with shared needles because he could no longer afford the cost of escalating doses of street oxycodone. Other findings on physical examination included lymphadenopathy, thrush (fungal infection of the oropharynx), and a faint, diffuse rash. Point-of-care tests for Epstein-Barr virus infection (monospot) and oropharyngeal streptococcal infection (rapid strep) were negative, as were blood cultures for bacteria or fungi. He was discharged with a presumed viral syndrome and given topical nystatin, an oral antifungal for his thrush.

Normal individual

HIV-infected patient

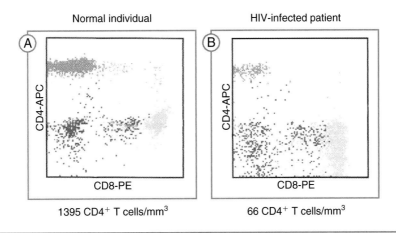

1395 CD4$^+$ T cells/mm^3

66 CD4$^+$ T cells/mm^3

FIGURE A-6 Flow cytometry analysis of CD4$^+$ and CD8$^+$ T cells in blood of patient with human immunodeficiency virus (HIV) infection. A suspension of the patient's white blood cells was incubated with monoclonal antibodies specific for CD4 and CD8. The anti-CD4 antibody was labeled with the fluorochrome allophycocyanin (APC), and the anti-CD8 antibody was labeled with the fluorochrome phycoerythrin (PE). These two fluorochromes emit light of different colors when excited by the appropriate wavelengths. The cell suspensions were analyzed in a flow cytometer, which can enumerate the number of cells stained by each of the differently labeled antibodies. In this way, the number of CD4$^+$ and CD8$^+$ T cells can be determined. Shown here are two-color plots of a control blood sample **(A)** and that of the patient **(B)**. The CD4$^+$ T cells are shown in orange (upper left quadrant), and the CD8$^+$ T cells are shown in green (lower right quadrant). (Note that these are not the colors of light emitted by the APC and PE fluorochromes.)

1. What is the significance of 3 weeks of low-grade fevers and lymphadenopathy?

J.C. was seen the next week in the Infectious Diseases clinic, where enzyme-linked immunosorbent assays (ELISA) performed on his blood were found to be negative for anti-HIV antibody but positive for human immunodeficiency virus (HIV) nucleocapsid p24. The concentration of HIV viral genomes in his blood (viral load) was determined to be 700,000/mL, and his blood CD4$^+$ T cell count was 300/mm^3 (Fig. A-6). Hepatitis B virus (HBV) ELISAs were negative for anti-HBV surface antigen and HBV surface antigen. HIV genotyping showed a lysine-to-asparagine mutation at codon 103 (K103N) of the HIV reverse transcriptase gene. Antiretroviral therapy (ART) was recommended, but the patient was lost to follow-up.

2. What was this patient's major risk factor for acquiring HIV infection? What are other risk factors for HIV infection?

3. Why do the HIV tests include testing for the presence of both HIV antibodies and p24 protein?

Six months later, J.C. was seen at an outside hospital for an abscess at an injection site. After incision and drainage, he left against medical advice. A CD4$^+$ T cell count obtained at that time was 200, and viral load was 15,000. He still refused ART therapy.

Six years later, J.C. was admitted to the hospital after a week of fevers and shortness of breath. A chest x-ray showed faint, diffuse infiltrates, and oxygen saturation was 90%. Initial microscopic examination of sputum stained for fungi (silver stain) was unrevealing, but he was started on antibiotics plus prednisone. PCR testing of sputum was positive for *Pneumocystis jirovecii*. J.C.'s condition initially worsened, but eventually he recovered fully. A repeat CD4$^+$ T cell count was now 150, with a viral load of 50,000/mL. At this point, J.C. was amenable to ART and was started on elvitegravir/cobicistat (an HIV integrase inhibitor with a boosting co-drug), plus two nucleoside/nucleotide analog inhibitors of the HIV reverse transcriptase (NRTIs), tenofovir/emtricitabine. He was also continued on trimethoprim/sulfa antibiotics. He was advised to stop smoking.

4. Why does ART therapy for HIV typically include three different antiviral drugs?

5. What caused the gradual decline in J.C.'s CD4+ T cell count?

6. Why were antibiotics and prednisone started in the patient before a diagnosis of *Pneumocystis jirovecii* infection was established by PCR?

One year later, his CD4 count was 800 and his viral load was undetectable, but he developed methicillin-resistant *Staphylococcal aureus* (MRSA) infection of his mitral valve (staph endocarditis), requiring surgical replacement with a bioprosthetic valve. Preoperative cardiac catheterization showed significant coronary artery disease. Postoperatively, he was able to discontinue heroin use with methadone maintenance. His antiretroviral drugs were continued, but the trimethoprim sulfa was stopped. He has remained in good health since. His long-term partner remains HIV negative.

7. What are the main risks to J.C.'s life at this point?

Answers to Questions for Case 5

1. This pattern is referred to as acute HIV syndrome. Although a very large number of infectious agents can cause this syndrome for a few days, the persistence in this case suggests one of a relatively small number of causes in a young, previously healthy person, including HIV infection.

2. Intravenous drug use is the major risk factor for HIV infection in this patient. Shared needles among drug addicts transmit blood-borne viral particles from one infected person to others. Other major risk factors for HIV infection include sexual intercourse with an infected person, transfusion of contaminated blood products, and birth from an infected mother (see Chapter 12).

3. In acute infection, there has often been insufficient time to develop an antibody response, but levels of virus are high, so viral proteins can readily be detected. This is a screening test that, to be deployed widely, must be highly sensitive but also simple and inexpensive.

New, so-called "fourth generation" tests were approved in the United States in 2010, several years later than in other countries. If the screening test was positive, it would be followed up with more specific (but more complex) assays for levels and genotype of viral nucleic acid.

4. HIV has a very high mutation rate. Mutations in the reverse-transcriptase gene that render the enzyme resistant to nucleoside inhibitors occur frequently in patients receiving these drugs. Resistance to protease inhibitors may come about by similar mechanisms. Triple-drug therapy greatly reduces the chances of viral drug resistance, but poor compliance permits the emergence of mutant strains resistant to several drugs. Non-nucleoside analog reverse transcriptase inhibitors (NNRTIs) are also effective anti-HIV drugs, but the lysine-to-asparagine mutation at codon 103 (K103N) of the HIV reverse transcriptase gene, discovered at the time of diagnosis, would make this patent resistant to NNRTIs. As of 2015, the integrase inhibitors were the last of the major anti-HIV drugs to be approved.

5. After initial infection, HIV rapidly enters various types of cells in the body, including CD4+ T lymphocytes, dendritic cells, mononuclear phagocytes, and others. Once it is in an intracellular location, the virus is safe from antibody neutralization. The gradual decline in CD4+ T cells in this patient was caused by repetitive cycles of HIV infection of CD4+ T cells in lymphoid organs, leading to death of the cells. The symptoms of acquired immunodeficiency syndrome (AIDS) do not usually occur until the blood count of CD4+ T cells is below 200/mm^3, reflecting a severe depletion of T cells in the lymphoid organs.

6. This presentation in a person with known HIV infection is so highly suggestive of *Pneumocystis jirovecii* pneumonia (PJP) that there was no need to wait for confirmatory diagnosis. The deficiencies in T cell–mediated immunity in patients with AIDS lead to impaired immunity to viruses, fungi, and protozoa, which otherwise are easily controlled by a normal immune system. *Pneumocystis jirovecii* is a fungal organ-

ism that can live within phagocytes, but usually it is eradicated by the action of activated CD4$^+$ T cells. In the first days of antifungal treatment, a potent inflammatory response to the dying microorganisms can cause dangerous clinical worsening, so steroid antiinflammatories are started immediately for severe cases.

7. With well-controlled HIV infection, patients can have a near-normal life expectancy, and most deaths are from causes not directly related to HIV infection. Both HIV infection it-self and some of the antiretroviral drugs seem to accelerate coronary artery disease; hence, infected persons who are effectively treated with antiretrovirals tend to die more frequently of disorders not directly related to the viral infection. The highest risk to this patient was active intravenous drug use, now discontinued. In addition, people with well-suppressed HIV infection very rarely transmit the virus to others, so treatment can both prevent and control infection.

Pages followed by *b, t,* or *f* refer to boxes, tables, or figures, respectively.

329